Myocardial Infarction: Advances in Cardiovascular Medicine

Myocardial Infarction: Advances in Cardiovascular Medicine

Edited by Megan Smith

hayle medical

New York

Hayle Medical,
750 Third Avenue, 9th Floor,
New York, NY 10017, USA

Visit us on the World Wide Web at:
www.haylemedical.com

ISBN: 978-1-63241-926-2

Cataloging-in-Publication Data

Myocardial infarction : advances in cardiovascular medicine / edited by Megan Smith.
p. cm.
Includes bibliographical references and index.
ISBN 978-1-63241-926-2
1. Myocardial infarction. 2. Cardiovascular system--Diseases.
3. Cardiovascular system--Diseases--Treatment. I. Smith, Megan.
RC685.I6 M96 2020
616.123 7--dc23

Table of Contents

Preface

I am honored to present to you this unique book which encompasses the most up-to-date data in the field. I was extremely pleased to get this opportunity of editing the work of experts from across the globe. I have also written papers in this field and researched the various aspects revolving around the progress of the discipline. I have tried to unify my knowledge along with that of stalwarts from every corner of the world, to produce a text which not only benefits the readers but also facilitates the growth of the field.

Myocardial infarction (MI), commonly called heart attack, is a cardiac condition characterized by reduction or termination of blood flow to a part of the heart causing damage to the heart muscle. MIs are classified into STEMI (ST elevation MI) and NSTEMI (non-ST elevation MI). Pain radiating to the right arm or shoulder is suggestive of myocardial infarction. The pain is usually diffuse and may last for more than 20 minutes. Sweating, nausea, vomiting, shortness of breath, abnormalities in blood pressure or heart rate, or heart palpitations may also occur. Loss of consciousness, cardiogenic shock and sudden death may also occur. ECG, myocardial perfusion imaging, stress echocardiography, cardiac and physical examination and cardiac biomarkers may support the diagnosis of myocardial infarction. MI is a medical emergency and requires quick medical response. The treatment is designed to unblock blood vessels, rescue ischemia, reduce blot clot enlargement and prevent future MIs. This book elucidates the concepts and innovative models around prospective developments with respect to myocardial infarction. Through this book, we attempt to further enlighten the readers about the modern concepts in cardiovascular medicine.

Finally, I would like to thank all the contributing authors for their valuable time and contributions. This book would not have been possible without their efforts. I would also like to thank my friends and family for their constant support.

Editor

1

Use of secondary prevention pharmacotherapy after first myocardial infarction in patients with diabetes mellitus

Casper H Jørgensen[1*], Gunnar H Gislason[1], Ole Ahlehoff[1], Charlotte Andersson[1], Christian Torp-Pedersen[1,2] and Peter R Hansen[1]

Abstract

Background: Despite recommended pharmacotherapies the use of secondary prevention therapy after myocardial infarction (MI) remains suboptimal. Patients with diabetes mellitus (DM) have worse prognosis after MI compared to patients without DM and aggressive secondary prevention pharmacotherapy in this population is therefore warranted. We examined the changes in use of evidence-based secondary prevention pharmacotherapy in patients with and without DM discharged after first MI.

Methods: All patients aged 30 years or older admitted with first MI in Denmark during 1997–2006 were identified by individual-level linkage of nationwide registries of hospitalizations. Univariate and multivariate logistic regression models were used to identify patient characteristics associated with initiation of acetylsalicylic acid, angiotensin-converting enzyme inhibitors or angiotensin receptor blockers, β-blockers, and clopidogrel within 90 days, and statins within 180 days of discharge, respectively.

Results: A total of 78,230 patients were included, the mean age was 68.3 years (SD 13.0), 63.5% were men and 9,797 (12.5%) had diabetes. Comparison of claimed prescriptions in the period 1997–2002 and 2003–2006 showed significant ($p < 0.001$) increases in claims for acetylsalicylic acid (38.9% vs. 69.7%), angiotensin-converting enzyme inhibitors or angiotensin receptor blockers (38.7% vs. 50.4%), β-blockers (69.2% vs. 77.9%), clopidogrel (16.7% vs. 66.3%), and statins (41.3% vs. 77.3%). During 2003–2006, patients with DM claimed significantly less acetylsalicylic acid (odds ratio [OR] 0.81 [95% confidence interval [CI] 0.74–0.88) and clopidogrel (OR 0.91 [95% CI 0.83–1.00]) than patients without DM.

Conclusions: Despite sizeable increase in use of evidence-based secondary prevention pharmacotherapy after MI from 1997 to 2006, these drugs are not used in a substantial proportion of subjects and patients with DM received significantly less antiplatelet therapy than patients without DM. Increased focus on initiation of secondary prevention pharmacotherapy after MI is warranted, especially in patients with DM.

Background

Optimal use of evidence-based secondary prevention pharmacotherapy in patients with myocardial infarction (MI) reduces the risk of subsequent cardiovascular events and mortality [1-5]. The internationally recommended pharmacotherapies based on confirmative trials for secondary prevention after MI during the study period 1997–2006 included treatment with platelet inhibitors (acetylsalicylic acid [ASA] and a thienopyridine, e.g. clopidogrel), β-blockers, and lipid-lowering agents for most patients without contraindications and irrespective of reperfusion therapy [6-12]. Furthermore, high-risk post-MI patients with diabetes mellitus (DM), clinical heart failure, and/or left ventricular dysfunction should additionally receive angiotensin-converting enzyme inhibitors/angiotensin 2 receptor blockers (ACEIs/ARBs) [5,13].

Patients with DM have worse prognosis after MI compared to patients without DM and aggressive secondary prevention pharmacotherapy is warranted in DM patients [14]. Despite substantial data, however, the use of secondary prevention therapy after MI remains

* Correspondence: casperj@dadlnet.dk
[1]Department of Cardiology, Copenhagen University Hospital Gentofte, Niels Andersens Vej 65, Copenhagen 2900, Denmark
Full list of author information is available at the end of the article

suboptimal [15]. To further examine this clinically important topic, the current study used population-based administrative databases to examine the temporal development in use of evidence-based secondary prevention pharmacotherapy in post-MI patients, with particular focus on patients with DM.

Methods

Health care system in Denmark

All permanent residents in Denmark can use the Danish health care system freely and are entitled to free treatment at a hospital. Data in the present study were obtained from admissions all of 82 existing public hospitals in Denmark in 1996. Expenses for the cost of drugs are partially reimbursed. The more expenses patients have for reimbursable drugs, the more reimbursement they will receive. Annual medical expenses >900 Danish Kroners (DKr) are reimbursed by 50%, >1,470 DKr by 75%, and >3,180 DKr by 85%. Moreover, general practitioners can apply (usually successfully) for 100% reimbursement of drug expenses payable to their patients with chronic conditions, i.e. DM.

Databases

In Denmark all citizens have a unique personal civil registration number, allowing individual linkage of information across nationwide registers. The Danish National Patient Register holds information of all admissions and invasive therapeutic procedures performed in Danish hospitals since 1978. Each admission is registered by one primary diagnosis and, if appropriate, one or more secondary diagnoses, coded according to the 8th or 10th revision of the International Classification of Diseases (ICD-8 code 410 for 1978–94 and ICD-10 codes I21–I22 from 1995 and onwards). The diagnosis of MI has previously been validated in the National Patient Registry with a specificity of 93% [16]. The Danish Register of Medicinal Product Statistics (National Prescription Register) holds information on all prescriptions dispensed from Danish pharmacies since 1995. Drugs are registered according to the international Anatomical Therapeutical Chemical (ATC) classification system. The national health care reimbursement scheme of drug expenses requires pharmacies in Denmark to register all dispensed prescriptions, which ensures complete registration [17]. Percutaneous coronary interventions (PCI) and coronary by-pass grafting (CABG) procedures performed <30 days after admission were detected by use of the Danish Health Care Classification System using the codes KFNG and KNFA-KNFE, respectively.

Study population

Patients aged ≥30 years admitted to Danish hospitals during 1997–2006 with a diagnosis of first MI (ICD-10 codes I21–I22) were identified from the Danish National Patient Registry. To certify the first hospitalization for MI, we traced the hospitalizations of all patients back to 1978. Patients with DM were identified in the Danish Register of Medicinal Product Statistics as individuals claiming at least one prescription for glucose-lowering drugs (GLDs; ATC A10), including all oral agents and insulin, in the period from 180 days before to 90 days after admission for MI. Although use of GLDs represents a conservative approach to identification of DM, this strategy has been shown to capture at least 85% of patients with DM in Denmark and it has a positive predictive value of 98% [18]. In 2002 the treatment strategy for ST-segment elevation myocardial infarction (STEMI) in Denmark was changed from fibrinolysis to primary PCI after results of the DANAMI II trial were presented [19]. Based on these treatment changes in 2002, we therefore specifically compared patients with first MI in the period 1997–2002 with patients admitted in 2003–2006.

Pharmacotherapy

We identified secondary prevention pharmacotherapy prescriptions claimed ≤90 days of discharge after first MI. The following drugs (ATC codes) were identified: ASA (B01AC06), ACEIs/ARBs (C09), β-blockers (C07), clopidogrel (B01AC04), and statins (A10A). Initiation of statin treatment has been shown to increase during the first 6 months after discharge after MI [20] and therefore prescription claims within the first 180 days after discharge were selected to identify patients that initiated statin therapy. Initiation of β-blockers and ACEIs/ARBs has been shown to occur primarily during the first 30 days after MI [20]. In addition, claims of loop-diuretics (C03C) and proton pump inhibitors (PPIs; A02B) were identified as proxies for heart failure (HF) and dyspeptic disease, respectively.

Comorbidity

Comorbidity was defined according to the modified Ontario Myocardial Infarction Mortality Prediction Rules by admission diagnoses at the index admission and 1 year previously [21]. The following diagnoses (ICD-10 codes) were used: HF (I42, I43, I50) cardiac dysrhythmias (I47-I49), pulmonary edema (J81), shock (R57), cerebrovascular disease (I60-I69), DM with chronic complications (E10-E14), acute renal failure (N17, N19, R34), chronic renal failure (N18, I12, I13) and malignancy (C00-C97).

Statistical analyses

All continuous variables were described as mean values ± SD. Comparisons between groups were made using unpaired t-test and χ^2 test for discrete variables. Multivariable logistic regression models were used to analyze differences in odds ratios (ORs) for drug use between patients with and without DM, women and men, different patient age groups and between the two study periods, respectively. Patients were stratified in 5 age groups, i.e., 30–49 years, 50–59 years, 60–69 years, 70–79 years, and ≥80 years, and in age-dependent analyses, patients aged 60–69 years were chosen as the reference. Analyses were adjusted for comorbidity and concomitant pharmacotherapy. The linearity of continuous variables and lack of interactions was tested and found valid unless otherwise reported. Statistical calculations were performed with the SAS statistical software package, version 9.1 (SAS Institute Inc., Cary, NC).

Ethics

The Danish Data Protection Agency approved the study (No. 2007-41-1667). Data were delivered with anonymized, unique personal identification numbers, enabling linkage between registers on an individual level. Retrospective register studies where individuals cannot be identified do not require ethical approval in Denmark [22].

Results

During the 10-year study period, 101,852 patients with MI were identified. Of these, 78,230 patients ≥30 years of age alive 30 days after discharge after their first MI were included in the study. The selection of the study population is shown in Figure 1. The study population comprised 49,665 (63.5%) men with a mean age of 65.7 years (SD 12.6), and 9,797 (12.5%) that claimed GLDs in the period 180 days before or 90 days after the index admission were identified as the study DM population. The prevalence of DM increased from 12.1% in 1997–2002 to 13.1% in 2003–2006. During the 30 to 90 days after discharge 3,951 (5.1%) died of which 628 (15.9%) had DM, leaving 74,279 patients to claim drug prescriptions for the entire period after discharge. For the entire period, patients with DM accounted for 12.3% of those surviving ≥ 90days. Patients with DM were older, i.e., 69.2 (SD 11.8) years vs. 68.1 (SD 13.2) years, more often women (39.4% vs. 36.1%; $p < 0.0001$) and had more comorbidity at baseline, especially HF (27.5% vs. 17.4%; $p < 0.0001$), cardiac dysrhythmias (11.1% vs. 10.2%; $p < 0.0001$), and cerebrovascular disease (7.2% vs. 4.4%; $p < 0.0001$), compared to patients without DM. The use of loop diuretics (a proxy for HF) in the late study period was significantly higher in DM patients than in patients without DM (52.7% vs. 32.4%; $p < 0.0001$). Women claimed more loop diuretics (OR 1.19 [95% CI 1.15-1.21]) than men. These findings were consistent for both study periods (1997–2002 and 2003–2006) and were independent of DM status. Baseline characteristics of the study population with and without DM are shown in Table 1.

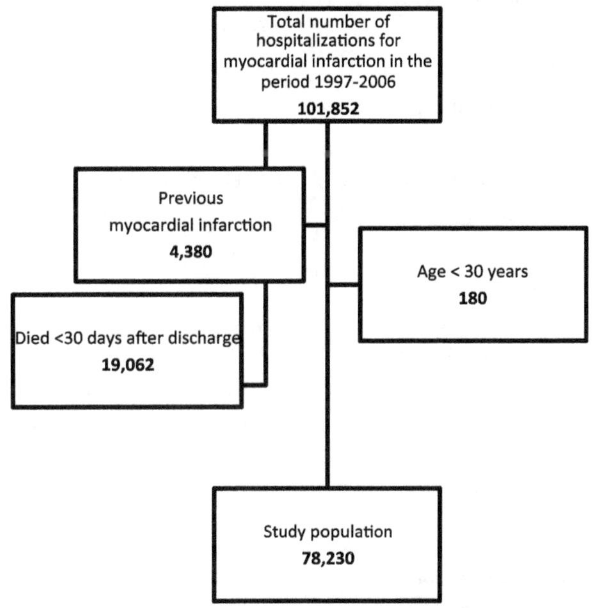

Figure 1 The selection of patients aged ≥30 years and alive 30 days after first myocardial infarction admitted to a Danish hospital during 1 January 1997–31 December 2006.

Initiation of secondary prevention pharmacotherapy

The proportion of patients that claimed secondary prevention therapy increased significantly over time, i.e., for patients with DM the following increase in drug use between 1997–2002 and 2003–2006 was observed: ASA from 37.4% to 64.3%, ACEIs/ARBs from 55.1% to 66.3%, β-blockers from 64.8% to 75.8%, clopidogrel from 14.1% to 62.2%, and statins from 39.1% to 77.5% (all $p<0.0001$). Similarly for patients without DM drug use increased as follows: ASA from 39.1% to 70.5%, ACEIs/ARBs from 36.4% to 48.0%, β-blockers from 69.8% to 78.2%, clopidogrel from 17.0% to 69.9%, and statins from 41.6% to 77.3% (all $p < 0.001$). During the entire study period 1997–2006 patients with DM claimed significantly less evidence-based secondary prevention pharmacotherapy compared with patients without DM, except for ACEIs/ARBs and statins in the late (2003–2006) study period. An unadjusted analysis showed that the ORs for receiving ASA, β-blockers, and clopidogrel were significantly lower in patients with DM compared to patients without DM, while OR for treatment with ACEIs/ARBs was increased in patients with DM (Table 2). Figure 2 shows multivariable logistic regression analyses with ORs for claims of secondary prevention pharmacotherapy in the period 2003–2006 after adjustments for age, gender, and comorbidity. In 2003–2006 patients with DM claimed less ASA (OR 0.81 [95% CI 0.74-0.88]) and clopidogrel (OR 0.91 [95% CI 0.83-1.00]) than patients without DM (Figure 2). Sensitivity analyses excluding patients with vs. without DM claiming ASA (26.5% vs. 15.0%) and

Table 1 Baseline characteristics

	No DM	DM	p-value
Number:	**68,433**	**9,797**	
Percentage of study population:	87.5	12.5	
Gender, female (%)	36.1	39.4	<0.0001
Age at hospitalization (years ± SD)	68.1 (±13.2)	69.2 (±11.8)	<0.0001
Period of hospitalization (%)			
1997–2002	87.9	12.1	
2003–2006	86.9	13.1	
Secondary prevention claimed 1997–2002 (%)	**40,982**	**5,649**	
ASA	39.1	37.4	<0.0149
ACEIs/ARBs	36.4	55.1	<0.0001
β-blockers	69.8	64.8	<0.0001
Clopidogrel	17.0	14.1	<0.0001
Statins	41.6	39.1	<0.0003
Secondary prevention claimed 2003–2006 (%)	**27,451**	**4,148**	
ASA	70.5	64.3	<0.0001
ACEIs/ARBs	48.0	66.3	<0.0001
β-blockers	78.2	75.8	<0.0005
Clopidogrel	66.9	62.2	<0.0001
Statins	77.3	77.5	0.8050
Comorbidity diseases (%)			
Cardiac dysrhythmias	10.2	11.1	<0.0038
Heart failure	17.4	27.5	<0.0001
Pulmonary edema	1.0	1.8	<0.0001
Shock	0.9	1.5	<0.0001
Cerebrovascular disease	4.4	7.2	<0.0001
Renal disease	1.5	3.5	<0.0001
Diabetes complications	0.5	33.1	<0.0001
Malignancy	0.5	0.5	0.2953
Concomitant pharmacotherapy			
Loop diuretics	35.1	54.4	<0.0001
Proton pump inhibitors	18.1	21.2	<0.0001
Reperfusion therapy			
Percutaneous coronary intervention	28.0	21.8	<0.0001
Coronary artery by-pass graft	4.8	5.9	<0.0001

DM: diabetes mellitus, SD: standard deviation, ASA: acetyl salicylic acid, ACEI: angiotensin-converting enzyme inhibitor, ARB: angiotensin receptor blocker, CI: confidence interval.

clopidogrel (1.5% vs. 2.2%) 90 days prior to admission provided similar results and in this analysis patients with DM claimed less ASA (OR 0.76 [95% CI 0.69-0.84]) and clopidogrel (OR 0.90 [95% CI 0.82-0.98]) than patients without DM. Statistically significant interactions were found between all examined secondary prevention pharmacotherapy agents and patient gender and age.

Table 2 Univariate analysis

	OR	95% CI	*p*
ASA	0.75	0.70–0.81	<0.0001
ACEIs/ARBs	2.13	1.99–2.28	<0.0001
β-blockers	0.87	0.80–0.94	<0.0001
Statins	1.01	0.93–1.09	0.8054
Clopidogrel	0.81	0.76–0.87	<0.0001

Odds ratio (OR) for claiming secondary prevention pharmacotherapy after first myocardial infarction during 2003–2006 in patients with vs. without diabetes mellitus. ASA: acetyl salicylic acid, ACEI: angiotensin-converting enzyme inhibitor, ARB: angiotensin receptor blocker, CI: confidence interval.

The ORs for claiming secondary prevention therapy were found to be significantly lower in women than in men for β-blockers (OR 0.84 [95% CI 0.79–0.89]), clopidogrel (OR 0.84 [95% CI 0.80–0.89]), and statins (OR 0.79 [95% CI 0.74–0.84]). The proportion of patients that claimed secondary prevention therapy decreased significantly with increasing age, except for claims of ASA, and this age-dependent decrease in secondary prevention therapy was most apparent for β-blockers and statins, i.e., patients aged >69 years had OR 0.86 (95% CI 0.79–0.93) for receiving β-blockers and OR 0.63 (95% CI 0.57–0.70) for receiving statins, compared to patients aged 60–69 years, respectively. Furthermore, as shown in Table 1, patients with DM underwent significantly fewer PCI procedures and significantly more CABG procedures (both $p < 0.0001$).

Combinations of secondary prevention pharmacotherapy agents

The ORs for claiming two or more secondary prevention drugs increased markedly between the two study periods. In the total study population the proportion of patients claiming a combination of 2, 3, 4 and 5 agents increased from 62.3% to 87.9%, 34.4% to 75.1%, 12.9% to 57.1% and 2.8% to 22.6 respectively, between 1997–2002 and 2003–2006. Patients with DM claimed more ACEIs/ARBs in any combination than patients without DM. A comparison of the use combinations of 2, 3, 4 and 5 agents, for patients with and without DM during 2003–2006, is shown in Figure 3.

Discussion

In this nationwide study of patients discharged after their first MI in Denmark, we found that the proportion of patients that claimed secondary prevention pharmacotherapies increased substantially from 1997–2002 to 2003–2006. Patients with DM, however, claimed less ASA and clopidogrel than patients without DM, and women and the elderly generally received less secondary prevention agents. In the total study population, the fraction of patients claiming a combination of two or more secondary prevention pharmacotherapy agents increased significantly during the

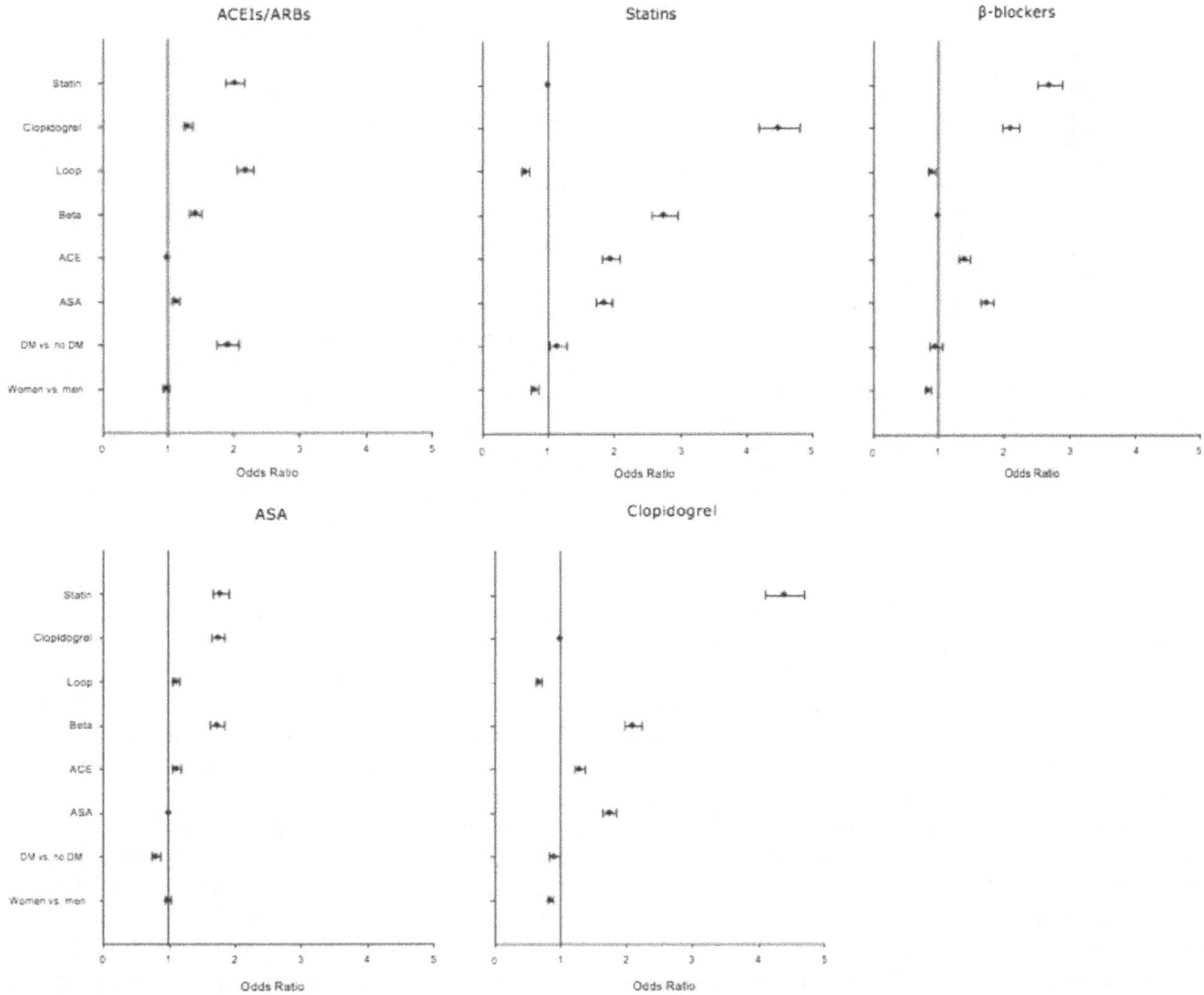

Figure 2 Multivariable logistic regression analyses showing odds ratios for claiming secondary prevention therapy after first myocardial infarction during 2003–2006 for acetylsalicylic acid (ASA), angiotensin-converting enzyme inhibitors or angiotensin-2 receptor blockers (ACEIs/ARBs), β-blockers, clopidogrel, and statins. DM: diabetes mellitus. Analyses were adjusted for age, gender, comorbidity, and concomitant pharmacotherapy.

study period but combination therapies appear to remain underused as compared to treatment guidelines [2,3,23]. Although previous studies have shown that even in the modern era patients with coronary artery disease generally receive suboptimal secondary prevention pharmacotherapy [15,24], our study adds important information on treatment differences between patients with and without DM, genders, and age groups, respectively, in an unselected nationwide post-MI population. Specifically, the data suggest that in post-MI patients with DM, there should be increased focus on increased provision of antiplatelet therapy with ASA and clopidogrel and of combinations of evidence-based secondary prevention drug therapies. In the general population, there also remains considerable room for improvement of secondary prevention pharmacotherapy, particularly in women and the elderly.

Antiplatelets

Platelet inhibitors, i.e., low dose ASA and clopidogrel are recommended for secondary prevention after MI irrespective of, for example, patient gender, age, and DM status [25-27]. In the current study, post MI patients with DM claimed significantly less ASA and clopidogrel than patients without DM. The reasons for this undertreatment are not readily apparent but patients with DM underwent more CABG than patients without DM (Table 1), and contrary to treatment guidelines, surgeons may discontinue clopidogrel after CABG in post MI patients [28]. Patients ≥70 years of age claimed significantly less clopidogrel than the younger population, whereas the use of ASA was not affected by increasing age. Results from the Can Rapid risk stratification of Unstable angina patients Suppress ADverse outcomes

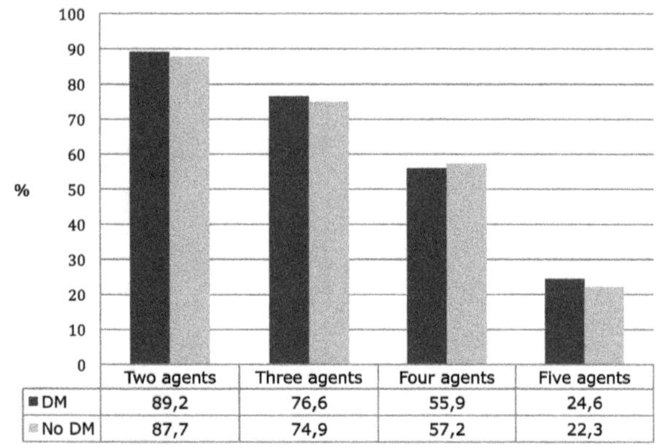

Figure 3 Use of secondary prevention drugs after first myocardial infarction in combinations of two, three, four or five agents including acetylsalicylic acid, angiotensin-converting enzyme inhibitors or angiotensin-2 receptor blockers, β-blockers, clopidogrel, and statins, respectively, claimed ≤90 days after discharge during the period 2003–2006. DM: diabetes mellitus.

with Early implementation of the American College of Cardiology/American Heart Association Guidelines (CRUSADE) initiative have showed that even very old (≥90 years) patients with acute coronary syndromes benefit from clopidogrel treatment [29]. Consistent with our findings, the use of ASA in patients with atherothrombotic disease was recently found to be lower in patients with DM than patients without DM in the international Reduction of Atherothrombosis for Continued Health (REACH) registry [30]. Patients with DM may have received less ASA due to clinicians' concern of retinal bleeding in patients with retinopathy. However, the Early Treatment Diabetic Retinopathy Study Report 14 results from 1992 support treatment with ASA in patients with diabetes at increased risk of cardiovascular disease and found no increased risk of retinal bleeding associated with the use [6]. Female gender has previously been associated with lower use of ASA [29], but in or study there were no significant differences in claims of ASA prescriptions between women and men. Unsurprisingly, we found that a greater proportion of patients with DM compared to patients without DM claimed ASA and clopidogrel prior to admission, probably reflecting, in part, the increased baseline rate of cerebrovascular disease. The possibility that decreased utilization of ASA and clopidogrel after first MI in patients with DM was caused by these patients using their remaining stocks of the antiplatelet agents after discharge was not supported by our comparable finding in a sensitivity analysis that excluded patients with prior use of ASA and clopidogrel. Patients with DM have increased prevalence of gastrointestinal discomfort, e.g., due to gastroparesis, which may reduce initiation of and compliance with pharmacologic treatment, especially ASA and clopidogrel [31]. After including claims of PPIs 90 days after discharge in the multivariable analyses, however, there remained a significant underuse in DM compared to non-DM patients. Mortality rates 30–90 days after MI, i.e., the period where prescription claims were retrieved according to our study design, did not differ significantly between patients with and without DM and are therefore unlikely to have contributed to the observed discrepancy in drug use between the two groups.

β-blockers

Secondary prevention with β-blockers after MI are recommended for all patients and is particularly important because immediate treatment can reduce mortality and risk of re-MI [2]. The absolute benefit of a given relative reduction of post-MI risk may be greater in patients with DM because of their higher absolute risk. In the current study, the univariate analysis demonstrated a significantly lower β-blocker use in DM patients (Table 2) and the multivariate analysis (Figure 2) showed a similar trend. Since β-blockers are also a mainstay in treatment of severe HF, this apparent under treatment is reinforced by the increased prevalence of HF in DM patients after MI during the late (2003–2006) study period. Among the reasons contributing to this finding may be the widespread misconception that β-blockers may mask symptoms of hypoglycemia and prolong recovery from hypoglycaemia [32], although the value of β-blocker is post MI DM patients has been firmly established [33]. Also, patients with DM in our study were slightly older than their non DM controls and the elderly are at an increased risk of adverse cardiac effects of β-blockers, e.g., low cardiac output and bradycardia, which together with their increased prevalence of chronic obstructive lung disease may have added to the underuse of β-blockers in patients with DM.

Angiotensin-converting enzyme inhibitors and angiotensin receptor blockers

The international guidelines generally recommend ACEI/ARB for secondary post MI prevention in patients with HF, left ventricular ejection fraction less than 45%, DM, hypertension, chronic renal disease, peripheral arterial disease, and/or when patients are otherwise considered as being at high risk [34,35]. In the current study, 50.4% of patients claimed ACEIs/ARBs, which is markedly lower than reported in the European Action on Secondary and Primary Prevention through Interventions to Reduce Events (EUROASPIRE) III survey where 71% reported use of these agents six months after an acute coronary syndrome [24]. Patients included in that study, however, were not exclusively those with first-time MI but also included subjects with a recurrent diagnosis of or treatment for coronary artery disease which could lead to more patients receiving treatment [24]. We found that patients with DM claimed significantly more ACEIs/ARBs than patients without DM, i,e., 66.3% vs. 48.0%, in agreement with the guideline recommendation, and the increased prevalence of HF and renal disease in these patients (Table 1) [36]. The risk of lactic acidosis relating to concomitant use of metformin in subjects with DM and renal impairment may also have contributed to the underuse of ARB/ACEI in patients with DM.

Statins

During the study period, the increase in the number of patients claiming statins was greater than the increase in the use of any of the other secondary prevention agents. Indeed, 77.4% of patients claimed statins in 2003–2006, and the increase in statin use was independent of DM status. During the study period several landmark studies and guidelines on primary and secondary prevention of cardiovascular disease with statins were published which probably contributed to the increased use [37-39]. Based on current evidence all patients with MI and in particular patients with DM should receive statins [40]. Even a higher fraction of patients with DM claiming statins may therefore have been expected in the present study. The proportion of women claiming statins was consistently lower than the proportion of men, regardless of subject age. Women have lower primary risk of coronary artery disease than men, but in the post-MI population there should be no differences in secondary prevention statin use between genders. In particular, the elderly (≥70 years) population claimed significantly fewer prescriptions for statins, even though results of the Prospective Study of Pravastatin in the Elderly at Risk (PROSPER) study published in 2002 clearly showed a reduced risk of coronary death and non-fatal MI in a population aged 70–82 years with a history of (or risk factors for), vascular disease.

Combinations of secondary prevention drugs

A combination of secondary prevention pharmacotherapies is frequently needed to optimize myocardial function post MI and prevent subsequent adverse events [25,35]. Based on the marked survival advantages associated with combination treatment of post MI patients the present results are disappointing [41]. In our study only 32.1% of patients with DM and 27.0% without DM claimed prescriptions for ASA, ACEIs/ARBs, β –blockers, and statins during the first 90 days post-MI. According to current evidence DM patients should receive more aggressive post MI therapy than patients without DM to reduce their increased risk and the fact that they received less combination therapy, apart from combinations containing ACEIs/ARBs, is disturbing. Our data essentially suggest a substantial underuse of combinations of recommended secondary prevention therapies after MI irrespective of DM status, not least since synergistic effects of co-administration of such therapies are reasonably well established. For example, in the Steno 2 trial published in 2003 [42] intensive multifactorial interventions including ACEIs/ARBs, β –blockers, and statins in patients with type 2 DM and microalbuminuria reduced the risk of cardiovascular and microvascular events by about 50%. The publication of this study may have increased awareness of clinicians of the effectiveness of both primary and secondary preventive therapies in patients with diabetes. Concerns about possible drug interactions leading to inadequate initiation of therapies and poor patient compliance in patients with chronic disease may also contribute to drug underuse [43].

Numerous previous studies have examined the proportion of hospitalized cardiac patients discharged with secondary prevention medications. A meta-analysis of data from 376,162 patients in 20 studies of primary and secondary prevention (9 studies) assessing adherence to aspirin, ACEIs, ARBs, *β*-blockers, calcium channel blockers, thiazides, and statins found a mean general adherence to secondary prevention therapies of 66% [44]. A registry study of a 2008–2009 population cohort in Spain of patients admitted with acute coronary syndrome found the proportions of drug adherence to be 69.9%, 45.4%, 43.3%, and 58.8%, for antiplatelet drugs, ACEIs/ARBs β-blockers and statins, respectively. In that study only 47.6% received 3 or more drugs and no association was found between low drug adherence and DM [45]. Although we did not specifically examine drug adherence but only used the correlate of claimed prescriptions the use of ACEIs/ARBs, *β*-blockers and statins in the late study period (2003–2006) in the present study is consistent with these more recent results albeit that the percentage of patients that used combinations of 3 or more drugs (75,1%) in our study was markedly higher.

Methods to improve adherence to secondary prevention therapies

Adherence is a key factor associated with the effectiveness of all pharmacological therapies not least for medications prescribed for chronic conditions like cardiovascular diseases and DM. Medical adherence is a complex issue and involves demographic, psychological, and social factors, as well as factors related to the health care provider, medical system, specific disease and treatments. Improved adherence may be achieved by targeted education of patients, involving patients in decisions regarding their treatments, changes of dosing regimens, reduction of adverse effects, and improvements of access to medication and medical consultations.

Limitations and strengths

The main study limitation is inherent in the observational study design. The registers did not include information on important confounders, e.g., left ventricular ejection fraction, renal function, and contraindications for treatment. Additionally, we did not know the number of patients who initiated secondary prevention therapy during hospitalization but did not tolerate treatment. Furthermore, the definition of DM was based on prescription claims for GLDs. Therefore DM patients treated with diet were identified as not having DM. The data collected in this study origin only from Denmark and the results should only be extrapolated to other countries with different health care systems with caution. The use of secondary prevention therapies after first MI according to the specific hospitals that patients were admitted to in Denmark has been investigated previously and was found to vary substantially [46]. In the present study, data from admissions to a total of 82 hospitals were included and clustering of prescription claims, e.g., with patients discharged from highly specialized cardiology clinics receiving more evidence-based drugs than those discharged from community hospitals, is likely to have influenced the results. Therefore, our results apply to an average of Danish hospitals and patients and cannot be extrapolated to represent the performance status of any specific institution. The data is now 5–15 years old but since the underlying fundamentals, e.g., the free-of-charge health care system and well-structured organisation of post-MI treatment in Denmark, have not changed we sincerely believe that today's situation in terms of suboptimal treatment of a considerable number of patients is unlikely to be markedly different from our 1997–2006 results. Indeed, in view of these favourable features of the Danish health care system it is likely that implementation of secondary prevention therapies after MI is even worse in other countries. Therefore, the overall message of our paper is likely to remain valid and the implicit call for a focused effort to increase use of evidence-based secondary prevention drugs is probably as relevant today as in 2006.

The main strength of this study was the nationwide consecutive patient registries, the contemporary data collection, the large sample size comprising approximately 78,000 patients, and the use of pharmacy dispensations and not prescriptions alone, which better reflected true as opposed to intended drug use. Selection bias arising from inclusion of only subgroups of patients or patients from selected hospitals, medical centers, or health care systems was avoided. Furthermore, the cohort comprised patients both in and out of the labor market. In Denmark, a government-financed health care system ensures practically equal access to health care for all inhabitants.

Conclusions

In patients with first MI, the proportion of subjects who claimed secondary prevention pharmacotherapies increased significantly over time during 1997–2006. However, patients with DM claimed significantly less ASA and clopidogrel and suboptimal use of drug combinations was found. Moreover, women and elderly patients were less treated with secondary prevention pharmacotherapy compared to men and younger individuals, respectively. A focused effort to increase use of evidence-based secondary prevention drugs in post MI patients with and without DM is likely to provide long-term benefit.

Competing interest

The authors declare that they have no competing interest.

Authors' contributions

CJ, GG, CTP and PRH conceived and designed the study. CJ, OA, CA, PRH and GG acquired and analyzed data. CJ drafted the first version of the manuscript. All authors interpreted data and critically revised the manuscript for important intellectual content and accepted the final version of the manuscript for submission.

Acknowledgement

This study was supported by research grants from the Danish Heart Foundation (Grant No. 08-4-R64-A1889-B898-22468) and The Danish Agency for Science, Technology and Innovation – The Danish Medical Research Council – 2008 (Grant No. 271-08-0944).

Author details

[1]Department of Cardiology, Copenhagen University Hospital Gentofte, Niels Andersens Vej 65, Copenhagen 2900, Denmark. [2]Department of Health Science and Technology, Aalborg University, Niels Jernes Vej 12, Aalborg 9220, Denmark.

References

1. Wald NJ, Law MR: **A strategy to reduce cardiovascular disease by more than 80%.** *BMJ* 2003, **326**(7404):1419.
2. Freemantle N, Cleland J, Young P, Mason J, Harrison J: **β Blockade after myocardial infarction: systematic review and meta regression analysis.** *BMJ* 1999, **318**(7200):1730–1737.
3. LaRosa JC, He J, Vupputuri S: **Effect of statins on risk of coronary disease: a meta-analysis of randomized controlled trials.** *JAMA* 1999, **282**(24):2340–2346.
4. Pfeffer MA, McMurray JJV, Velazquez EJ, Rouleau J-L, Køber L, Maggioni AP, *et al*: **Valsartan, captopril, or both in myocardial infarction complicated by heart failure, left ventricular dysfunction, or both.** *N Engl J Med* 2003, **349**(20):1893–1906.
5. Mehta RH, Eagle KA: **Secondary prevention in acute myocardial infarction.** *BMJ* 1998, **316**(7134):838–842. Epub 1998/04/29.
6. **Aspirin effects on mortality and morbidity in patients with diabetes mellitus: early treatment diabetic retinopathy study report 14: ETDRS investigators.** *JAMA* 1992, **268**(10):1292–1300. Epub 1992/09/09.
7. **Collaborative overview of randomised trials of antiplatelet therapy–I: prevention of death, myocardial infarction, and stroke by prolonged antiplatelet therapy in various categories of patients: antiplatelet trialists' collaboration.** *BMJ* 1994, **308**(6921):81–106. Epub 1994/01/08.
8. Yusuf S, Peto R, Lewis J, Collins R, Sleight P: **Beta blockade during and after myocardial infarction: an overview of the randomized trials.** *Progress in cardiovascular diseases* 1985, **27**(5):335–371. Epub 1985/03/01.
9. Lancet: **A randomised, blinded, trial of clopidogrel versus aspirin in patients at risk of ischaemic events (CAPRIE): CAPRIE steering committee.** *Lancet* 1996, **348**(9038):1329–1339. Epub 1996/11/16.
10. Yusuf S, Zhao F, Mehta SR, Chrolavicius S, Tognoni G, Fox KK: **Effects of clopidogrel in addition to aspirin in patients with acute coronary syndromes without ST-segment elevation.** *N Engl J Med* 2001, **345**(7):494–502. Epub 2001/08/25.

11. Investigators THOPES: **Effects of an angiotensin-converting–enzyme inhibitor, ramipril, on cardiovascular events in high-risk patients.** *N Engl J Med* 2000, **342**(3):145–153.
12. Randomised trial of cholesterol lowering in 4444 patients with coronary heart disease: the Scandinavian Simvastatin Survival Study (4S): **Randomised trial of cholesterol lowering in 4444 patients with coronary heart disease: the scandinavian simvastatin survival study (4S).** *Lancet* 1994, **344**(8934):1383–1389. Epub 1994/11/19.
13. Deedwania PC, Amsterdam EA, Vagelos RH: **Evidence-based, cost-effective risk stratification and management after myocardial infarction: California cardiology working group on post-MI management.** *Archives of internal medicine* 1997, **157**(3):273–280. Epub 1997/02/10.
14. AmericanDiabetesAssociation: **Standards of medical care in diabetes - 2008.** *Diabetes Care* 2008, **31**(1):S12–S54.
15. Newby LK, Allen LaPointe NM, Chen AY, Kramer JM, Hammill BG, DeLong ER, *et al*: **Long-term adherence to evidence-based secondary prevention therapies in coronary artery disease.** *Circulation* 2006, **113**(2):203–212.
16. Madsen M, Davidsen M, Rasmussen S, Abildstrom SZ, Osler M: **The validity of the diagnosis of acute myocardial infarction in routine statistics: a comparison of mortality and hospital discharge data with the Danish MONICA registry.** *J Clin Epidemiol* 2003, **56**(2):124–130.
17. Gaist D, Sorensen HT, Hallas J: **The Danish prescription registries.** *Dan Med Bull* 1997, **44**(4):445–448.
18. Drivsholm TB, Frederiksen K, Olivarius NF, Odegaard B, Kristensen JK: **The prevalence of diabetes in Denmark: development of a method for a registry-based assessment.** *Ugeskrift for laeger* 2003, **165:**2887–2891.
19. Andersen HR, Nielsen TT, Rasmussen K, Thuesen L, Kelbaek H, Thayssen P, *et al*: **A comparison of coronary angioplasty with fibrinolytic therapy in acute myocardial infarction.** *N Engl J Med* 2003, **349**(8):733–742.
20. Gislason GH, Rasmussen JN, Abildstrøm SZ, Gadsbøll N, Buch P, Friberg J, *et al*: **Long-term compliance with beta-blockers, angiotensin-converting enzyme inhibitors, and statins after acute myocardial infarction.** *Eur Heart J* 2006, **27**(10):1153–1158.
21. Tu JV, Austin PC, Walld R, Roos L, Agras J, McDonald KM: **Development and validation of the ontario acute myocardial infarction mortality prediction rules.** *J Am Coll Cardiol* 2001, **37**(4):992–997.
22. Daasnes C: **The personal data act, clinical trials and data privacy: rules for treatment of personal data in clinical trials and scientific research projects.** *Ugeskrift for laeger* 2003, **165**(16):1683–1685. Epub 2003/05/22. Persondataloven, laegemiddelforsog og datasikkerhed. Reglerne for behandling af personoplysninger i laegemiddelforsog og laegevidenskabe lige forskningsprojekter.
23. Fox KM, EURopean trial On reduction of cardiac events with Perindopril in stable coronary Artery disease Investigators: **Efficacy of perindopril in reduction of cardiovascular events among patients with stable coronary artery disease: randomised, double-blind, placebo-controlled, multicentre trial (the EUROPA study).** *Lancet* 2003, **362**(9386):782–788.
24. Kotseva K, Wood D, De Backer G, De Bacquer D, Pyorala K, Keil U, *et al*: **EUROASPIRE III: a survey on the lifestyle, risk factors and use of cardioprotective drug therapies in coronary patients from 22 European countries.** *Eur J Cardiovasc Prev Rehabil* 2009, **16**(2):121–137.
25. Ryden L, Standl E, Bartnik M, Van den Berghe G, Betteridge J, de Boer M-J, *et al*: **Guidelines on diabetes, pre-diabetes, and cardiovascular diseases: executive summary.** *Eur Heart J* 2007, **28**(1):88–136.
26. Antithrombotic TC: **Aspirin in the primary and secondary prevention of vascular disease: collaborative meta-analysis of individual participant data from randomised trials.** *Lancet* 2009, **373**(9678):1849–1860.
27. Yusuf S, Zhao F, Mehta SR, Chrolavicius S, Tognoni G, Fox KK, Clopidogrel in Unstable Angina to Prevent Recurrent Events Trial Investigators: **Effects of clopidogrel in addition to aspirin in patients with acute coronary syndromes without ST-segment elevation.** *N Eng J Med* 2001, **345**(7):494–502.
28. Sørensen R, Abildstrøm SZ, Hansen PR, Hvelplund A, Andersson C, Charlot M, *et al*: **Efficacy of post-operative clopidogrel treatment in patients revascularized with coronary artery bypass grafting after myocardial infarction.** *J Am Coll Cardiol* 2011, **57**(10):1202–1209.
29. Adam HS, Karen PA, Anita YC, Matthew TR, Charles VP, Ohman EM, *et al*: **Characteristics, management, and outcomes of 5,557 patients age ≥90 years with acute coronary syndromes: results from the CRUSADE initiative.** *J Am Coll Cardiol* 2007, **49**(17):1790–1797.
30. Cannon CP, Rhee KE, Califf RM, Boden WE, Hirsch AT, Alberts MJ, *et al*: **Current use of aspirin and antithrombotic agents in the united states among outpatients with atherothrombotic disease (from the REduction of atherothrombosis for continued health [REACH] registry).** *Am J Cardiol* 2010, **105**(4):445–452.
31. Ma J, Rayner CK, Jones KL, Horowitz M: **Diabetic gastroparesis: diagnosis and management.** *Drugs* 2009, **69**(8):971–986.
32. Lang N, Fox K: **Current drug therapies for the secondary prevention of MI.** *Prescriber* 2008, **19**(1):14–25.
33. UK Prospective Diabetes Study Group: **Efficacy of atenolol and captopril in reducing risk of macrovascular and microvascular complications in type 2 diabetes: UKPDS 39.** *BMJ* 1998, **317**(7160):713–720.
34. Skinner JS, Cooper A, Feder GS: **Secondary prevention for patients following a myocardial infarction: summary of NICE guidance.** *Heart* 2007, **93**(7):862–864.
35. Antman EM, Hand M, Armstrong PW, Bates ER, Green LA, Halasyamani LK, *et al*: **2007 Focused update of the ACC/AHA 2004 guidelines for the management of patients with ST-elevation myocardial infarction.** *Circulation* 2008, **117**(2):296–329.
36. Estep J, Aguilar D: **Diabetes and heart failure in the post-myocardial infarction patient.** *Curr Heart Fail Rep* 2006, **3**(4):164–169.
37. The Long-Term Intervention with Pravastatin in Ischaemic Disease (LIPID) Study Group: **Prevention of cardiovascular events and death with pravastatin in patients with coronary heart disease and a broad range of initial cholesterol levels.** *N Engl J Med* 1998, **339**(19):1349–1357.
38. Snow V, Aronson MD, Hornbake ER, Mottur-Pilson C, Weiss KB: **Lipid control in the management of type 2 diabetes mellitus: a clinical practice guideline from the American college of physicians.** *Ann Intern Med* 2004, **140**(8):644–649.
39. **MRC/BHF heart protection study of cholesterol-lowering with simvastatin in 5963 people with diabetes: a randomised placebo-controlled trial.** *Lancet* 2003, **361**(9374):2005–2016.
40. Baigent CKA, Kearney PM, *et al*: **Efficacy and safety of cholesterol-lowering treatment: prospective meta-analysis of data from 90.056 participants in 14 randomised trials of statins.** *Lancet* 2005, **366**(9493):1267–1278.
41. Mukherjee D, Fang J, Chetcuti S, Moscucci M, Kline-Rogers E, Eagle KA: **Impact of combination evidence-based medical therapy on mortality in patients with acute coronary syndromes.** *Circulation* 2004, **109**(6):745–749.
42. Gaede P, Vedel P, Larsen N, Jensen GVH, Parving H-H, Pedersen O: **Multifactorial intervention and cardiovascular disease in patients with type 2 diabetes.** *N Engl J Med* 2003, **348**(5):383–393.
43. Grant RW, Meigs JB: **Overcoming barriers to evidence-based diabetes care.** *Curr Diabetes Rev* 2006, **2:**261–269.
44. Naderi SH, Bestwick JP, Wald DS: **Adherence to drugs that prevent cardiovascular disease: meta-analysis on 376,162 patients.** *Am J Med* 2012, **125**(9):882–887. e1.
45. Sanfelix-Gimeno G, Peiro S, Ferreros I, Perez-Vicente R, Librero J, Catala-Lopez F, *et al*: **Adherence to evidence-based therapies after acute coronary syndrome: a retrospective population-based cohort study linking hospital, outpatient, and pharmacy health information systems in Valencia, Spain.** *J Manag Care Pharm* 2013, **19**(3):247–257. Epub 2013/03/30.
46. Rasmussen S, Abildstrom SZ, Rasmussen JN, Gislason GH, Schramm TK, Folke F, *et al*: **Hospital variation in use of secondary preventive medicine after discharge for first acute myocardial infarction during 1995–2004.** *Med Care* 2008, **46**(1):70–77. Epub 2007/12/29.

2

Statin use associated with a reduced risk of pneumonia requiring hospitalization in patients with myocardial infarction

Chao-Feng Lin[1,5,6], Ya-Hui Chang[2], Ju-Chi Liu[1], Ming-Tsang Chuang[3] and Li-Nien Chien[4*]

Abstract

Background: Statins have been reported to prevent adverse cardiovascular events in patients with myocardial infarction (MI). However, the association of statin use and the risk of pneumonia requiring hospitalization in MI patients remains unclear.

Methods: A nested case-control study was conducted by using data from the National Health Insurance Research Database of Taiwan. Among 24,975 patients with MI, 2686 case patients with pneumonia requiring hospitalization were age- and sex-matched with 10,726 control patients using the incidence density sampling approach. Duration and dosage of statin use were obtained from pharmaceutical claims. Conditional logistic regression analyses were used to estimate the risk of hospitalization for pneumonia associated with statin use adjusted for patient's demographics, medical conditions and prescribed medications.

Results: Statin use was associated with a 15 % reduced risk of pneumonia requiring hospitalization among MI patients (adjusted odds ratio [aOR] = 0.85, 95 % confidence interval [CI] = 0.77–0.95, $P = 0.004$). The association was more significant for MI patients unexposed to statin pretreatment (aOR = 0.76, 95 % CI = 0.64–0.90, $P = 0.001$). Statins also exhibited favorable benefits in a time- and dose-dependent manner. The results were consistent in various subgroup analysis of the patients who were female, age ≥ 65 years, a low $CHADS_2$ (i.e. congestive heart failure, hypertension, diabetes mellitus, previous stroke and age > 75 years old) score, and fewer comorbidities. Atorvastatin, fluvastatin and simvastatin were the most common prescribed statins and had similar effects.

Conclusions: Statins might be considered as an adjunctive therapy to reduce the risk of hospitalization for pneumonia for MI patients under thorough evaluation of individual comorbidities, previous statin use and optimal dosage.

Keywords: Myocardial infarction, Pneumonia, Statins, Incidence-density sampling

Background

Myocardial infarction (MI) is the most acute and severe presentation of ischemic heart disease. Approximately 620,000 people have a new coronary attack each year in the United States, and 15 % of those do not survive the event [1, 2]. Besides, survivors of MI have a higher chance of illness and death from cardiac or noncardiac causes compared with the general population [1–3]. Patients with MI had a 79 % increased risk of incident infection compared with those without an MI history, and the most frequent infection was pneumonia [3]. Additionally, MI patients had a significantly higher rate of all-cause mortality during the course of pneumonia than that of patients without a history of MI [4]. Therefore, strategies for preventing the development of adverse cardiovascular events and incident pneumonia among patients with MI are crucial.

* Correspondence: lnchien@tmu.edu.tw
[4]School of Health Care Administration, College of Management, Taipei Medical University, Taipei, Taiwan
Full list of author information is available at the end of the article

Statins are competitive inhibitors of 3-hydroxy-3-methylglutaryl-coenzyme A (HMG-CoA) reductase, a rate-limiting enzyme of the cholesterol biosynthesis pathway [5], and are commonly used in the primary and secondary prevention of atherosclerotic cardiovascular diseases [6]. Previous researches have also demonstrated that statin pretreatment improves the clinical outcomes of MI [7, 8]. Recently, epidemiological studies have shown that statins have pleiotropic effects, resulting in a reduced risk of incident pneumonia in the general population as well as patients with diabetes [9–12]. However, whether statin use is associated with a reduced risk of pneumonia in MI patients who are at high cardiovascular risk and susceptible to pneumonia remains unclear.

The aim of this study was to investigate the association between statin use and pneumonia hospitalization among patients with a history of MI. We conducted a nested case–control study by using data from the National Health Insurance Research Database (NHIRD) of Taiwan. Subgroup analysis was performed to identify the aforementioned association among patients with different characteristics and those who were unexposed to statin pretreatment.

Methods

Ethics statement

This retrospective observational research was approved by the Joint Institutional Review Board of Taipei Medical University (TMU-JIRB No. 201404055). Data from the NHIRD was provided by the National Health Insurance Administration (NHIA) of Taiwan that covers 99 % of residents in Taiwan under the legislation of National Health Insurance (NHI). To protect the privacy of beneficiaries, individual identifiers have been encrypted before data are released to researchers. Consequently, informed consent of the participants was exempted under the full review process of the Joint Institutional Review Board of Taipei Medical University.

Study design and data source

This nested case-control study was conducted by using data from NHIRD which were collected between 2000 and 2011. The NHIRD files contained International Classification of Diseases, Ninth Revision, Clinical Modification (ICD-9-CM) disease diagnosis codes, treatment procedures, date of service, reimbursement amounts, demographic information on beneficiaries and beneficiary- and provider-encrypted identifiers. Claims for prescribed drugs were also provided and could be classified according to the Anatomical Therapeutic Chemical (ATC) classification system. To verify the accuracy of diagnoses and the rationale for treatments, the NHIA routinely samples a proportion of the NHI claims. Additionally, hospitals and clinics are penalized if they provide any unnecessary medical treatment to patients [13].

Study cohort

The study cohort consisted of patients who were first admitted for a primary diagnosis of MI (ICD-9-CM: 410) between the year of 2002 and 2010, and received prescriptions of statins during MI hospitalization. We excluded participants who were < 20 years old or > 80 years old, for whom the sex was unidentified, and had a history of MI or pneumonia (ICD-9-CM: 480–486) in the preceding 2 years. Figure 1 presents the patient selection process.

Case ascertainment and control selection

The case patients were those who were readmitted for the primary diagnosis of incident pneumonia (ICD-9-CM: 480–486) requiring hospitalization after MI admission. In Taiwan, the diagnosis of pneumonia at least must comply with the positive findings of the patient's chest X-ray. The date of hospitalization for pneumonia was defined as the index date. The control patients were randomly selected by using incidence density sampling of all patients with MI who were alive and free of pneumonia at the time of being observed. Each case patient was matched to 4 control patients by sex, age ± 1 year, year of hospitalization for MI, and follow-up period. The control patients were assigned a pseudo index date of pneumonia admission, which corresponded to the index date of their matched cases.

Statin exposure

Statin use was determined based on prescription claims in the NHIRD. The duration of statin use was defined as the period between the latest date of prescription and the index date of pneumonia of case patients or the pseudo index date of control patients (hereafter, "index date"). For each patient, the drug prescriptions were traced back from the index date up to 1 year. Both case and control patients were categorized into "users" if they had any statin claim and "nonusers" if they had no statin claims 1 year before the index date. Subsequently, the users were further classified into "current users" for 0–90 days, "recent users" for 91–180 days, or "former users" for >180 days. The dose-response effect was assessed based on the defined daily dose (DDD), which is the assumed maintenance dose per day for adults recommended by the World Health Organization [14], and was classified as < 0.5, 0.5–1.0, and > 1.0 of the DDD within a 90-day period (DDD_{90}). Additionally, we performed analyses to compare the effects of different statins among the patients with statin prescription within a 90-day period before the index date. A specific statin was defined if it was the nearest and longest statin to

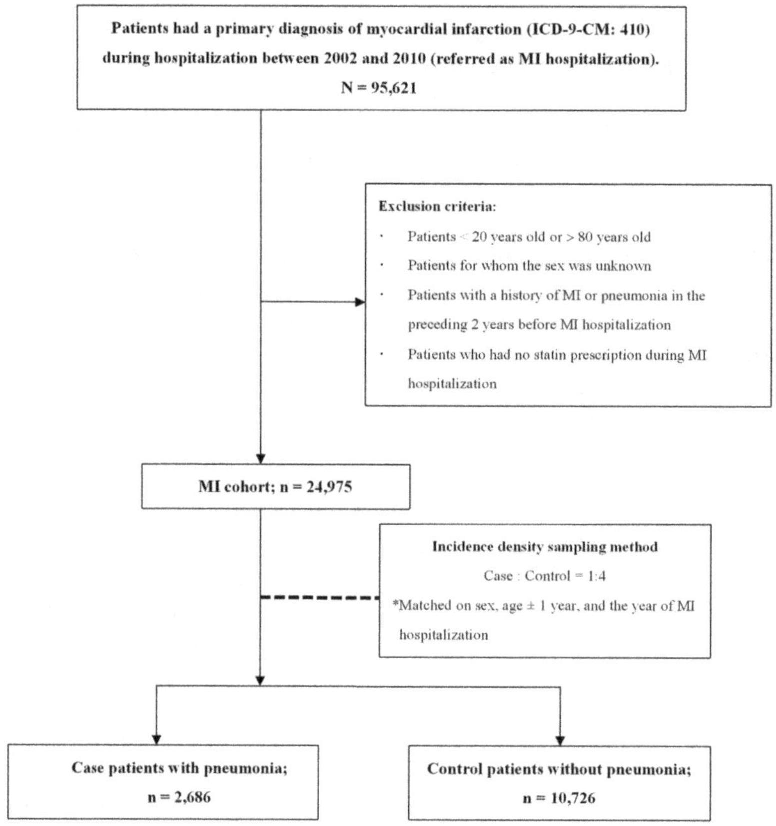

Fig. 1 Flow diagram of patient selection. MI = myocardial infarction

the index date. The DDDs of the statins considered in our study are provided in Additional file 1: Table S1.

Potential confounding variables

Previous or coexisting medical conditions were recorded if the patients had ≥ 2 diagnostic claims for diabetes mellitus (DM), hypertension (HTN), congestive heart failure (CHF), stroke, asthma, chronic obstructive pulmonary disease (COPD), chronic kidney disease (CKD), chronic liver disease (CLD), Parkinson disease or dementia. We also considered and controlled for the $CHADS_2$ score, which is the sum of the risk factors for CHF, HTN, DM and stroke as well as the age > 75 years at the diagnosis of MI. The $CHADS_2$ score was initially used to predict the risk of stroke in patients with nonvalvular atrial fibrillation [15], and has been proposed recently for predicting the prognosis of patients with acute coronary syndrome [16, 17]. The history of influenza and pneumonia vaccination and prescribed medications before the index date were further adjusted. For each patient, the records of medical conditions and medications were traced from the index date up to 1 year. Detailed information on ICD-9-CM diagnosis codes and the ATC classification system codes are provided in Additional file 2: Table S2 and Additional file 3: Table S3, respectively.

Statistical analyses

The primary analysis was to examine the association between statin use and the risk of pneumonia requiring hospitalization. To investigate the effect of statin pretreatment before an MI event, the secondary analysis was limited to MI patients unexposed to statin pretreatment. The stratified analysis of the patients with a specific characteristic was also performed. For all variables of interest, risk estimates were computed as both univariate and multivariate analyses, with additional adjustments for potential confounders. Conditional logistic regression was used to estimate unadjusted and adjusted odds ratios (ORs) and 95 % confidence intervals (CIs) for the association of statin exposure and the risk of hospitalization for pneumonia; and the incidence density sampling yields ORs that are interpretable as unbiased estimates of the incidence ORs [18, 19]. All analyses were performed using SAS/STAT 9.3 (SAS Institute Inc., Cary, NC, USA) and STATA 12 (Stata Corp LP, College Station, TX, USA); $P < 0.05$ was considered significant.

Results

Of the 24,975 patients with a history of MI, we identified 2686 case patients who were hospitalized for pneumonia and 10,726 control patients who were not hospitalized for pneumonia (Fig. 1). Compared with the control patients, the case patients had higher $CHADS_2$ scores ($CHADS_2$ scores ≥ 1: case 36.6 %; control 17.7 %), and higher rates of previous or coexisting DM, HTN, CHF, stroke, asthma, COPD, CKD, CLD and dementia. In addition, the case patients were more likely to use antineoplastic drugs, proton pump inhibitors (PPIs), steroids, angiotensin converting enzyme inhibitor and angiotensin receptor blockade (ACEI/ARBs), immunosuppressants, immunostimulants and nitrates compared with the control patients (Table 1).

The percentage of any use of statins among the case and control patients was 68.9 and 71.6 %, respectively. Statin use was associated with a 15 % reduced risk of incident pneumonia requiring hospitalization after we controlled for all risk factors (aOR 0.85, 95 % CI 0.77–0.95, $P = 0.004$) (Table 2). Additionally, the timing of statin use for the case patients significantly differed from that for the control patients (Table 2). The odds of current users for the case patients were lower than that for the control patients (aOR 0.75, 95 % CI 0.67–0.85, $P < 0.001$). We also observed that the DDD_{90} was associated with a dose-dependent manner that the benefits of statin to prevent the occurrence of pneumonia were determined when the DDD_{90} was ≥ 0.5. However, the protective effect of a DDD_{90} of 0.5–1.0 (aOR 0.75, 95 % CI 0.66–0.84, $P < 0.001$) was closed to that of a DDD_{90} ≥ 1.0 (aOR 0.74, 95 % CI 0.63–0.87, $P = 0.002$) (Table 2).

Table 1 Baseline characteristics of case patients with pneumonia and control patients

		Controls		Cases				
Variables		N	(%)	N	(%)	Crude OR	(95 % CI)	*P*
Sample size		10,726	(100.0)	2,686	(100.0)			
Female		3,280	(30.6)	824	(30.7)			
Age (y)	Mean (± SD)	67.1	(±10.0)	67.1	(±10.0)			
$CHADS_2$ score								
0		8,830	(82.3)	1,703	(63.4)	1.00	(Ref.)	
1–2		1,695	(15.8)	838	(31.2)	3.33	(2.99–3.71)	<0.001
> 2		201	(1.9)	145	(5.4)	5.85	(5.03–6.79)	<0.001
Comorbidities, yes (Ref. = No)								
Diabetes mellitus		800	(7.5)	552	(20.6)	3.33	(2.94–3.76)	<0.001
Hypertension		418	(3.9)	268	(10)	2.77	(2.36–3.26)	<0.001
Congestive heart failure		800	(7.5)	570	(21.2)	3.43	(3.04–3.87)	<0.001
Stroke		1,372	(12.8)	654	(24.3)	2.21	(1.98–2.45)	<0.001
Asthma		133	(1.2)	74	(2.8)	2.28	(1.70–3.04)	<0.001
COPD		246	(2.3)	196	(7.3)	3.43	(2.82–4.18)	<0.001
Chronic kidney disease		118	(1.1)	108	(4)	3.76	(2.88–4.91)	<0.001
Chronic liver disease		28	(0.3)	16	(0.6)	2.29	(1.23–4.22)	0.008
Parkinson disease		20	(0.2)	8	(0.3)	1.60	(0.70–3.63)	0.260
Dementia		49	(0.5)	24	(0.9)	1.96	(1.20–3.19)	0.007
Medication use, yes (Ref. = No)								
Antineoplastic drug		67	(0.6)	71	(2.6)	4.35	(3.10–6.10)	<0.001
PPI		1,127	(10.5)	665	(24.8)	2.86	(2.56–3.19)	<0.001
Steroid		1,756	(16.4)	736	(27.4)	1.96	(1.77–2.16)	<0.001
ACEI/ARB		5,983	(55.8)	1,674	(62.3)	1.33	(1.21–1.45)	<0.001
Antiviral drug		143	(1.3)	47	(1.7)	1.32	(0.95–1.84)	0.100
Immunosuppressants		19	(0.2)	12	(0.4)	2.53	(1.22–5.20)	0.010
Immuostimulants		7	(0.1)	8	(0.3)	5.01	(1.72–14.5)	0.003
Nitrate		6,277	(58.5)	1,847	(68.8)	1.62	(1.47–1.78)	<0.001
Antiplatelet		9,151	(85.3)	2,330	(86.7)	1.13	(0.99–1.28)	0.050
Vaccine (influenza or pneumococcal)		2,551	(23.8)	631	(22.8)	0.94	(0.85–1.05)	0.280

ACEI/ARB angiotensin-converting enzyme inhibitor/angiotensin receptor blockade, *$CHADS_2$* congestive heart failure, hypertension, age > 75 years, diabetes, previous stroke, *CI* confidence interval, *COPD* chronic obstructive pulmonary disease, *OR* odds ratio, *PPI* proton pump inhibitor, *Ref* reference group, *SD* standard deviation

Table 2 Association between statin use and the risk of pneumonia requiring hospitalization

	Controls		Cases		Crude OR		Adjusted[a] OR	
	N	(%)	N	(%)	(95 % CI)	*P*	(95 % CI)	*P*
Sample size	10,726	(100.0)	2,686	(100.0)	-		-	
Statin measurement								
Any statin ≤ 365 d								
Non-user	3,041	(28.4)	835	(31.1)	1.00 (Ref.)		1.00 (Ref.)	
User	7,685	(71.6)	1,851	(68.9)	0.87 (0.78–0.95)	0.003	0.85 (0.77–0.95)	0.004
By recency								
Non-user	3,041	(28.4)	835	(31.1)	1.00 (Ref.)		1.00 (Ref.)	
≤ 90 d (current)	4,778	(44.5)	963	(35.9)	0.72 (0.64–0.80)	<0.001	0.75 (0.67–0.85)	<0.001
91–180 d (recent)	697	(6.5)	229	(8.5)	1.17 (0.98–1.39)	0.080	1.06 (0.87–1.28)	0.570
>180 d (former)	2,210	(20.6)	659	(24.5)	1.08 (0.96–1.23)	0.190	0.98 (0.86–1.12)	0.810
By DDD_{90}								
Non-user	3,041	(28.4)	835	(31.1)	1.00 (Ref.)		1.00 (Ref.)	
≤ 0.5 DDD_{90}	1,278	(11.9)	388	(14.4)	1.05 (0.92–1.19)	0.510	0.98 (0.85–1.13)	0.760
0.5-1 DDD_{90}	2,808	(26.2)	539	(20.1)	0.66 (0.59–0.74)	<0.001	0.75 (0.66–0.84)	<0.001
> 1 DDD_{90}	1,389	(12.9)	265	(9.9)	0.66 (0.57–0.76)	<0.001	0.74 (0.63–0.87)	0.002

ACEI/ARB angiotensin-converting enzyme inhibitor/angiotensin receptor blockade, *$CHADS_2$* congestive heart failure, hypertension, age > 75 years, diabetes, previous stroke, *CI* confidence interval, *COPD* chronic obstructive pulmonary disease, *DDD* defined daily dose, *DDD_{90}* average defined daily dose within 90 days, *OR* odds ratio, *PPI* proton pump inhibitor, *Ref* reference group, *SD* standard deviation

[a] Adjusted for $CHASD_2$ score, medical conditions (diabetes mellitus, hypertension, chronic heart failure, stroke, COPD, chronic kidney disease, chronic liver disease, Parkinson disease, and dementia) and medication use (antineoplastic drug, PPI, ACEI/ARB, antiviral drug, immunosuppressants, immunostimulants, nitrate, antiplatelet and influenza or pneumococcal vaccine)

Of the patients who were unexposed to statin pretreatment at the time of being diagnosed with MI, we identified 1313 case patients who were hospitalized for pneumonia and 6321 control patients who were not hospitalized for pneumonia. The percentage of any use of statins among the case and control patients was 60.4 and 66.3 %, respectively. Among patients unexposed to pretreatment, statin users had a 24 % decreased risk of pneumonia hospitalization (aOR 0.76, 95 % CI 0.64–0.90, $P = 0.001$). The results of current users and dosage manner were consistent with the findings of the primary analysis, but the association was stronger (Table 3).

We performed a stratified analysis and redefined "statin users" if patients had a statin of $DDD_{90} \geq 0.5$. Our results showed a negative association between statin exposure and the risk of pneumonia requiring hospitalization in the patients who were female, were aged ≥ 65 years, had lower $CHADS_2$ scores (0 or 1), or had no history of DM, HTN, CHF, asthma or COPD (Fig. 2).

The major statins used within a 90-day period prior to the index date were atorvastatin, fluvastatin and simvastatin (Table 4). For all patients with MI, fluvastatin and simvastatin had similar associations with the risk of pneumonia requiring hospitalization compared to atorvastatin (fluvastatin: aOR 1.14, 95 % CI 0.85–1.52, $P = 0.390$; simvastatin: aOR 1.19, 95 % CI 0.87–1.64, $P = 0.283$). For patients unexposed to statin pretreatment, the results were consistent with the findings of overall MI patients.

Discussion

In this nested case-control study, we observed that statin use in MI patients was associated with a 15-25 % reduced risk of pneumonia requiring hospitalization. We also observed that the benefits of statins were particularly marked for current users who used statins within 90 days and for those who used statins of ≥ 0.5 DDD_{90}. In addition, the favorable effect was shown in the patients who were female, were aged ≥ 65 years, and had no history of cardiovascular and respiratory diseases. Atorvastatin, fluvastatin and simvastatin were the most common prescribed statins and had similar effects on reducing the risk of pneumonia requiring hospitalization.

The effect of statin use on reducing the occurrence of pneumonia has been shown in the general population [10, 11]. In this present study, we additionally found that statin use might also have a favorable effect on decreasing pneumonia hospitalization in MI patients who were more susceptible to pneumonia and had more comorbidities compared to general population. However, this favorable effect was not significant when the analysis was limited to MI patients with a higher $CHADS_2$ score ($CHADS_2$ score ≥ 2). Some unmeasured differences in baseline characteristics might still exist in statin users and nonusers, resulting in overestimating the benefits of

Table 3 Subgroup analysis of patients unexposed to statin pretreatment

	Controls		Cases		Crude OR		Adjusted[a] OR	
	N	(%)	N	(%)	(95 % CI)	*P*	(95 % CI)	*P*
Sample size	6,321	(100.0)	1,313	(100.0)	-		-	-
Statin Measurement								
Any statin ≤ 365 d								
Non-user	2,130	(33.7)	520	(39.6)	1.00 (Ref.)		1.00 (Ref.)	
User	4,191	(66.3)	793	(60.4)	0.75 (0.65–0.87)	<0.001	0.76 (0.64–0.90)	0.001
By recency								
Non-user	2,130	(33.7)	520	(39.6)	1.00 (Ref.)		1.00 (Ref.)	
≤ 90 d (current)	2,683	(42.4)	403	(30.7)	0.60 (0.51–0.71)	<0.001	0.65 (0.54–0.79)	<0.001
91–180 d (recent)	376	(5.9)	110	(8.4)	1.16 (0.88–1.52)	0.290	1.20 (0.88–1.64)	0.240
> 180 d (former)	1,132	(17.9)	280	(21.3)	0.97 (0.80–1.18)	0.770	0.84 (0.68–1.05)	0.130
By DDD_{90}								
Non-user	2,130	(33.7)	520	(39.6)	1.00 (Ref.)		1.00 (Ref.)	
≤ 0.5 DDD_{90}	757	(12.0)	178	(13.6)	0.99 (0.80–1.22)	0.900	0.99 (0.78–1.27)	0.960
0.5–1 DDD_{90}	1,574	(24.9)	233	(17.7)	0.61 (0.51–0.73)	<0.001	0.73 (0.59–0.89)	0.002
> 1 DDD_{90}	728	(11.5)	102	(7.8)	0.55 (0.43–0.69)	<0.001	0.65 (0.50–0.85)	0.001

ACEI/ARB angiotensin-converting enzyme inhibitor/angiotensin receptor blockade, *$CHADS_2$* congestive heart failure, hypertension, age > 75 years, diabetes, previous stroke, *CI* confidence interval, *COPD* chronic obstructive pulmonary disease, *DDD* defined daily dose, *DDD_{90}* average defined daily dose within 90 days, *OR* odds ratio, *PPI* proton pump inhibitor, *Ref* reference group, *SD* standard deviation

[a] Adjusted for $CHASD_2$ score, medical conditions (diabetes mellitus, hypertension, chronic heart failure, stroke, COPD, chronic kidney disease, chronic liver disease, Parkinson disease, and dementia) and medication use (antineoplastic drug, PPI, ACEI/ARB, antiviral drug, immunosuppressants, immunostimulants, nitrate, antiplatelet and influenza or pneumococcal vaccine)

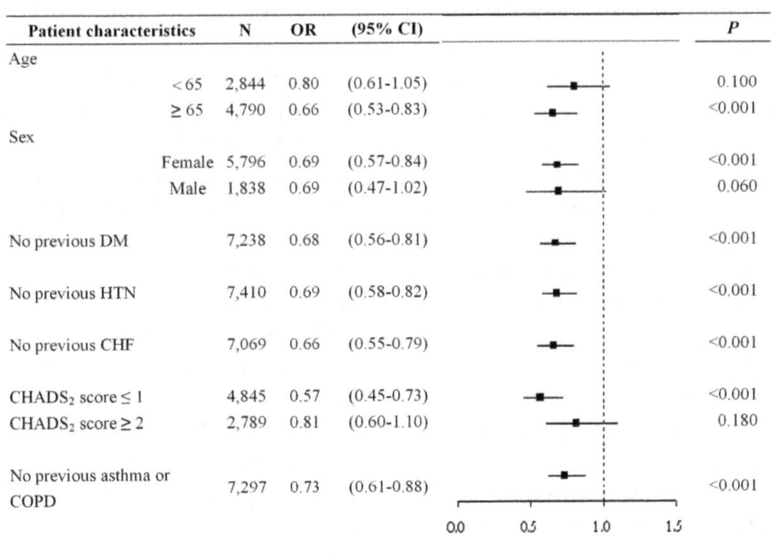

Fig. 2 Subgroup analysis of patients in different comorbidity subgroups. $CHADS_2$ = congestive heart failure, hypertension, age > 75 years, diabetes mellitus and previous stroke; CHF = congestive heart failure; CI = confidence interval; COPD = chronic obstructive pulmonary disease; DM = diabetes mellitus; HTN = hypertension; OR = odds ratio

Table 4 Statin type and the risk of pneumonia requiring hospitalization within a 90-day exposure

	Controls N	Cases N	Crude OR (95 % CI)	*P*	Adjusted[a] OR (95 % CI)	*P*
Overall MI patients	4,778	963	-		-	
Statin type						
Artovastatin	3,242	639	1.00 (Ref.)		1.00 (Ref.)	
Fluvastatin	556	132	1.21 (0.94–1.56)	0.136	1.14 (0.85–1.52)	0.390
Simvastatin	510	109	1.04 (0.79–1.38)	0.781	1.19 (0.87–1.64)	0.283
Other	470	83	0.87 (0.65–1.17)	0.363	0.73 (0.51–1.03)	0.075
MI patients unexposed to statin pretreatment	2,683	403				
Statin type						
Atorvastatin	1,863	270	1.00 (Ref.)		1.00 (Ref.)	
Fluvastatin	297	55	1.16 (0.71–1.90)	0.549	1.11 (0.6–2.04)	0.743
Simvastatin	278	54	0.80 (0.49–1.32)	0.386	1.12 (0.59–2.10)	0.729
Other	245	24	0.65 (0.36–1.17)	0.153	0.66 (0.31–1.41)	0.286

ACEI/ARB angiotensin-converting enzyme inhibitor/angiotensin receptor blockade, *$CHADS_2$* congestive heart failure, hypertension, age > 75 years, diabetes, previous stroke, *CI* confidence interval; COPD, chronic obstructive pulmonary disease, *DDD* defined daily dose, *DDD_{90}* average defined daily dose within 90 days, *OR* odds ratio, *PPI* proton pump inhibitor, *Ref* reference group, *SD* standard deviation

[a] Adjusted for $CHASD_2$ score, medical conditions (diabetes mellitus, hypertension, chronic heart failure, stroke, COPD, chronic kidney disease, chronic liver disease, Parkinson disease, and dementia) and medication use (antineoplastic drug, PPI, ACEI/ARB, antiviral drug, immunosuppressants, immunostimulants, nitrate, antiplatelet and influenza or pneumococcal vaccine)

statins on pneumonia hospitalization. For example, patients who adhered to statin therapy might have other related preventive behaviors (eg, exercising, avoiding tobacco and accessing medical help). Thus, rigorous and randomized controlled clinical trials are required to minimize the potential confounding bias and confirm the preventive effect of statin use on pneumonia hospitalization.

Our analyses showed some discrepancies about the recency of the benefits of statins compared with the previous studies. Nielsen demonstrated that statin use within 125 days before index pneumonia had a protective effect [10]. In another case-control study [11], Vinogradova demonstrated that the benefit was observed only in patients who used statin within 28 days before pneumonia. In the present study, we observed the protective effect on MI patients lasted for 90 days. The possible mechanisms underlying these discrepancies might be related to the differences of study designs, prescription rates of statin, commonly prescribed statins and patient characteristics between studies. Although discrepancies existed, the observations from our and previous research revealed that statin use might be associated with prevention of pneumonia in different patient groups.

Regarding prevention of adverse cardiovascular events, it remains controversial whether statin therapy before an MI event is beneficial. Some studies have reported that chronic statin pretreatment resulted in a small infarct area, more preserved ventricular function [7], and low hospital mortality [8] when patients developed acute MIs. However, Feurnau et al. recently showed that chronic statin pretreatment was not associated with minimal myocardial damage during MI events [20]. The differences of baseline risk profiles between patients exposed to statin pretreatment and those unexposed to pretreatment might have affected the effects of statin therapy [7, 8, 20]. Based on our results, statin use has superior benefits for patients unexposed to statin pretreatment than for all patients with MI. The major reason might be that MI patients exposed to statin pretreatment might have a significantly greater risk profile (e.g. hyperlimpidia) than patients unexposed to pretreatment [7, 8, 20]. Other potential reasons such as exact type, dose, duration and compliance of statin pretreatment might have also contributed to the heterogeneity [20]. These findings provide implications for further research on the pleiotropic effects of statins.

In our stratified analysis, statin users who were female or had fewer comorbidities had a significantly low risk of pneumonia. Our observations are similar to those of van de Garde, who reported that statin use was associated with a reduced risk of pneumonia in patients with diabetes who were female and had no previous pulmonary diseases [12]. Both findings suggested that the clinical presentation of pleiotropic effects of statins might be influenced by the individual's risk profiles of patients. The specific conditions that might affect the effects of statins on the occurrence of pneumonia provide crucial information on how a randomized controlled trial should be designed to clarify the role of statins as an adjunctive treatment for the prevention of pneumonia in patients with MI.

In addition to time-dependent effect of statin use, our results showed a dose-dependent relationship of the benefits of statins that were similar to those reported by Wang et al., who demonstrated that statins prescribed at a medium or high DDD led to a 40–67 % reduction in the risk of COPD exacerbation, including concurrent pneumonia [21]. Additionally, two randomized controlled trials showed that statins exerted an anti-inflammatory effect in a dose-dependent manner [22, 23]. These findings raise a concern of optimal dosage of statins regarding their anti-inflammatory and pleiotropic effects. The exact mechanisms behind the effect of statin use on reducing the occurrence of pneumonia have not been completely elucidated. Statins have been shown to exert variable antimicrobial activity against various bacterial strains [24] and control the bacilli burden by enhancing host-induced autophagy and phagosomal maturation during pathogen invasion [25]. In addition, statins promote the clearance of microparticles from lung tissues to regional lymph nodes, attenuate recruitment and activation of alveolar macrophages, thereby reducing local proinflammatory cytokine production in the lungs [26]. The results from these aforementioned studies might provide possible mechanisms for the protective benefits of statin therapy. It still remains unclear whether different lipid-lowering abilities of statins can be correlated to their different anti-inflammatory abilities. In the present study, we observed that atorvastatin, fluvastatin and simvastatin had similar effects on reducing the risk of pneumonia among MI patients. Our findings were consistent with those of Vinogradova, who demonstrated that atorvastatin and simvastatin had similar associations with the risk of pneumonia in the general population [11]. These observations might provide implications for further clinical trials to compare the effects of different statins on the risk of pneumonia.

We observed that the percentage of any use of statins after MI in present study was only 60–70 %. Another study which was also conducted from an administrative database in the United States showed that 46.9 % of patients with high risk of cardiovascular disease were no longer taking a statin at a mean time of 3 months after drug initiation [27]. Adherence rates of statins in most observational studies have been low, with approximately 50 % at 6 months and 25 % at 1 year [28]. Even in clinical studies, adherence with statins is suboptimal, with 5-year discontinuation rate of 33 and 18 % in primary and secondary prevention trials, respectively [29, 30]. The most common reasons contributing to discontinuation and non-adherence are statin-related muscle side effects [31]. To increase the adherence rate and benefits of statins, especially in patients with MI and high risk of cardiovascular disease, statins should be prescribed after thoroughly evaluating the patient's comorbidities, types and dosage of statins, and concomitant medications [31]. In this study, we considered the risk of COPD and found that COPD was associated with an increased risk of pneumonia requiring hospitalization (crude OR = 3.43, 95 % CI = 2.82–4.18, $P < 0.001$). The adherence rate of inhaled therapy in patients with COPD has been reported about 41.357 % and underuse of medications was common [32–34]. We did not analyze the adherence of medications for COPD because the numbers of MI patients with coexisting COPD were relatively small. Further clinical research is needed to investigate whether concomitant adherence to statins use and COPD treatment in MI patients with COPD could be an effective treatment in reducing the incidence of pneumonia requiring hospitalization.

Limitations

Our findings are subject to certain limitations. First, the data on drug exposure were based on prescription claims, which might not reflect actual use. Second, the NHIRD does not have certain patient information, such as tobacco use and ambulatory status, which might contribute to the occurrence of pneumonia. Third, the NHIRD was derived from the administrative claims database that did not consider certain clinical information, such as the severity and etiology of pneumonia. Fourth, we did not further investigate the effects of specific statins. Fifth, we did not analyze the effect of concomitant use of statins and medications for coexisting pulmonary comorbidities. Finally, this study was conducted using a cohort of Taiwanese patients. The results might not be generalized to other populations. Future prospective, randomized studies on the effects of statins are warranted to confirm our findings.

Conclusions

Statin use among patients with MI might be associated with a decreased risk of hospitalization for pneumonia in time- and dose-dependent manners, particularly for patients who were unexposed to statin pretreatment or had fewer comorbidities. Our results suggest that statin use might be used in an adjunctive therapy in preventing pneumonia hospitalization for patients with MI under thorough evaluation of individual comorbidities, previous statin use and optimal dosage.

Abbreviations

ACEI/ARBs: Angiotensin converting enzyme inhibitor and angiotensin receptor blockade; ATC: Anatomical therapeutic chemical; CHF: Congestive heart failure; CIs: Confidence intervals; CKD: Chronic kidney disease; CLD: Chronic liver disease; COPD: Chronic obstructive pulmonary disease; DDD: Defined daily dose; DDD_{90}: Defined daily dose within a 90-day period; DM: Diabetes mellitus; HMG-CoA: 3-hydroxy-3-methylglutaryl-coenzyme A; HTN: Hypertension; ICD-9-CM: International Classification of Diseases, Ninth Revision, Clinical Modification; MI: Myocardial infarction; NHI: National Health Insurance; NHIA: National Health Insurance Administration; NHIRD: National Health Insurance Research Database; ORs: Odds ratios; PPIs: Proton pump inhibitors.

Competing interests
The authors declare that they have no competing interests.

Authors' contributions
CFL and LNC carried out the studies, participated in the design of the study and drafted the manuscript. YHC and MTC participated in the design of the study and performed the statistical analysis. JCL conceived of the study, and participated in its design and coordination and helped to draft the manuscript. All authors read and approved the final manuscript.

Acknowledgements
This study was supported by the Health and Clinical Data Research Center of Taipei Medical University.

Author details
[1]Division of Cardiology, Department of Internal Medicine, Shuang Ho Hospital, Taipei Medical University, New Taipei City, Taiwan. [2]Pharmacy Department of Mackay Memorial Hospital, Taipei, Taiwan. [3]School of Public Health, College of Public Health and Nutrition, Taipei Medical University, Taipei, Taiwan. [4]School of Health Care Administration, College of Management, Taipei Medical University, Taipei, Taiwan. [5]Division of Cardiology, Department of Internal Medicine, MacKay Memorial Hospital, Taipei, Taiwan. [6]Department of Medicine, Mackay Medical College, New Taipei, Taiwan.

References
1. Go AS, Mozaffarian D, Roger VL, Benjamin EJ, Berry JD, Blaha MJ, et al. American Heart Association Statistics Committee and Stroke Statistics Subcommittee: Executive summary: Heart disease and stroke statistics–2014 update: a report from the American Heart Association. Circulation. 2014;129:399–410.
2. Ankam J, Feldman DI, Blaha MJ, Martin SS. Improving lipid control following myocardial Infarction. Curr Opin Cardiol. 2014;29:454–66.
3. Wang HE, Shapiro NI, Griffin R, Safford MM, Judd S, Howard G. Chronic Medical Conditions and Risk of Sepsis. PLoS One. 2012;7:e48307.
4. Mortensen EM, Coley CM, Singer DE, Marrie TJ, Obrosky DS, Kapoor WN, et al. Causes of death for patients with community-acquired pneumonia: results from the Pneumonia Patient Outcomes Research Team cohort study. Arch Intern Med. 2002;162:1059–64.
5. Endo A. The discovery and development of HMG-CoA reductase inhibitors. J Lipid Res. 1992;33:1569–82.
6. Baigent C, Keech A, Kearney PM, Blackwell L, Buck G, Pollicino C, et al. Cholesterol Treatment Trialists' (CTT) Collaborators. Efficacy and safety of cholesterol-lowering treatment: prospective meta-analysis of data from 90,056 participants in 14 randomised trials of statins. Lancet. 2005;366:1267–78.
7. Oduncu V, Tanalp AC, Erkol A, Sırma D, Dündar C, Akgün T, et al. Impact of chronic pre-treatment of statins on the level of systemic inflammation and myocardial perfusion in patients undergoing primary angioplasty. Am J Cardiol. 2011;107:179–85.
8. Bauer T, Böhm M, Zahn R, Jünger C, Koeth O, Gitt A, et al. Acute Coronary Syndromes Registry Investigators. Effect of chronic statin pretreatment on hospital outcome in patients with acute non-ST-elevation myocardial infarction. J Cardiovasc Pharmacol. 2009;53:132–6.
9. Liao JK, Laufs U. Pleiotropic effects of statins. Annu Rev Pharmacol Toxicol. 2005;45:89–118.
10. Nielsen AG, Nielsen RB, Riis AH, Johnsen SP, Sørensen HT, Thomsen RW. The impact of statin use on pneumonia risk and outcome: a combined population-based case-control and cohort study. Crit Care. 2012;16:R122.
11. Vinogradova Y, Coupland C, Hippisley-Cox J. Risk of pneumonia in patients taking statins: population-based nested case–control study. Br J Gen Pract. 2011;61:e742–8.
12. van de Garde EMW, Hak E, Souverein PC, Hoes AW, van den Bosch JM, Leufkens HG. Statin treatment and reduced risk of pneumonia in patients with diabetes. Thorax. 2006;61:957–61.
13. National Health Insurance: Review Legislations of Medical Institutes, 2011; [http://www.nhi.gov.tw/Resource/webdata/19428_1_6-NATIONAL%20HEALTH%20INSURANCE%20ACT_1030425更新(修15條1項3款).pdf] (Accesed 30 Apr 2014).
14. WHO Collaborating Centre for Drug Statistics Methodology. ATC/DDD Index 2014. http://www.whocc.no/atcddd/
15. Gage BF, Waterman AD, Shannon W, Boechler M, Rich MW, Radford MJ. Validation of clinical classification schemes for predicting stroke: results from the National Registry of Atrial Fibrillation. JAMA. 2001;285:2864–70.
16. Poçi D, Hartford M, Karlsson T, Herlitz J, Edvardsson N, Caidahl K. Role of the $CHADS_2$ Score in Acute Coronary Syndromes: Risk of Subsequent Death or Stroke in Patients With and Without Atrial Fibrillation. Chest. 2012;141:1431–40.
17. Huang SS, Chen YH, Chan WL, Huang PH, Chen JW, Lin SJ. Usefulness of the $CHADS_2$ Score for Prognostic Stratification of Patients With Acute Myocardial Infarction. Am J Cardiol. 2014;114:1309–14.
18. Morabia A, Ten Have T, Landis JR. Empirical Evaluation of the Influence of Control Selection Schemes on Relative Risk Estimation: The Welsh Nickel Workers Study. Occup Environ Med. 1995;52:489–93.
19. Lubin JH, Gail MH. Biased selection of controls for case-control analyses of cohort studies. Biometrics. 1984;40:63–75.
20. Fuernau G, Eitel I, Wöhrle J, Kerber S, Lauer B, Pauschinger M, et al. Impact of long-term statin pretreatment on myocardial damage in ST elevation myocardial infarction (from the AIDA STEMI CMR Substudy). Am J Cardiol. 2014;114:503–9.
21. Wang MT, Lo YW, Tsai CL, Chang LC, Malone DC, Chu CL, et al. Statin Use and Risk of COPD Exacerbation Requiring Hospitalization. Am J Med. 2013;126:598–606.
22. Nohria A, Prsic A, Liu PY, Okamoto R, Creager MA, Selwyn A, et al. Statins inhibit Rho kinase activity in patients with atherosclerosis. Atherosclerosis. 2009;205:517–21.
23. Subramanian S, Emami H, Vucic E, Singh P, Vijayakumar J, Fifer KM, et al. High-dose atorvastatin reduces periodontal inflammation: a novel pleiotropic effect of statins. J Am Coll Cardiol. 2013;62:2382–91.
24. Masadeh M, Mhaidat N, Alzoubi K, Al-azzam S, Alnasser Z. Antibacterial activity of statins: a comparative study of Atorvastatin, Simvastatin, and Rosuvastatin. Ann Clin Microbiol Antimicrob. 2012;11:13.
25. Parihar SP, Guler R, Khutlang R, Lang DM, Hurdayal R, Mhlanga MM, et al. Statin Therapy Reduces the Mycobacterium tuberculosis Burden in Human Macrophages and in Mice by Enhancing Autophagy and Phagosome Maturation. J Infec Dis. 2014;209:754–63.
26. Miyata R, Bai N, Vincent R, Sin DD, Van Eeden SF. Statins Reduce ambient particulate matter-induced lung inflammation by promoting the clearance of particulate matter < 10 μm from lung tissues. Chest. 2013;143:452–60.
27. Simpson Jr RJ, Tunceli K, Ramey DR, Neff DR, Kern DM, Hsieh HM, et al. Treatment pattern changes in high-risk patients newly initiated on statin monotherapy in a managed care setting. J Clin Lipidol. 2013;7:399–407.
28. Benner JS, Glynn RJ, Mogun H, Neumann PJ, Weinstein MC, Avorn J. Long-term persistence in use of statin therapy in elderly patients. JAMA. 2002;288:455–61.
29. Downs JR, Clearfield M, Weis S, Whitney E, Shapiro DR, Beere PA, et al. Primary prevention of acute coronary events with lovastatin in men and women with average cholesterol levels. Results of AFCAPS/TexCAPS. JAMA. 1998;279:1615–22.
30. Heart Protection Study Collaborative Group. MRC/BHF heart protection study of cholesterol lowering with simvastatin in 20,536 high-risk individuals: a randomized placebo-controlled trial. Lancet. 2002;360:7–22.
31. Wei MY, Ito MK, Cohen JD, Brinton EA, Jacobson TA. Predictors of statin adherence, switching, and discontinuation in the USAGE survey: understanding the use of statins in America and gaps in patient education. J Clin Lipidol. 2013;7:472–83.
32. Osterberg L, Blaschke T. Adherence to medication. N Engl J Med. 2005;353:487–97.
33. Bosley C, Corden Z, Rees P, Cochrane G. Psychological factors associated with the use of home nebulized therapy for COPD. Eur Respir J. 1996;9:2346–50.
34. Taylor DR, Kinney CD, McDevitt DC. Patient compliance with oral theophylline therapy. Br J Clin Pharmacol. 1984;17:15–20.

3

Whole-exome sequencing in an extended family with myocardial infarction unmasks familial hypercholesterolemia

Ingrid Brænne[1,2], Benedikt Reiz[1,2], Anja Medack[1], Mariana Kleinecke[1,2], Marcus Fischer[3], Salih Tuna[6], Christian Hengstenberg[4,5], Panos Deloukas[6,7,8], Jeanette Erdmann[1,2*†], Heribert Schunkert[4,5†] and Cardiogenics consortium

Abstract

Background: Familial hypercholesterolemia (FH) is an autosomal-dominant disease leading to markedly elevated low-density lipoprotein (LDL) cholesterol levels and increased risk for premature myocardial infarction (MI). Mutation carriers display variable LDL cholesterol levels, which may obscure the diagnosis. We examined by whole-exome sequencing a family in which multiple myocardial infarctions occurred at a young age with unclear etiology.

Methods: Whole-exome sequencing of three affected family members, validation of the identified variant with Sanger-sequencing, and subsequent co-segregation analysis in the family.

Results: The index patient (LDL cholesterol 188 mg/dL) was referred for molecular-genetic investigations. He had coronary artery bypass graft (CABG) at the age of 59 years; 12 out of 15 1st, 2nd and 3rd degree relatives were affected with coronary artery disease (CAD) and/or premature myocardial infarction (MI). We sequenced the whole-exome of the patient and two cousins with premature MI. After filtering, we were left with a potentially disease causing variant in the LDL receptor (*LDLR*) gene, which we validated by Sanger-sequencing (nucleotide substitution in the acceptor splice-site of exon 10, c.1359-1G > A). Sequencing of all family members available for genetic analysis revealed co-segregation of the variant with CAD (LOD 3.0) and increased LDLC (>190 mg/dL), following correction for statin treatment (LOD 4.3). Interestingly, mutation carriers presented with highly variable corrected (183–354 mg/dL) and on-treatment LDL levels (116–274 mg/dL) such that the diagnosis of FH in this family was made only after the molecular-genetic analysis.

Conclusion: Even in families with unusual clustering of CAD FH remains to be underdiagnosed, which underscores the need for implementation of systematic screening programs. Whole-exome sequencing may facilitate identification of disease-causing variants in families with unclear etiology of MI and enable preventive treatment of mutation carriers in a more timely fashion.

Keywords: Familial hypercholesterolemia, Myocardial infarction, Whole-exome sequencing

* Correspondence: jeanette.erdmann@iieg.uni-luebeck.de
†Equal contributors
[1]Institute for Integrative and Experimental Genomics, University of Lübeck, 23562 Lübeck, Germany
[2]DZHK (German Research Centre for Cardiovascular Research), partner site Hamburg/Lübeck/Kiel, 23562 Lübeck, Germany
Full list of author information is available at the end of the article

Background

Familial hypercholesterolemia (FH) may explain as much as 20 percent of familial cases with premature coronary artery disease (CAD) [1,2]. Despite well-established criteria for clinical diagnosis and the proven benefits of medical treatment FH remains to be largely under-diagnosed and untreated [3]. In most European populations between 5-15% of cases are diagnosed [4,5]. It has been considered that many FH cases are simply overlooked in the large number of CAD patients, a disease usually caused multifactorially by the interplay of common risk factors and common risk alleles [4,6]. Moreover, with significant impact, the fact that nowadays most families are small may mask the inherited nature of the disease [7,8].

In cases with suspected FH, family-based cascade screening by either clinical or molecular-genetic instruments is guideline recommended to unravel the autosomal-dominant mode of inheritance and to facilitate medical treatment at a young age (European Society of Cardiology [9], British National Institute for Clinical Excellence (NICE) [10], US Centres for Disease Control and Prevention [11]).

Yet, such testing either using lipid panels paired with clinical diagnostic criteria or molecular-genetic DNA sequencing of the currently known disease-causing genes is vastly under-used [4,12,13]. Exceptions are found in the Netherlands and Norway, where national screening programs for mutations in the disease-causing genes *LDLR, APOB* and *PCSK9* have been initiated [4,14,15].

Here, we report on an extended MI-family, which remained without diagnosis until whole-exome sequencing was performed. The index patient was referred to us because of premature MI (CABG at the age of 59) and positive family history for CAD (rather than for elevated LDL-cholesterol levels, LDL-C). His LDL-C was 188 mg/dL, which initially detracted from a clinical suspicion of FH. The family with 15 CAD cases (plus two that are related by marriage) and several untreated mutation carriers illustrates the need for a more systematic employment of molecular FH testing to increase the awareness and timely initiation of medical treatment.

Methods

MI family

The index patient had suffered from CABG at the age of 59 years. Figure 1A depicts the pedigree of the MI family used for whole-exome sequencing. Clinical and angiographic characteristics of the family members available for analysis are described in detail in Table 1. All subjects analyzed in this study gave written informed consent before participating. The local Ethical Committee (University Regensburg, Germany) approved the study.

Exome sequencing

Whole-exome sequencing was performed as 54 bp paired-end runs on a Genome Analyzer IIx system (Illumina) after in-solution enrichment of exonic sequences (SureSelect Human All Exon 50 Mb kit, Agilent). Reads are mapped to the reference genome, duplicate fragments are marked using Picard and GATK is then used to recalibrate base

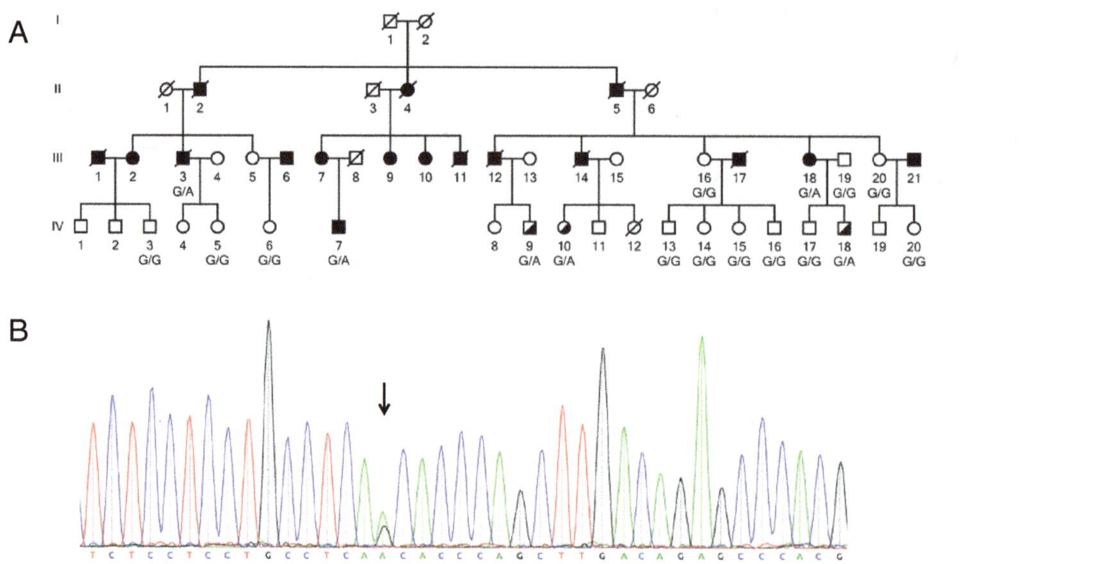

Figure 1 Pedigree of the analyzed family and confirmation of mutation by Sanger sequencing. A) The index patient is IV.7. The family members selected for whole-exome sequencing are III.3, III.18, and IV.7. Elevated LDL-C levels are shown as half filled symbols. Mutation carriers are shown as G/A and non-carriers as G/G. **B)** Confirmation of the nucleotide substitution in the acceptor splice-site of exon 10, c.1359-1G > A by Sanger sequencing. Shown is the sequence of the index patient IV.7. The black arrow points to the heterozygote position.

Table 1 Clinical characteristics of family 6652

Family ID	Pedigre ID	Sex[$]	BMI (kg/m^2)	Age at first MI (years)	Age at first CAD (years)	LDL-C (mg/dL)	Statin therapy	Daily dose	Hyper-cholesterol-emia[1#]	Hyper-tension[2#]	Diabetes[3#]	Smoking[4#]
6652501	III.2	2	28.5		58	252	Atorvastatin	20	1	1	2	1
6652502	III.3	1	26.5		55	214	Atorvastatin	60	1	1	2	2
6652505	III.16	2	22.8			186			2	1	2	2
6652506	III.18	2	25.0		55	233	Atorvastatin	80	1	2	2	1
6652509	IV.6	2	26.4			184			2	2	2	1
6652511	III.6	1	25.9	44	67	189	Atorvastatin	10	1	1	2	1
6652512	III.20	1	30.5			136	Cerivastatin	0.3	1	1	2	2
6652513	IV.3	1	24.2			96			2	2	2	2
6652515	IV.5	2	23.4			171			2	2	2	1
6652516	**IV.7**	**1**	**25.2**		**59**	**188**	**Atorvastatin**	**40**	**1**	**2**	**2**	**2**
6652518	III.13	2	27.3			156			2	2	2	1
6652520	IV.9	1	22.5			142	Simvastatin	10	1		2	2
6652522	IV.13	1	29.4			166			2	2	2	1
6652523	IV.14	2	24.2			168			2	2	2	2
6652524	IV.15	2	23.5			130			2		2	2
6652525	IV.16	1	22.7			145			2	2	2	2
6652527	IV.20	2	23.4			143			2		2	1
6652531	IV.10	2	20.9			116	Atorvastatin	60	1	2	2	2
6652533	IV.12	2	21.3							2	2	2
6652534	III.19	1	23.1			115			2	1	2	2
6652535	IV.17	1	23.2			184			2	2	2	2
6652536	IV.18	1	22.8			274	Atorvastatin	20	1	2	2	2

$:1 = male, 2 = female; #: 1 = yes, 2 = no; [1]Blood pressure >140/90 mm Hg; [2]LDL cholesterol > 190 mg/dL or statin therapy; [3]History of diabetes mellitus; [4]History of smoking. Index patient IV.7 in bold.

qualities. We used the human genome assembly hg19 (GRCh37) as reference.

Mutation validation

We annotated the single nucleotide variants (SNVs) with Annovar [16] using the UCSC database, Exome sequencing project and 1000 Genomes. Protein altering effect was predicted using SnpEFF [17] and avsift (Annovar). Mutation validation was performed by PCR and Sanger-sequencing of candidate gene region identified by whole-exome sequencing. After confirmation of the variant (Figure 1B), additional affected and unaffected family members were screened considering co-segregation. Primers used for mutation validation and PCR conditions are as following. A set of primers (Left Primer 5′-tgtaaaacgacggccagtGAGGCACTCTTGGTTCCATC-3′ and Right Primer 5′-caggaaacagctatgaccGTGGATACGCACCCATGAAC-3′) was chosen to amplify the region of the LDLR gene encompassing the c.1359-1G > A variant (562 bp length). Standard PCR was carried out in a 10 μl volume containing 10 ng genomic DNA, 5 pmol of each primer and 4 μl of Mastermix (VWR International GmbH, Darmstadt, Germany). Samples were processed in a Sensoquest labcycler with a standard touchdown PCR program (annealing temperature from 61°C-55°C).

Results and discussion

We analyzed an extended German MI-family consisting of 53 members of whom 13 were affected with CAD and/or MI (Figure 1A). Of these, 18 family members were available for genetic analysis. Based on the phenotypic presentation in this family, we suspected an autosomal dominant mode of inheritance. Therefore, we decided to carry out whole-exome sequencing of three affected family members to unravel the genetic cause of CAD/MI in this family.

The amount of disease-unspecific variants present in the downstream analysis of whole-exome sequencing is largely influenced by the subset of family members that are selected for the initial analysis [18,19]. To optimize the variant search, one strategy is to select distantly related family members. Whereas siblings share 50% of the genetic variants, cousins share only 12.5% [20]. Hence, we selected cousins instead of siblings to reduce the number of disease-unspecific variants and to increase the chance for identifying the truly disease-causing variants (Figure 1A; III.3, III.18, and IV.7) [21,22].

To identify the causal variant in this family, we based our filtering on three assumptions: (1) the variant is inherited in an autosomal dominant mode of inheritance; (2) the variant is very rare (<0.1%) in the general population; and (3) most affected family members carry the variant (high penetrance).

The sequencing was performed on a Genome Analyzer llx system (Illumina) after in-solution enrichment of exonic sequences. The exome sequencing revealed an average read depth of 155 with minimum 84% of the target regions covered at least 20X.

Whole-exome sequencing revealed around 39,000 variants in total and approximately 20,000 located in exonic regions. We filtered the variants using the frequencies stated in 1000 Genomes (1 kG, Annovar version 1000g2012apr), Exome Sequencing Project (ESP, Annovar version 6500) and in internal exome data (8 samples sequenced with the same platform). Around 1,800 variants were found with a frequency less than 0.1% in ESP and 1 kG. In a next filtering step, we kept only variants that were conserved and outside regions of segmental duplication, leaving ~825 variants. To identify variants with potentially severe function-altering effects, we filtered all variants based on avsift score >0.05 and "HIGH" effect predicted using Annovar and SnpEFF. These variants are either amino acid changes, stop gain, stop loss or splice-site mutations (more details can be found in Table 2). Only one variant, a G > A substitution in the acceptor splice-site of exon 10 in the *LDLR* gene (IVS9-1G > A or c.1359-1G > A), was shared by the three sequenced family members and was validated by Sanger-sequencing.

This G > A substitution results in the loss of a splice-site with a predicted splice-site score of –4.2 for the variant versus 6.8 for the reference allele [http://rulai.cshl.edu]. We genotyped this variant in all family members available for genetic analysis to check for co-segregation with the disease. There were 18 (one related by marriage) family members available for genotyping. Of these, three were affected and these carried the *LDLR*-variant. Of the 14 unaffected family members, which were not related by marriage, three carried the variant. The three unaffected mutation carriers were, at the time included in this analysis, 48, 54 and 54 years old. Since MI is a late-onset disease, we expect the disease to occur late in life. Hence, the affection status regarding MI must be considered unknown at this point.

Table 2 Bioinformatic filtering of the family members that were exome sequenced

Filter	III.3	III.18	IV.7	Mean
Total aligned variants	38,702	38,408	38,775	38,628
Variants (exome)	20,344	20,387	20,173	20,301
Not in internal controls	1,995	2,123	2,097	2,072
Variants with frequency <0.1% in 1000G and ESP	1,643	1,885	1,864	1,797
Conserved and no segmental duplication	713	900	862	825
snpEFF = HIGH and AVSIFT <0.05	7	18	19	15
Shared variants				1

The data was annotated using annovar [16] (Version August 2013). Functional prediction was performed with snpEFF [17] (build 2014-01-16) and AVSIFT (Annovar).

Since the 1990s, it is well established that mutations in the *LDLR* gene are the major cause for familial hypercholesterolemia [1,23]. Around 90% of all known disease-causing mutations (more than 1,800 mutations are listed in HGMD (version 2013.4)) for FH are found in the *LDLR* gene [3,24,25]. FH is also caused by mutations in the *APOB* and *PCSK9* genes, with frequencies of around 5% and ~1% respectively [4,26].

We compared the LDL-C levels of the family members that carry the variant with those that do not carry the variant. The results showed that the variant co-segregates with increased LDL-C levels (LOD 4.3). The average LDL-C levels were significantly increased in mutation carriers compared with non-mutation carriers (279 mg/dL versus 155 mg/dL). However, the plasma levels were highly variable ranging from 183 mg/dL to 354 mg/dL; this fact misled the clinical diagnosis in the index patient (188, corrected for statin use 279 mg/dL). To estimate the functional implication of the identified variant, we systematically searched the literature. This revealed that the LDLR variant has been previously described as disease-causing in families with FH [27,28].

This variant is reported to originate from the south of the Netherlands and to significantly increase the LDL-C levels and hence cause a higher risk of premature CVD. The risk increase was found to be 15.95% for mutation carriers compared to unaffected relatives [29]. In our analyzed family, all but one mutation carrier have LDL-C levels above 190 mg/dL. This result clearly underlines the previous reported significant risk increase.

The variant cause an abnormally spliced transcript, which results in a deletion of 7 bp and a frame shift with premature termination [30]. The deletion affects the normal acceptor splice site in the 9th intron. This leads to a cryptic splice site that consist of the 6th and 7th nucleotide of exon 10.

The variant is likely to cause haploinsufficiency because of the truncated transcript and hence nonsense-mediated decay. However, even a protein product would lead to a loss-of-function of the receptor since several important domains of the receptor would be missing, such as the crucial transmembrane region, the C-terminal part of the epidermal growth factor precursor homology domain, the

O-linked sugar domain, the membrane-spanning domain, and the cytoplasmic domain. Other variants lacking these domains have been reported to have reduced activity (around 2%) and are classified as null allele (class 1) mutations [31]. These mutations produce normal mRNA transcripts, however, in reduced concentration [32], which explains the increased risk of FH caused by this mutation.

With FH as the underlying cause of MI in this family, we could have anticipated a mutation in the LDLR gene. However, the index patient was referred to us and included in our study with the diagnosis of premature MI/CABG and positive family history for CAD.

The varying LDL-C levels in this family had initially hindered the diagnosis of FH. It is, however, well known, that the LDL-C levels may vary remarkably even among individuals with the same mutation. One explanation for this is that other modifying factors are present [31]. One such mutation was described by Hobbs et al. [31]. They reported a family in which one-third of the mutation carriers have LDL concentrations below the 90th percentile. They suggested the existence of a dominant gene that suppresses the effect of the LDL receptor mutation. Hence, the fact that one of our mutation carriers have LDL-C levels below 190 mg/dL might have similar explanation and demonstrate the complexity of even expected monogenic disease variants.

The result of this study underlines the power of whole-exome sequencing approaches to identify disease-causing variants. Whole-exome sequencing is a promising tool to identify the cause of a disease in families with unclear etiology of MI.

Conclusion

We strongly suggest that whole-exome sequencing can be used for stratified medicine. If we know the disease-causing variant in affected families, we can enable specific preventive treatment of so-far unaffected mutation carriers and this may prevent or delay the onset of the disease. In addition, having overseen FH in the family at hand, we believe that the systematic sequencing of *LDLR* pathway genes may accelerate the diagnostic work-up.

Competing interests

The authors declare no competing interests.

Authors' contributions

JE, HS, and PD designed the study; IB, BR, AM, ST, and MK performed the analysis; MF and CH collected the family data; IB, JE, and HS wrote the manuscript. All authors read and approved the final manuscript.

Acknowledgements

We thank all the family members who participated in this research. Without the continuous support of these patients over more than fifteen years, the present work would not have been possible. We like to thank Sandra Wrobel for technical assistance. We also would like to thank Drs. Björn Mayer, Ute Hubauer, and Anika Großhennig for help with the German Myocardial Infarction Study.

The study was supported by the FP6/FP7 EU funded integrated projects *Cardiogenics* (LSHM-CT-2006-037593) and *CVgenes@target* (HEALTH-F2-2013-601456), and the local focus program "Medizinische Genetik" of the Universität zu Lübeck. IB is funded by the DFG-funded Excellence Cluster *Inflammation at interfaces*. Principle investigators of the Cardiogenics Consortium not included in the authors list are Willem H. Ouwehand[1], Alison Goodall[2], Nilesh J Samani[2], and Francois Cambien[3]. 1 Department of Haematology, University of Cambridge, Long Road, Cambridge, CB2 2PT, UK and National Health Service Blood and Transplant, Cambridge Centre, Long Road, Cambridge, CB2 2PT, UK; 2 Department of Cardiovascular Sciences, University of Leicester, Glenfield Hospital, Groby Road, Leicester, LE3 9QP, UK; 3 INSERM UMRS 937, Pierre and Marie Curie University (UPMC, Paris 6) and Medical School, 91 Bd de l'Hôpital 75013, Paris, France.

Author details

[1]Institute for Integrative and Experimental Genomics, University of Lübeck, 23562 Lübeck, Germany. [2]DZHK (German Research Centre for Cardiovascular Research), partner site Hamburg/Lübeck/Kiel, 23562 Lübeck, Germany. [3]Klinik und Poliklinik für Innere Medizin II, Universitätsklinikum Regensburg, 93053 Regensburg, Germany. [4]Deutsches Herzzentrum München and Medizinische Klinik, Klinikum rechts der Isar, Technische Universität München, 80636 München, Germany. [5]DZHK (German Centre for Cardiovascular Research), partner site Munich Heart Alliance, 80636 Munich, Germany. [6]Wellcome Trust Sanger Institute, Wellcome Trust Genome Campus, Hinxton CB10 1SA, UK. [7]William Harvey Research Institute, Barts and The London School of Medicine and Dentistry, Queen Mary University of London, London, UK. [8]Princess Al-Jawhara Al-Brahim Centre of Excellence in Research of Hereditary Disorders (PACER-HD), King Abdulaziz University, Jeddah 21589, Saudi Arabia.

References

1. Goldstein JL, Schrott HG, Hazzard WR, Bierman EL, Motulsky AG: **Hyperlipidemia in coronary heart disease. II. Genetic analysis of lipid levels in 176 families and delineation of a new inherited disorder, combined hyperlipidemia.** *J Clin Invest* 1973, **52:**1544–1568.
2. Neefjes LA, Ten Kate GJ, Alexia R, Nieman K, Galema-Boers AJ, Langendonk JG, Weustink AC, Mollet NR, Sijbrands EJ, Krestin GP, de Feyter PJ: **Accelerated subclinical coronary atherosclerosis in patients with familial hypercholesterolemia.** *Atherosclerosis* 2011, **219:**721–727.
3. Talmud PJ, Shah S, Whittall R, Futema M, Howard P, Cooper JA, Harrison SC, Li K, Drenos F, Karpe F, Neil HA, Descamps OS, Langenberg C, Lench N, Kivimaki M, Whittaker J, Hingorani AD, Kumari M, Humphries SE: **Use of low-density lipoprotein cholesterol gene score to distinguish patients with polygenic and monogenic familial hypercholesterolaemia: a case-control study.** *Lancet* 2013, **381:**1293–1301.
4. Nordestgaard BG, Chapman MJ, Humphries SE, Ginsberg HN, Masana L, Descamps OS, Wiklund O, Hegele RA, Raal FJ, Defesche JC, Wiegman A, Santos RD, Watts GF, Parhofer KG, Hovingh GK, Kovanen PT, Boileau C, Averna M, Boren J, Bruckert E, Catapano AL, Kuivenhoven JA, Pajukanta P, Ray K, Stalenhoef AF, Stroes E, Taskinen MR, Tybjaerg-Hansen A, European Atherosclerosis Society Consensus P: **Familial hypercholesterolaemia is underdiagnosed and undertreated in the general population: guidance for clinicians to prevent coronary heart disease: consensus statement of the European Atherosclerosis Society.** *Eur Heart J* 2013, **34:**3478.
5. Brice P, Burton H, Edwards CW, Humphries SE, Aitman TJ: **Familial hypercholesterolaemia: a pressing issue for European health care.** *Atherosclerosis* 2013, **231:**223–226.
6. CARDIoGRAMplusC4D-Consortium, Deloukas P, Kanoni S, Willenborg C, Farrall M, Assimes TL, Thompson JR, Ingelsson E, Saleheen D, Erdmann J, Goldstein BA, Stirrups K, Konig IR, Cazier JB, Johansson A, Hall AS, Lee JY, Willer CJ, Chambers JC, Esko T, Folkersen L, Goel A, Grundberg E, Havulinna AS, Ho WK, Hopewell JC, Eriksson N, Kleber ME, Kristiansson K, Lundmark P, *et al*: **Large-scale association analysis identifies new risk loci for coronary artery disease.** *Nat Genet* 2013, **45:**25–33.
7. Pötzsch O, Weinmann J, Haustein T: **Geburtentrends und familiensituation in deutschland.** 2012. Available from Statistisches Bundesamt: www.destatis.de.
8. Office-for-National-Statistics: *Family size in 2012*; 2013. Available from: http://www.ons.gov.uk/.

9. Reiner Z, Catapano AL, De Backer G, Graham I, Taskinen MR, Wiklund O, Agewall S, Alegria E, Chapman MJ, Durrington P, Erdine S, Halcox J, Hobbs RH, Kjekshus JK, Perrone Filardi P, Riccardi G, Storey RF, David W, Clinical Practice Guidelines Committee of the Spanish Society of C: **[ESC/EAS Guidelines for the management of dyslipidaemias].** *Rev Esp Cardiol* 2011, **64:**1168 e1161–1168 e1160.
10. Minhas R, Humphries SE, Qureshi N, Neil HA, Group NGD: **Controversies in familial hypercholesterolaemia: recommendations of the NICE Guideline Development Group for the identification and management of familial hypercholesterolaemia.** *Heart* 2009, **95:**584–587. discussion 587-591.
11. **Third Report of the Expert Panel on Detection, Evaluation, and Treatment of High Blood Cholesterol in Adults (Adult Treatment Panel III).** [http://www.cdc.gov/]
12. Benn M, Watts GF, Tybjaerg-Hansen A, Nordestgaard BG: **Familial hypercholesterolemia in the danish general population: prevalence, coronary artery disease, and cholesterol-lowering medication.** *J Clin Endocrinol Metab* 2012, **97:**3956–3964.
13. Goldberg AC, Hopkins PN, Toth PP, Ballantyne CM, Rader DJ, Robinson JG, Daniels SR, Gidding SS, de Ferranti SD, Ito MK, McGowan MP, Moriarty PM, Cromwell WC, Ross JL, Ziajka PE, National Lipid Association Expert Panel on Familial H: **Familial hypercholesterolemia: screening, diagnosis and management of pediatric and adult patients: clinical guidance from the National Lipid Association Expert Panel on Familial Hypercholesterolemia.** *J Clin Lipidol* 2011, **5:**S1–8.
14. Umans-Eckenhausen MA, Defesche JC, Sijbrands EJ, Scheerder RL, Kastelein JJ: **Review of first 5 years of screening for familial hypercholesterolaemia in the Netherlands.** *Lancet* 2001, **357:**165–168.
15. Leren TP, Manshaus T, Skovholt U, Skodje T, Nossen IE, Teie C, Sorensen S, Bakken KS: **Application of molecular genetics for diagnosing familial hypercholesterolemia in Norway: results from a family-based screening program.** *Semin Vasc Med* 2004, **4:**75–85.
16. Wang K, Li M, Hakonarson H: **ANNOVAR: functional annotation of genetic variants from high-throughput sequencing data.** *Nucleic Acids Res* 2010, **38:**e164.
17. Cingolani P, Platts A, Wang le L, Coon M, Nguyen T, Wang L, Land SJ, Lu X, Ruden DM: **A program for annotating and predicting the effects of single nucleotide polymorphisms, SnpEff: SNPs in the genome of Drosophila melanogaster strain w1118; iso-2; iso-3.** *Fly (Austin)* 2012, **6:**80–92.
18. Campbell N, Sinagra G, Jones KL, Slavov D, Gowan K, Merlo M, Carniel E, Fain PR, Aragona P, Di Lenarda A, Mestroni L, Taylor MR: **Whole exome sequencing identifies a troponin T mutation hot spot in familial dilated cardiomyopathy.** *PLoS One* 2013, **8:**e78104.
19. Bras J, Guerreiro R, Hardy J: **Use of next-generation sequencing and other whole-genome strategies to dissect neurological disease.** *Nat Rev Neurosci* 2012, **13:**453–464.
20. Houwen RH, Baharloo S, Blankenship K, Raeymaekers P, Juyn J, Sandkuijl LA, Freimer NB: **Genome screening by searching for shared segments: mapping a gene for benign recurrent intrahepatic cholestasis.** *Nat Genet* 1994, **8:**380–386.
21. Erdmann J, Stark K, Esslinger UB, Rumpf PM, Koesling D, de Wit C, Kaiser FJ, Braunholz D, Medack A, Fischer M, Zimmermann ME, Tennstedt S, Graf E, Eck S, Aherrahrou Z, Nahrstaedt J, Willenborg C, Bruse P, Braenne I, Nothen MM, Hofmann P, Braund PS, Mergia E, Reinhard W, Burgdorf C, Schreiber S, Balmforth AJ, Hall AS, Bertram L, Steinhagen-Thiessen E, *et al*: **Dysfunctional nitric oxide signalling increases risk of myocardial infarction.** *Nature* 2013, **504:**432–436.
22. Gilissen C, Hoischen A, Brunner HG, Veltman JA: **Disease gene identification strategies for exome sequencing.** *Eur J Hum Genet* 2012, **20:**490–497.
23. Usifo E, Leigh SE, Whittall RA, Lench N, Taylor A, Yeats C, Orengo CA, Martin AC, Celli J, Humphries SE: **Low-density lipoprotein receptor gene familial hypercholesterolemia variant database: update and pathological assessment.** *Ann Hum Genet* 2012, **76:**387–401.
24. Futema M, Plagnol V, Whittall RA, Neil HA, Simon Broome Register G, Humphries SE, Uk10K: **Use of targeted exome sequencing as a diagnostic tool for Familial Hypercholesterolaemia.** *J Med Genet* 2012, **49:**644–649.
25. Soutar AK, Naoumova RP: **Mechanisms of disease: genetic causes of familial hypercholesterolemia.** *Nat Clin Pract Cardiovasc Med* 2007, **4:**214–225.
26. Austin MA, Hutter CM, Zimmern RL, Humphries SE: **Genetic causes of monogenic heterozygous familial hypercholesterolemia: a HuGE prevalence review.** *Am J Epidemiol* 2004, **160:**407–420.
27. Peeters AV, Van Gaal LF, du Plessis L, Lombardi MP, Havekes LM, Kotze MJ: **Mutational and genetic origin of LDL receptor gene mutations detected in both Belgian and Dutch familial hypercholesterolemics.** *Hum Genet* 1997, **100:**266–270.
28. Lombardi P, Sijbrands EJ, van de Giessen K, Smelt AH, Kastelein JJ, Frants RR, Havekes LM: **Mutations in the low density lipoprotein receptor gene of familial hypercholesterolemic patients detected by denaturing gradient gel electrophoresis and direct sequencing.** *J Lipid Res* 1995, **36:**860–867.
29. Kusters DM, Huijgen R, Defesche JC, Vissers MN, Kindt I, Hutten BA, Kastelein JJ: **Founder mutations in the Netherlands: geographical distribution of the most prevalent mutations in the low-density lipoprotein receptor and apolipoprotein B genes.** *Neth Heart J* 2011, **19:**175–182.
30. Rodningen OK, Tonstad S, Saugstad OD, Ose L, Leren TP: **Mutant transcripts of the LDL receptor gene: mRNA structure and quantity.** *Hum Mutat* 1999, **13:**186–196.
31. Hobbs HH, Brown MS, Goldstein JL: **Molecular genetics of the LDL receptor gene in familial hypercholesterolemia.** *Hum Mutat* 1992, **1:**445–466.
32. Hobbs HH, Leitersdorf E, Goldstein JL, Brown MS, Russell DW: **Multiple crm- mutations in familial hypercholesterolemia. Evidence for 13 alleles, including four deletions.** *J Clin Invest* 1988, **81:**909–917.

4

Interaction of type 2 diabetes mellitus with Chromosome 9p21 rs10757274 polymorphism on the risk of myocardial infarction

Liu-wei Zhang[1], Jian-ping Li[2*], Fang-fang Duan[1], Zhi-ke Liu[1], Si-yan Zhan[1], Yong-hua Hu[1], Jie Jiang[2], Yan Zhang[2], Yong Huo[2] and Da-fang Chen[1*]

Abstract

Background: Myocardial infarction (MI) is a serious complication of Coronary Artery Disease (CAD). Previous studies have identified genetic variants on chromosome 9p21 and 6p24 that are associated with CAD, but further studies need to be conducted to investigate whether these genetic variants are associated with the pathogenesis of MI. We therefore performed this study to assess the association between the risk of MI and SNP rs10757274 on chromosome 9p21 and SNP rs6903956 on chromosome 6p24, and to explore the gene-environment interactions in a Chinese population.

Methods: A hospital-based case–control study, consisting of 502 MI patients and 308 controls, was conducted in a Chinese population. Demographic, behavioral information and clinical characteristics were collected, and genotyping of the two SNPs was performed using single base primer extension genotyping technology. The unconditional logistic regression (ULR) method was adopted to assess the association of the two SNPs with MI risk. Both generalized multifactor dimensionality reduction (GMDR) and ULR methods were applied to explore the effect of gene-environment interactions on the risk of MI.

Results: After adjusting for covariates, it was observed that SNP rs10757274 on chromosome 9p21 was significantly associated with MI. Compared with subjects carrying the AA genotype, subjects carrying the GA or GG genotypes had a higher MI risk ($OR_a = 1.52$, 95% CI:1.06–2.19, $p_a = 0.0227$; $OR_a = 2.40$, 95% CI:1.51–3.81, $p_a = 0.0002$, respectively). Furthermore, a two-factor gene-environment interaction model of CDKN2A/B (rs10757274) and type 2 diabetes mellitus (T2DM) was identified to be the best model by GMDR ($p = 0.0107$), with a maximum prediction accuracy of 59.18%, and a maximum Cross-validation Consistency of 10/10. By using the ULR method, additive interaction analysis found that the combined effect resulted in T2DM-positive subjects with genotype GG/GA having an MI risk 4.38 times that of T2DM-negative subjects with genotype AA ($OR_{add} = 4.38$, 95% CI:2.56–7.47, $p_{add} < 0.0001$).

Conclusions: These results show that gene polymorphism of CDKN2A/B (rs10757274) is associated with MI risk in a Chinese population. Furthermore, T2DM is likely to have an interaction with CDKN2A/B (rs10757274) that contributes to the risk of MI.

* Correspondence: lijianping@medmail.com.cn; dafangchen@bjmu.edu.cn
[2]Department of Cardiology, Peking University First Hospital, Beijing 100034, China
[1]Department of Epidemiology and Biostatistics, School of Public Health, Peking University Health Science Center, Beijing 100191, China

Background

It has been reported that the global endemic of Coronary Artery Disease (CAD) is the leading cause of morbidity and mortality worldwide, due to serious complications such as myocardial infarction (MI) [1,2]. Most researchers agree that, similarly to other complex diseases, multiple environmental factors, genetic factors and gene-environment interactions play important roles in determining the onset and development of CAD/MI [3]. There are many well-recognized environmental risk factors such as smoking, physical activity and body mass index (BMI). Genetic factors have also been considered to be substantial risk contributors to the pathogenesis of CAD/MI [4,5]. Although previous studies have shown that the heritability of CAD ranges from approximately 40 to 60%, the genetic mechanism underlying the inherited component of CAD/MI is still not fully characterized [6].

In the past decade, there have been many studies on linkage and candidate gene association, however, these have only identified a limited number of genetic variants involved in the pathogenesis of CAD/MI. Genome-wide association studies (GWAS) have been a new approach since the completion of the Human Genome Project and the International HapMap Project, and have provided improved resolution in identifying genetic factors in relation to complex diseases. To date, many genome-wide studies have revealed that several genomic regions are strongly associated with an increased risk of CAD/MI [7-14], and it has been generally accepted that the association between genetic variants on chromosome 9p21 and the risk of CAD is the most robustly replicated finding in different ethnic populations [15-18]. However, several other studies have shown inconsistent results when the association between these genetic variants and MI was examined [19,20]. Recently, a Chinese GWAS reported that chromosome 6p24 contains a novel susceptibility locus associated with CAD [14]. Some previous single studies have also suggested that genetic variants associated with cardiovascular disease might interact with hypertension or glycemic control [21,22]. Therefore, we chose to study SNP rs10757274 on chromosome 9p21 and SNP rs6903956 on chromosome 6p24, to identify the association between these two susceptible genes and the risk of MI, and to explore gene-environment interactions in a Chinese population.

Methods

Study population

This project was designed as a hospital-based case–control study. Between June 2012 and May 2013, a total of 810 consecutive unrelated adult patients at Peking University First Hospital (Beijing, China) were enrolled in the study. Of these subjects, 502 patients undergoing coronary angiography for suspected or known coronary atherosclerosis were diagnosed with MI according to the universal definition of myocardial infarction [23], while 308 subjects were considered as the control group, who underwent coronary angiography for other reasons (mainly valvular heart disease) and had completely normal coronary arteries. Quanto software was used to measure the statistical power of this study; according to the frequencies of the minor allele (listed on NCBI) and the genetic effects that have been reported for these two SNPs, the statistical power of this study based on the current sample size is more than 0.90. The study was approved by the Ethics Committee of the Peking University Health Science Center, and all the subjects provided written informed consent for participation.

Information collection

Demographic, behavioral information and clinical characteristics were collected from physicians and hospital records, including age, gender, ethnicity, smoking and drinking habits and some medical history information. A smoking habit was defined as current active smokers or those with a smoking history of at least10 packs per year, while a drinking habit was defined as consuming more than 50 g of alcohol per week for at least 6 months. Weight and height were measured when the subjects were lightly clothed and barefoot, and the BMI was calculated as the weight divided by the square of the height (kg/m^2)). Overnight fasting blood samples were obtained from all participants, and measurements of the plasma concentrations of glucose, total cholesterol (TC, mmol/L), low density lipoprotein cholesterol (LDL-C, mmol/L), high density lipoprotein cholesterol (HDL-C, mmol/L) and triglyceride (TG, mmol/L) were conducted in the clinical laboratory of the Peking University First Hospital according to the standard biochemical methods. Combined with laboratory findings, type two diabetes mellitus (T2DM) was diagnosed according to the WHO diagnostic criteria from 1999 [24]; hypertension was defined as systolic blood pressure ≥140 mmHg and/or diastolic blood pressure ≥90 mmHg based on the average of two separate measurements, or current antihypertensive treatment; hyperlipidemia was diagnosed as fasting total cholesterol ≥200 mg/dL or low-density lipoprotein cholesterol ≥130 mg/dL.

DNA preparation

EDTA anti-coagulated blood samples were drawn from every participant, and genomic DNA was extracted from the participants' peripheral blood leucocytes by using the protein precipitation method following standard procedures. Each DNA sample was quantified using a Nanophotometer (Implen, Germany) and was diluted to a final concentration of 50 ng/uL.

SNP genotyping

Genotyping of two SNPs (rs6903956 and rs10757274) was performed using the single base primer extension genotyping technology with the GenomeLab SNPstream genotyping system (Beckman Coulter Inc, Fullerton, CA, USA) following the manufacturer's protocol [25]. Both of the SNPs had a call rate of greater than 95%, 10% of the blind duplicate samples were genotyped repeatedly and the rate of consistency was 100%.

Statistical analysis

The descriptive and association analyses were performed using the SAS 9.1 software (SAS Institute Inc., Cary, NC). The continuous variables were shown as Mean ± SD, a two-sample *t*-test was adopted to compare their means. The comparison of categorical variables and testing of the Hardy-Weinberg Equilibrium (HWE) at each polymorphic locus in the control group was conducted using Pearson's χ^2 test. Unconditional logistic regression (ULR) was performed to estimate the association (Odds ratios (ORs) and 95% confidence intervals (CIs)) between individual polymorphisms and MI, adjusting for potential confounders, including gender, age, ethnicity, BMI, smoking and drinking habits. High dimensional gene-environment interactions were examined using the generalized multifactor dimensionality reduction method (GMDR, version 0.7, obtained from http://www.medicine.virginia.edu/clinical/departments/psychiatry/sections/neurobiologicalstudies/genomics/gmdr-software-request) [26], adjusting for age, gender, ethnicity, BMI, smoking and drinking habits as covariates. GMDR is a nonparametric method reducing high-dimensional data into one dimension. In this study, one- to five-factor models were constructed and the model with the highest prediction accuracy was defined as the "best model". If the model was considered to be significant using the sign statistical test ($p < 0.05$), then a 1000 times permutation test was performed to validate the results. One dimensional multiplicative interaction was detected by ULR, adjusting for the potential confounders mentioned above. One dimensional additive interaction was estimated using the "Biological interaction calculating Excel" provided by Andersson et al. [27]. For two dichotomized risk factors, let OR_{01}/OR_{10} represent exposure of each risk factor alone, let OR_{11} represent exposure of both risk factors, and let OR_{00} represent absence of both risk factors, which was used as the reference category. Three statistical indicators were calculated: relative excess risk of interaction ($RERI = OR_{11} - (OR_{01} + OR_{10} - 1)$), attributable proportion of interaction ($API = RERI/OR_{11}$), and the synergy index ($S = (OR_{11} - 1)/[(OR_{01} - 1) + (OR_{10} - 1)]$), along with their 95% CIs, to measure the additive interaction. If the 95% CIs of RERI and API did not include 0 and the 95% CI of the S index did not include 1, it can be considered that an additive interaction exists.

Results

Demographic, behavioral information and clinical characteristics of participants

A total of 810 unrelated Chinese subjects were enrolled in this study. The minimum and maximum ages among the participants were 28 and 88, respectively. The average age of the 502 cases was (63.66 ± 11.57) years, and the average age of the 308 controls was (61.87 ± 10.39) years. 64.92% of participants were male and 35.08% were female. The distributions of demographic, behavioral information and clinical characteristics of the subjects are listed in Table 1. There were no significant differences between the MI group and the control group in terms of mean BMI and distributions of ethnicity, hypertension and hyperlipidemia, while the mean age and frequencies of male gender, T2DM-positive, and smoking and drinking habits-positive were significantly higher in MI patients than in controls.

Association analysis of genetic polymorphisms with MI

Two SNPs, ADTRP (rs6903956) and CDKN2A/B (rs10757274) were studied in our association analysis. Both of their genotype distributions in the control group conformed to the HWE ($\chi^2 = 2.756$, $p = 0.097$; $\chi^2 = 0.968$, $p = 0.325$; respectively), which indicated these participants were from a homogeneous group. The genotype distributions of the two SNPs between MI patients and controls and their association with MI risk are available in Table 2, while the univariate associations between each of the two SNPs and the clinical characteristics listed in Table 1 for cases and controls are included in the Additional file 1: Table S1 and S2. Taking the subjects carrying the GG genotype for ADTRP (rs6903956) as a reference, the subjects carrying genotype AA/GA showed an increased risk of MI (OR = 1.51, 95% CI:1.01–2.23, $p = 0.0423$), but after adjusting for confounding factors including age, gender, ethnicity, BMI, smoking and drinking habits, the association between ADTRP (rs6903956) and MI risk was insignificant (OR = 1.49, 95% CI:0.97–2.29, $p = 0.0678$). According to the genetic effect and minor allele frequency of rs6903956 observed in this study, the statistical power based on the current sample size is 0.73. For CDKN2A/B (rs10757274), both before and after adjusting for confounding factors mentioned above, the subjects carrying GA or GG genotypes were all associated with MI risk ($OR_a = 1.52$, 95% CI:1.06–2.19, $p_a = 0.0227$; $OR_a = 2.40$, 95% CI:1.51–3.81, $p_a = 0.0002$; respectively), compared with subjects with the AA genotype. For rs10757274, the statistical power based on the current sample size is 0.97.

Gene-environment interactions analysis

First, GMDR was used to explore the gene-environment interactions. ADTRP (rs6903956), CDKN2A/B (rs10757274)

Table 1 Demographic, behavioral information and clinical characteristics of participants

Variable	Variable frequencies (%)			
	Controls (N = 308)	MI patients (N = 502)	t/χ2	p-value
Age	61.87 ± 10.39	63.66 ± 11.57	2.2823	0.0228
BMI (kg/m²)	25.84 ± 3.53	25.73 ± 3.09	0.4673	0.6404
Gender				
Male	47.73	77.09	73.2707	<.0001
Female	52.27	22.91		
Ethnicity				
Chinese Han	94.48	96.81	2.6567	0.1031
Ethnicity minority	5.52	3.19		
Smoking habit				
No	63.96	36.65	57.1381	<.0001
Yes	36.04	63.35		
Drinking habit				
No	74.68	61.75	14.3438	0.0002
Yes	25.32	38.25		
T2DM				
No	75.97	61.35	18.4275	<.0001
Yes	24.03	38.65		
Hypertension				
No	35.71	32.07	1.1376	0.2862
Yes	64.29	67.93		
Hyperlipidemia				
No	60.06	61.55	0.1778	0.6732
Yes	39.94	38.45		

and clinical characteristics (T2DM, hypertension and hyperlipidemia) were included in the gene-environment interactions analysis, adjusting for age, gender, ethnicity, BMI, and smoking and drinking habits as covariates. The results of the GMDR analysis for one-factor to five-factor models are shown in Table 3. Among these results, the two-factor interaction model of CDKN2A/B (rs10757274) and T2DM was identified to be the best model, with a maximum prediction accuracy of 59.18%, and a maximum Cross-validation Consistency (CVC) of 10/10. This model was identified as significant using the sign test ($p = 0.0107$) and validated by a 1000 times permutation test ($p < 0.001$). These results indicate that a potential gene-environment interaction is likely to exist between T2DM and CDKN2A/B (rs10757274) affecting MI risk in this study.

Second, to further reveal the potential gene-environment interaction mentioned above, ULR analysis was conducted to explore the possible multiplicative or additive gene-environment interactions between T2DM and CDKN2A/B (rs10757274) affecting MI risk. As shown in Table 4, there were no gene-environment multiplicative interactions between T2DM and CDKN2A/B (rs10757274) affecting MI risk ($OR_{multi} = 1.63$, 95% CI:0.78–3.44, $p_{multi} = 0.197$). After adjusting for age, gender, ethnicity, BMI, smoking and drinking habits as covariates, T2DM-negative subjects with the genotype GG/GA had a MI risk of 1.60 times that of T2DM-negative subjects carrying the genotype AA ($OR_{add} = 1.60$, 95% CI:1.04–2.46), and it was statistically significant ($p_{add} = 0.0329$); T2DM-positive subjects with genotype AA had a MI risk of 1.68 times that of T2DM-negative subjects carrying genotype AA ($OR_{add} = 1.68$, 95% CI:0.92 – 3.08), but it was not statistically significant ($p_{add} = 0.0943$). The combined effect resulted in T2DM-positive subjects with genotype GG/GA having an MI risk of 4.38 times that of T2DM-negative subjects carrying genotype AA ($OR_{add} = 4.38$, 95% CI:2.56 – 7.47), and this was statistically significant ($p_{add} < 0.0001$). Because the 95% CIs of RERI and API did not include 0, and the 95% CI of S did not include 1 (RERI = 2.10, 95% CI:0.18 – 4.03; API = 0.48, 95% CI:0.19 – 0.77; and S = 2.65, 95% CI:1.01 – 6.94, respectively), it can be considered that an additive gene-environment interaction exists between T2DM and CDKN2A/B (rs10757274) affecting the risk of MI.

Table 2 Association analysis of genetic polymorphisms with MI risk

Chromosome location	Closest gene	SNPs	Genotypes	Genotype frequencies (%)		Without adjustment		With adjustment	
				Controls (N = 308)	MI patients (N = 502)	OR (95% CI)	p	OR_a (95% CI)	p_a
6P24	ADTRP	rs6903956	GG	85.23	79.30	reference			
			GA	13.40	18.74	1.50 (1.00,2.27)	0.0525	1.55 (0.99,2.43)	0.0556
			AA	1.37	1.96	1.53 (0.47,5.03)	0.4813	1.04 (0.30,3.59)	0.9522
			AA/GA	14.78	20.70	1.51 (1.01,2.23)	0.0423	1.49(0.97,2.29)	0.0678
9P21	CDKN2A/B	rs10757274	AA	32.78	23.54	reference			
			GA	51.32	52.52	1.43 (1.02,1.99)	0.0374	1.52(1.06,2.19)	0.0227
			GG	15.89	23.94	2.10 (1.37,3.22)	0.0007	2.40 (1.51,3.81)	0.0002
			GG/GA	67.22	76.46	1.58 (1.15,2.18)	0.0045	1.72 (1.22,2.43)	0.0020

a: Adjusting for age, gender, ethnicity, BMI, smoking and drinking habits as covariates.

Table 3 GMDR models of gene-environmental interactions on MI risk

Models[a]	Prediction accuracy	CVC	p_{sign}	p_{perm}
T2DM	0.5815	10/10	0.0010	<0.001
T2DM, rs10757274	0.5918	10/10	0.0107	<0.001
T2DM, rs10757274, rs6903956	0.5796	10/10	0.0107	<0.001
T2DM, hyperlipidemia, rs10757274, rs6903956	0.5815	9/10	0.0547	<0.001
T2DM, hyperlipidemia, hypertension, rs10757274, rs6903956	0.5692	10/10	0.0547	0.008

[a]Adjusting for age, gender, ethnicity, BMI, smoking and drinking habits as covariates.
p_{sign}: p-value from sign test.
p_{perm}: p-value from 1000 times permutation test.

Discussion

Due to the fact that MI is the main complication of CAD and both of these diseases share common risk factors, both genetic variants and environmental risk factors associated with CAD are expected candidates affecting the risk of MI. In this case–control study, we chose two previously reported SNPs representing the genetic variants on 9p21 and 6p24 to investigate the association with MI. Our results indicate that a genetic variant of CDKN2A/B (rs10757274) on 9p21 is associated with MI after adjusting for conventional confounding factors, which consistently supports former results [10,28,29]. Further gene-environment interactions for ADTRP (rs6903956), CDKN2A/B (rs10757274), hypertension, dyslipidemia and T2DM were explored by GMDR and ULR methods, and the results from GMDR indicate that a gene-environment interaction is likely to exist between CDKN2A/B (rs10757274) and T2DM affecting the risk of MI. Further analytic results from ULR consistently support the existence of potential additive gene-environment interactions between CDKN2A/B (rs10757274) and T2DM, with a combined effect of increasing the risk of MI for T2DM-positive subjects with genotype GG/GA by 4.38 times that of T2DM-negative subjects carrying genotype AA. It had been previously reported that diabetes is a positive factor contributing to CAD/MI [30,31]. T2DM, accounting for the majority of forms of diabetes, has also been considered a common disorder and an important risk factor for cardiovascular disease [32]. Recently, a report in a Chinese population also found that another genomic variant on 9p21 is associated with a risk of T2DM [33]. This is thought to be due to the CDKN2A and CDKN2B genes in this genomic region inhibiting CDK4 and CDK6, which has been demonstrated to influence β cell proliferation and mass, eventually leading to diabetes [34-36]. Meanwhile, a study published in 2008 reported an interaction between poor glycemic control and a 9p21 variant that increased the risk of CAD in T2DM [21]. Therefore, it is reasonable to consider that CDKN2A/B (rs10757274) not only increases the risk of MI, but also enhances the effects of T2DM on the risk of MI in this study.

In contrast to CDKN2A/B (rs10757274), we found that the genetic variant of ADTRP (rs6903956) on 6p24 was not associated with MI after adjusting for conventional confounding factors, which is inconsistent with recent research results reported in a Japanese population [37]. To our knowledge, only this solo Japanese research report has investigated the association between ADTRP (rs6903956) and MI to date, and the risk allele identified in this Japanese study differs from our study and two other studies conducted in Han Chinese and Japanese populations [14,38]. Most former studies have focused on the identification of associations between ADTRP and CAD, but the results are controversial even in the same racial population [14,39,40]. It has been indicated that the underlying mechanism is due to regulation of the mRNA expression of the tissue factor pathway inhibitor (TFPI) by the ADTRP gene. Decreased TFPI expression would result in an increased rate of thrombosis and thus increase the risk of CAD [41]. Therefore,

Table 4 Multiplicative and additive gene-environmental interactions analysis between T2DM and CDKN2A/B (rs10757274) on MI risk

		Frequencies (%)					
Genotype	T2DM	Controls (N = 308)	MI patients (N = 502)	OR_{add}[a] (95% CI)	p_{add}	OR_{multi}[a] (95% CI)	p_{multi}
rs10757274						1.63(0.78,3.44)	0.197
AA	No	22.52	12.67	reference			
GG/GA		53.31	48.69	1.60 (1.04,2.46)	0.0329		
AA	Yes	10.26	10.87	1.68 (0.92,3.08)	0.0943		
GG/GA		13.91	27.77	4.38 (2.56,7.47)	<0.0001		
RERI				2.10 (0.18,4.03)			
API				0.48 (0.19,0.77)			
S				2.65(1.01,6.94)			

[a]Adjusting for age, gender, ethnicity, BMI, smoking and drinking habits as covariates.
p_{add}: p-value from additive gene-environmental interactions analysis.
p_{multi}: p-value from multiplicative gene-environmental interactions analysis.

further studies are needed to completely reveal whether genetic variants on 6p24 are associated with the risk of MI.

There are inevitably some limitations to this study. First, as our study is based on a case–control design, it was difficult to avoid recall bias completely, and the results should be confirmed in prospective cohort studies. Second, our study investigated only a limited number of genetic variants related to MI, whereas many other genes and SNPs have been reported to contribute to MI susceptibility. Therefore, this study is not sufficient to evaluate genetic susceptibility to MI, and it would be useful for further studies to investigate more genetic polymorphisms associated with MI.

Conclusion

In conclusion, the results of this study suggest that a gene polymorphism of CDKN2A/B (rs10757274) is associated with MI risk in a Chinese population. Furthermore, T2DM is likely to interact with CDKN2A/B (rs10757274) and contribute to the risk of MI.

Abbreviations

ULR: Unconditional logistic regression; GMDR: Generalized multifactor dimensionality reduction; CAD: Coronary Artery Disease; MI: Myocardial infarction; T2DM: Type two diabetes mellitus; BMI: Body mass index; GWAS: Genome-wide association studies; HWE: Hardy-Weinberg Equilibrium; ORs: Odds ratios; CIs: Confidence intervals.

Competing interests

The authors declare that they have no competing interests.

Authors' contributions

LZ carried out the experiments, performed the data analysis and drafted the manuscript. DC, JL, YH, SZ and YH conceived and designed the study and helped to draft the manuscript. JJ and YZ participated in the recruitment of subjects and acquisition of data. FD, ZL participated in the genotyping and interpretation of the data. All authors read and approved the final manuscript.

Acknowledgements

We acknowledge that this study was supported by the National Natural Science Foundation of China (81172768). We also need to thank the staff of the Department of Cardiology of Peking University First Hospital for their support in recruiting the study subjects.

References

1. Go AS, Mozaffarian D, Roger VL, Benjamin EJ, Berry JD, Blaha MJ, Dai S, Ford ES, Fox CS, Franco S, Fullerton HJ, Gillespie C, Hailpern SM, Heit JA, Howard VJ, Huffman MD, Judd SE, Kissela BM, Kittner SJ, Lackland DT, Lichtman JH, Lisabeth LD, Mackey RH, Magid DJ, Marcus GM, Marelli A, Matchar DB, McGuire DK, Mohler ER 3rd, Moy CS, *et al*: **Heart disease and stroke statistics–2014 update: a report from the American Heart Association.** *Circulation* 2014, **129**(3):e28–e292.
2. Lopez AD, Mathers CD, Ezzati M, Jamison DT, Murray CJ: **Global and regional burden of disease and risk factors, 2001: systematic analysis of population health data.** *Lancet* 2006, **367**(9524):1747–1757.
3. Kathiresan S, Srivastava D: **Genetics of human cardiovascular disease.** *Cell* 2012, **148**(6):1242–1257.
4. Topol EJ, Smith J, Plow EF, Wang QK: **Genetic susceptibility to myocardial infarction and coronary artery disease.** *Hum Mol Genet* 2006, **15**(Spec No 2):R117–R123.
5. Wang Q: **Advances in the genetic basis of coronary artery disease.** *Curr Atheroscler Rep* 2005, **7**(3):235–241.
6. Girelli D, Martinelli N, Peyvandi F, Olivieri O: **Genetic architecture of coronary artery disease in the genome-wide era: implications for the emerging "golden dozen" loci.** *Semin Thromb Hemost* 2009, **35**(7):671–682.
7. Consortium WTCC: **Genome-wide association study of 14,000 cases of seven common diseases and 3,000 shared controls.** *Nature* 2007, **447**(7145):661–678.
8. Helgadottir A, Thorleifsson G, Manolescu A, Gretarsdottir S, Blondal T, Jonasdottir A, Sigurdsson A, Baker A, Palsson A, Masson G, Gudbjartsson DF, Magnusson KP, Andersen K, Levey AI, Backman VM, Matthiasdottir S, Jonsdottir T, Palsson S, Einarsdottir H, Gunnarsdottir S, Gylfason A, Vaccarino V, Hooper WC, Reilly MP, Granger CB, Austin H, Rader DJ, Shah SH, Quyyumi AA, Gulcher JR, *et al*: **A common variant on chromosome 9p21 affects the risk of myocardial infarction.** *Science* 2007, **316**(5830):1491–1493.
9. Lee JY, Lee BS, Shin DJ, Woo Park K, Shin YA, Joong Kim K, Heo L, Young Lee J, Kyoung Kim Y, Jin Kim Y, Bum Hong C, Lee SH, Yoon D, Jung Ku H, Oh IY, Kim BJ, Lee J, Park SJ, Kim J, Kawk HK, Lee JE, Park HK, Nam HY, Park HY, Shin C, Yokota M, Asano H, Nakatochi M, Matsubara T, Kitajima H, *et al*: **A genome-wide association study of a coronary artery disease risk variant.** *J Hum Genet* 2013, **58**(3):120–126.
10. McPherson R, Pertsemlidis A, Kavaslar N, Stewart A, Roberts R, Cox DR, Hinds DA, Pennacchio LA, Tybjaerg-Hansen A, Folsom AR, Boerwinkle E, Hobbs HH, Cohen JC: **A common allele on chromosome 9 associated with coronary heart disease.** *Science* 2007, **316**(5830):1488–1491.
11. Samani NJ, Erdmann J, Hall AS, Hengstenberg C, Mangino M, Mayer B, Dixon RJ, Meitinger T, Braund P, Wichmann HE, Barrett JH, Konig IR, Stevens SE, Szymczak S, Tregouet DA, Iles MM, Pahlke F, Pollard H, Lieb W, Cambien F, Fischer M, Ouwehand W, Blankenberg S, Balmforth AJ, Baessler A, Ball SG, Strom TM, Braenne I, Gieger C, Deloukas P, *et al*: **Genomewide association analysis of coronary artery disease.** *N Engl J Med* 2007, **357**(5):443–453.
12. Schunkert H, Konig IR, Kathiresan S, Reilly MP, Assimes TL, Holm H, Preuss M, Stewart AF, Barbalic M, Gieger C, Absher D, Aherrahrou Z, Allayee H, Altshuler D, Anand SS, Andersen K, Anderson JL, Ardissino D, Ball SG, Balmforth AJ, Barnes TA, Becker DM, Becker LC, Berger K, Bis JC, Boekholdt SM, Boerwinkle E, Braund PS, Brown MJ, Burnett MS, *et al*: **Large-scale association analysis identifies 13 new susceptibility loci for coronary artery disease.** *Nat Genet* 2011, **43**(4):333–338.
13. Takeuchi F, Yokota M, Yamamoto K, Nakashima E, Katsuya T, Asano H, Isono M, Nabika T, Sugiyama T, Fujioka A, Awata N, Ohnaka K, Nakatochi M, Kitajima H, Rakugi H, Nakamura J, Ohkubo T, Imai Y, Shimamoto K, Yamori Y, Yamaguchi S, Kobayashi S, Takayanagi R, Ogihara T, Kato N: **Genome-wide association study of coronary artery disease in the Japanese.** *Eur J Hum Genet* 2012, **20**(3):333–340.
14. Wang F, Xu CQ, He Q, Cai JP, Li XC, Wang D, Xiong X, Liao YH, Zeng QT, Yang YZ, Cheng X, Li C, Yang R, Wang CC, Wu G, Lu QL, Bai Y, Huang YF, Yin D, Yang Q, Wang XJ, Dai DP, Zhang RF, Wan J, Ren JH, Li SS, Zhao YY, Fu FF, Huang Y, Li QX, *et al*: **Genome-wide association identifies a susceptibility locus for coronary artery disease in the Chinese Han population.** *Nat Genet* 2011, **43**(4):345–349.
15. Assimes TL, Knowles JW, Basu A, Iribarren C, Southwick A, Tang H, Absher D, Li J, Fair JM, Rubin GD, Sidney S, Fortmann SP, Go AS, Hlatky MA, Myers RM, Risch N, Quertermous T: **Susceptibility locus for clinical and subclinical coronary artery disease at chromosome 9p21 in the multi-ethnic ADVANCE study.** *Hum Mol Genet* 2008, **17**(15):2320–2328.
16. Schunkert H, Gotz A, Braund P, McGinnis R, Tregouet DA, Mangino M, Linsel-Nitschke P, Cambien F, Hengstenberg C, Stark K, Blankenberg S, Tiret L, Ducimetiere P, Keniry A, Ghori MJ, Schreiber S, El Mokhtari NE, Hall AS, Dixon RJ, Goodall AH, Liptau H, Pollard H, Schwarz DF, Hothorn LA, Wichmann HE, Konig IR, Fischer M, Meisinger C, Ouwehand W, Deloukas P, *et al*: **Repeated replication and a prospective meta-analysis of the association between chromosome 9p21.3 and coronary artery disease.** *Circulation* 2008, **117**(13):1675–1684.

17. Shen GQ, Li L, Rao S, Abdullah KG, Ban JM, Lee BS, Park JE, Wang QK: **Four SNPs on chromosome 9p21 in a South Korean population implicate a genetic locus that confers high cross-race risk for development of coronary artery disease.** *Arterioscler Thromb Vasc Biol* 2008, **28**(2):360–365.
18. Zhou L, Zhang X, He M, Cheng L, Chen Y, Hu FB, Wu T: **Associations between single nucleotide polymorphisms on chromosome 9p21 and risk of coronary heart disease in Chinese Han population.** *Arterioscler Thromb Vasc Biol* 2008, **28**(11):2085–2089.
19. Virani SS, Brautbar A, Lee VV, MacArthur E, Morrison AC, Grove ML, Nambi V, Frazier L, Wilson JM, Willerson JT, Boerwinkle E, Ballantyne CM: **Chromosome 9p21 single nucleotide polymorphisms are not associated with recurrent myocardial infarction in patients with established coronary artery disease.** *Circ J* 2012, **76**(4):950–956.
20. Horne BD, Carlquist JF, Muhlestein JB, Bair TL, Anderson JL: **Association of variation in the chromosome 9p21 locus with myocardial infarction versus chronic coronary artery disease.** *Circ Cardiovasc Genet* 2008, **1**(2):85–92.
21. Doria A, Wojcik J, Xu R, Gervino EV, Hauser TH, Johnstone MT, Nolan D, Hu FB, Warram JH: **Interaction between poor glycemic control and 9p21 locus on risk of coronary artery disease in type 2 diabetes.** *JAMA* 2008, **300**(20):2389–2397.
22. Hu WL, Li SJ, Liu DT, Wang Y, Niu SQ, Yang XC, Zhang Q, Yu SZ, Jin L, Wang XF: **Genetic variants on chromosome 9p21 and ischemic stroke in Chinese.** *Brain Res Bull* 2009, **79**(6):431–435.
23. Thygesen K, Alpert JS, White HD: **Universal definition of myocardial infarction.** *Eur Heart J* 2007, **28**(20):2525–2538.
24. World Health Organisation: *Definition Diagnosis and Classification of Diabetes Mellitus and its Complications: Report of a WHO Consultation. Part 1. Diagnosis and Classification of Diabetes Mellitus.* Geneva: WHO; 1999.
25. Bell PA, Chaturvedi S, Gelfand CA, Huang CY, Kochersperger M, Kopla R, Modica F, Pohl M, Varde S, Zhao R, Zhao X, Boyce-Jacino MT, Yassen A: **SNPstream UHT: ultra-high throughput SNP genotyping for pharmacogenomics and drug discovery.** *Biotechniques* 2002, **Suppl**:70–72. 74, 76–77.
26. Lou XY, Chen GB, Yan L, Ma JZ, Zhu J, Elston RC, Li MD: **A generalized combinatorial approach for detecting gene-by-gene and gene-by-environment interactions with application to nicotine dependence.** *Am J Hum Genet* 2007, **80**(6):1125–1137.
27. Andersson T, Alfredsson L, Kallberg H, Zdravkovic S, Ahlbom A: **Calculating measures of biological interaction.** *Eur J Epidemiol* 2005, **20**(7):575–579.
28. Motterle A, Pu X, Wood H, Xiao Q, Gor S, Ng FL, Chan K, Cross F, Shohreh B, Poston RN, Tucker AT, Caulfield MJ, Ye S: **Functional analyses of coronary artery disease associated variation on chromosome 9p21 in vascular smooth muscle cells.** *Hum Mol Genet* 2012, **21**(18):4021–4029.
29. Xie F, Chu X, Wu H, Sun W, Shen M, Yang L, Wang Y, Shi J, Huang W: **Replication of putative susceptibility loci from genome-wide association studies associated with coronary atherosclerosis in Chinese Han population.** *PLoS ONE* 2011, **6**(6):e20833.
30. Go AS, Mozaffarian D, Roger VL, Benjamin EJ, Berry JD, Blaha MJ, Dai S, Ford ES, Fox CS, Franco S, Fullerton HJ, Gillespie C, Hailpern SM, Heit JA, Howard VJ, Huffman MD, Judd SE, Kissela BM, Kittner SJ, Lackland DT, Lichtman JH, Lisabeth LD, Mackey RH, Magid DJ, Marcus GM, Marelli A, Matchar DB, McGuire DK, Mohler ER 3rd, Moy CS, *et al*: **Executive summary: heart disease and stroke statistics–2014 update: a report from the American Heart Association.** *Circulation* 2014, **129**(3):399–410.
31. Yusuf S, Hawken S, Ounpuu S, Dans T, Avezum A, Lanas F, McQueen M, Budaj A, Pais P, Varigos J, Lisheng L: **Effect of potentially modifiable risk factors associated with myocardial infarction in 52 countries (the INTERHEART study): case–control study.** *Lancet* 2004, **364**(9438):937–952.
32. Fox CS: **Cardiovascular disease risk factors, type 2 diabetes mellitus, and the Framingham Heart Study.** *Trends Cardiovasc Med* 2010, **20**(3):90–95.
33. Wen J, Ronn T, Olsson A, Yang Z, Lu B, Du Y, Groop L, Ling C, Hu R: **Investigation of type 2 diabetes risk alleles support CDKN2A/B, CDKAL1, and TCF7L2 as susceptibility genes in a Han Chinese cohort.** *PLoS ONE* 2010, **5**(2):e9153.
34. Krishnamurthy J, Ramsey MR, Ligon KL, Torrice C, Koh A, Bonner-Weir S, Sharpless NE: **p16INK4a induces an age-dependent decline in islet regenerative potential.** *Nature* 2006, **443**(7110):453–457.
35. Rane SG, Dubus P, Mettus RV, Galbreath EJ, Boden G, Reddy EP, Barbacid M: **Loss of Cdk4 expression causes insulin-deficient diabetes and Cdk4 activation results in beta-islet cell hyperplasia.** *Nat Genet* 1999, **22**(1):44–52.
36. Tsutsui T, Hesabi B, Moons DS, Pandolfi PP, Hansel KS, Koff A, Kiyokawa H: **Targeted disruption of CDK4 delays cell cycle entry with enhanced p27 (Kip1) activity.** *Mol Cell Biol* 1999, **19**(10):7011–7019.
37. Dechamethakun S, Ikeda S, Arai T, Sato N, Sawabe M, Muramatsu M: **Associations between the CDKN2A/B, ADTRP and PDGFD Polymorphisms and the Development of Coronary Atherosclerosis in Japanese Patients.** *J Atheroscler Thromb* 2014, [Epub ahead of print].
38. Tayebi N, Ke T, Foo JN, Friedlander Y, Liu J, Heng CK: **Association of single nucleotide polymorphism rs6903956 on chromosome 6p24.1 with coronary artery disease and lipid levels in different ethnic groups of the Singaporean population.** *Clin Biochem* 2013, **46**(9):755–759.
39. Lu X, Wang L, Chen S, He L, Yang X, Shi Y, Cheng J, Zhang L, Gu CC, Huang J, Wu T, Ma Y, Li J, Cao J, Chen J, Ge D, Fan Z, Li Y, Zhao L, Li H, Zhou X, Chen L, Liu D, Duan X, Hao Y, Lu F, Liu Z, Yao C, Shen C, Pu X, *et al*: **Genome-wide association study in Han Chinese identifies four new susceptibility loci for coronary artery disease.** *Nat Genet* 2012, **44**(8):890–894.
40. Guo CY, Gu Y, Li L, Jia EZ, Li CJ, Wang LS, Yang ZJ, Cao KJ, Ma WZ: **Association of SNP rs6903956 on chromosome 6p24.1 with angiographical characteristics of coronary atherosclerosis in a Chinese population.** *PLoS ONE* 2012, **7**(8):e43732.
41. Lupu C, Zhu H, Popescu NI, Wren JD, Lupu F: **Novel protein ADTRP regulates TFPI expression and function in human endothelial cells in normal conditions and in response to androgen.** *Blood* 2011, **118**(16):4463–4471.

5

Fractional flow reserve of non-culprit vessel post-myocardial infarction: is it reliable?

Luís Leite*, Joana Moura Ferreira, João Silva Marques, Elisabete Jorge, Vítor Matos, Jorge Guardado, João Calisto and Mariano Pego

Abstract

Background: Multi-vessel disease is frequent in patients presenting with myocardial infarction and have an important prognostic impact. The decision to proceed to revascularization in non-culprit vessels can be postponed until ischemia is proven in non-invasive stress tests. On the other hand, there is an increasing evidence to support the role of fractional flow reserve (FFR) in acute coronary syndrome setting.

Case presentation: We report a case in which a FFR-guided strategy for non-culprit vessels, 3 weeks after an ST-segment elevation myocardial infarction, was followed by a short-term sub-occlusion of the evaluated vessel.

Conclusion: The timing of the coronary microcirculation recovery post-myocardial infarction, avoiding a possible false negative FFR, and the diagnostic gaps between ischemia and plaque vulnerability are under discussion. An FFR-guided strategy in this setting should be interpreted with caution.

Keywords: Multi-vessel disease, Myocardial infarction, Fractional flow reserve, Ischemia, Plaque vulnerability

Background

The prevalence of multi-vessel disease (MVD) in patients presenting with acute ST-segment elevation myocardial infarction (STEMI) approaches 40 % [1]. This subgroup of STEMI patients has a higher risk of major adverse cardiac events (MACE) in the first year after primary percutaneous coronary intervention (PCI) [2]. Therefore, the assessment of the actual severity of the non-culprit coronary artery stenosis and its optimal treatment is clinically important soon after primary PCI.

Case presentation

A 79-year-old female with a history of hypertension and dyslipidaemia, was admitted for an inferior STEMI and underwent primary angioplasty of the right coronary artery with implantation of a 3.0 × 33 mm Xience™ everolimus-eluting stent. The emergency coronary angiography also showed three intermediate stenosis in the mid-segment of the left anterior descending artery (LAD) – Fig. 1. Transthoracic echocardiogram demonstrated normal biventricular systolic function with a left ventricular ejection fraction of 60 %. The patient was clinically stable and was discharged 4 days later with optimized medical therapy (aspirin 100 mg qd, ticagrelor 90 mg bid, atorvastatin 40 mg qd, carvedilol 6.25 mg bid, ramipril 1.25 mg qd, pantoprazol 40 mg qd).

In order to assess the hemodynamic relevance of the LAD lesions, a 3 week scheduled coronary angiography with fractional flow reserve (FFR) measurements of LAD was performed (Fig. 2), using a 0.014″ pressure guide wire (PressureWire Aeris™, St Jude Medical, Uppsala, Sweden). Resting distal coronary pressure to aortic pressure ratio (Pd/Pa) was 0.94. FFR was 0.87, indicating physiologically non-significant stenosis. There was no damping of the proximal aortic pressure trace, ensuring an accurate FFR measurement.

Two months later, the patient was admitted for an anterior STEMI and the emergency coronary angiography revealed a sub-occlusion of the mid-LAD (Fig. 3). The lesion was treated with a 3.0 × 15 mm Xience™ everolimus-eluting stent. Right coronary angiography showed neither restenosis in the previously implanted stent nor other significant coronary lesions. The patient assured having good compliance with the therapeutic regimen since the first cardiovascular event.

* Correspondence: luispcleite@gmail.com
Departament of Cardiology, Centro Hospitalar e Universitário de Coimbra, Praceta Prof. Mota Pinto, Coimbra 3000-075, Portugal

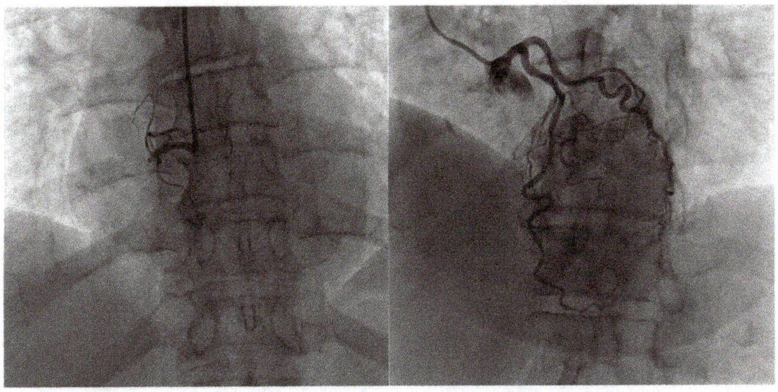

Fig. 1 Coronary angiography in the inferior STEMI. Total occlusion of the proximal-segment of the right coronary artery and three intermediate stenosis in the mid-segment of the LAD

Discussion

In patients with STEMI and MVD, the current recommendations state that primary PCI should be limited to the culprit vessel with the exception of cardiogenic shock in the presence of multiple, critical stenosis or highly unstable lesions, and if there is persistent ischemia after PCI on the supposed culprit lesion [3]. If staged PCI to non-culprit vessels is being considered, non-invasive stress testing (myocardial perfusion scintigraphy, stress echocardiography, positron emission tomography or magnetic resonance imaging) should be used for ischemia and viability testing prior to a decision to proceed with PCI [4].

Fractional flow reserve is a well-validated technique to guide coronary intervention by identification of lesion-level ischemia. In the DEFER study, the prognosis of intermediate lesions with an FFR of > 0.75 was excellent if treated medically, with a < 1 % risk of any AMI after 5 years of follow-up [5]. However, studies to date have mainly involved stable patients outside of acute myocardial infarction (AMI) [5–8]. The use of FFR to assess culprit and non-culprit lesions in the setting of acute ischemia represents a controversial area, although there is an increasing evidence base to support the role of FFR-guided strategy in acute coronary syndrome (ACS) [9].

The physiological principles underlying FFR are critically dependent on the ability to achieve maximal hyperaemia. In patients with AMI, pathophysiological disturbances in the microvasculature can have a potential impact on the ability to induce maximal hyperaemia, and thereby compromise the accuracy of FFR assessments in non-culprit vessels, theoretically leading to false negative results [10]. The 2011 ESC Guidelines for the management of ACS without ST-segment elevation [11] recommend that FFR should be ideally performed more than 5 days after the acute event in order to minimize the impact of any microvascular disturbance. The 2012 ESC Guidelines for the management

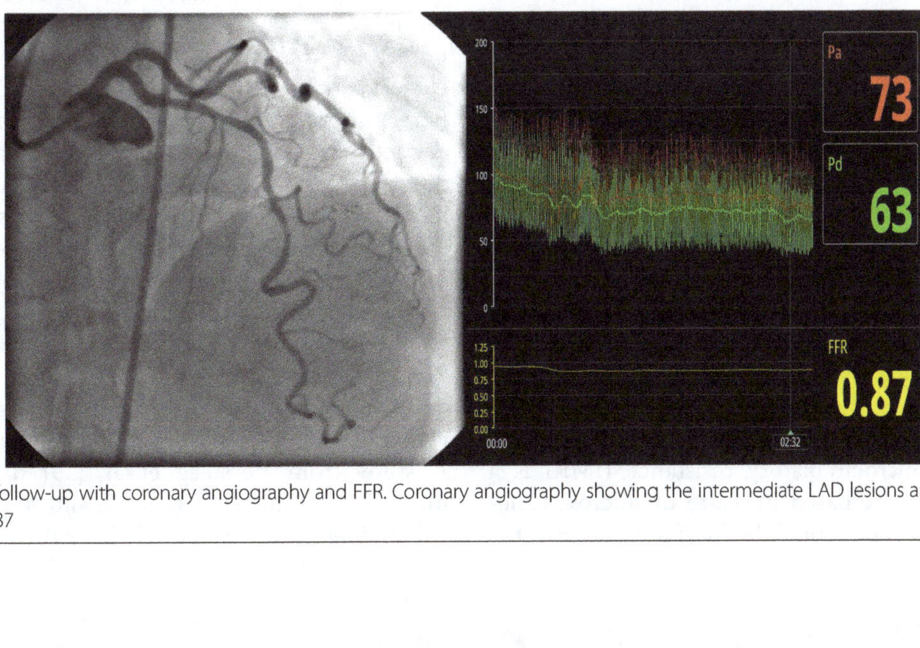

Fig. 2 Three-week follow-up with coronary angiography and FFR. Coronary angiography showing the intermediate LAD lesions and FFR evaluation with the result of 0.87

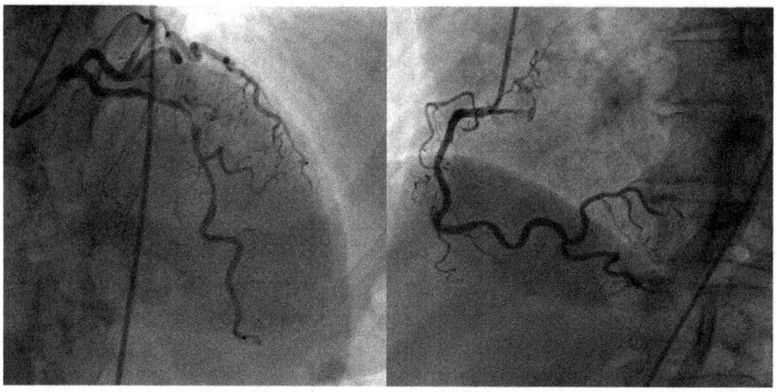

Fig. 3 Coronary angiography in the anterior STEMI. Sub-occlusion of the mid-LAD and right coronary artery without significant lesions

of STEMI [4] state the staged revascularization approach for STEMI with MVD can be guided by FFR if performed several days or weeks after primary PCI. In the case report presented, the functional assessment of the mid-LAD lesions was made 3 weeks later than the primary PCI, in concordance to the current guidelines.

One of the most important studies about the use of FFR in ACS was from Ntalianis et al. [12] who studied 75 acute STEMI patients and 26 NSTEMI patients (<72 h post onset) and measured FFR in the non-culprit stenosis immediately following PCI of the culprit vessel and then repeated the FFR at 35 ± 4 days post initial procedure. The FFR value remained unchanged between the acute and follow-up phases in patients with STEMI (0.78 ± 0.10 vs. 0.76 ± 0.10, p = NS) and NSTEMI (0.77 ± 0.10 vs. 0.77 ± 0.20, p = NS). In only 2 patients, the FFR value was higher than 0.80 at the acute phase and lower than 0.75 at follow-up. The authors stated the data support that FFR measurements are safe and reliable for evaluating the severity of non-culprit stenosis in the acute phase of ACS, even during primary PCI.

A more recent study from Cuculi et al. [13] performed an invasive assessment of coronary physiology in 82 STEMI patients, immediately following PCI of the culprit vessel and 6 months later, associated with a contrast-enhanced cardiac magnetic resonance imaging evaluation of microvascular obstruction. Baseline Pd/Pa remained stable over time, but FFR reduced significantly between primary PCI and 6 months ($p = 0.008$); this reduction was mainly observed in patients with microvascular obstruction. Therefore, the authors stated that coronary microcirculation recovery progresses further by 6 months, suggesting that using FFR soon after STEMI might underestimate the degree of non-culprit vessel stenosis in almost half of patients.

The index of microcirculatory resistance (IMR) is a validated invasive wire-based measure of microvasculature function [14] and could be useful to assess the status of the coronary microcirculation in the setting of AMI [15], which may be used to validate an FFR result. The other potential caveat in a FFR-guided strategy in ACS patients, as it was done in our case report, is the possible existence of vulnerable coronary plaques in absence of flow limitation [9]. In the Providing Regional Observations to Study Predictors of Events in the Coronary Tree (PROSPECT) study [16], patients presenting with ACS in whom PCI was successful, underwent 3-vessel radiofrequency intravascular ultra-sound (IVUS) imaging, and were followed for a median of 3.4 years for the incidence of MACE. In this study, the non-culprit lesions that led to MACE were frequently mild on angiographic assessment, but most were characterized by a large plaque burden, a small luminal area and were thin-cap fibroatheromas (TCFA); no MACE arose from untreated segments with a plaque burden resulting in less than 40 % loss of cross-sectional luminal area. Using data from PROSPECT study, some authors stated that clinical and angiographic characteristics had poor predictive accuracy in identifying patients with untreated high-risk plaques, at least not enough to obviate the need for intracoronary-imaging, although they assume that it is unrealistic to applicate 3-vessel invasive imaging in every clinical setting [17]. Others authors divided the same cohort into quartiles according to baseline angiographic diameter stenosis and concluded that the triad of predictors of future MACE increased in frequency with increasing angiographic diameter stenosis [18].

Some points of controversy involve the risk assessment of future MACE: do we have a cross-link between ischemia and plaque vulnerability? Can we expect that plaques with higher FFR values are stable and that lower FFR, with repetitive ischemia and high shear stress, induce vulnerability? Or do we have a diagnostic gap of vulnerable plaque between physiology and morphology? A study from Versteeg et al. [19] demonstrated that monocyte toll-like receptors 2 and 4 related to plaque vulnerability were significantly higher in patients with

FFR < 0.75 than in patients with an FFR measurement of > 0.80, suggesting that vulnerability may be preceded by ischemia. In the Fractional Flow Reserve and Intravascular Ultrasound Relationship Study (FIRST) [20], the aim was to evaluate the correlation between FFR, IVUS, and virtual histology (VH) in intermediate coronary lesions. Minimal lumen area obtained by IVUS showed a moderate correlation with FFR measurements and the optimal cut-off for a FFR of < 0.80 varied depending on the vessel size. Plaque composition assessed by VH-IVUS identified only plaque burden as having any correlation with FFR values. Lesions without TCFA had better correlation with FFR compared with lesions with TCFA. A study from Hüseyinova et al. [21] evaluated 48 non-ST-elevation ACS patients having paired hemodynamic and morphological data of the culprit vessel. It was demonstrated that for a given stenosis, FFR values decrease with an increase in necrotic core and dense calcium contents of the physiologically significant coronary plaques. However, plaque composition did not exert any influence on the hemodynamic effect generated by physiologically non-significant stenosis.

The COMPARE ACUTE trial is an ongoing study enrolling MVD patients undergoing primary PCI and randomly allocates patients to receive either FFR-guided PCI or culprit vessel-only PCI in the setting of STEMI [22]. This trial may help to define the role of FFR in STEMI patients with MVD.

Conclusions

The use of FFR to assess non-culprit lesions in AMI patients is useful to guide treatment if strongly indicative of ischemia. A negative FFR is this setting should be interpreted with caution and may be appropriate to access plaque vulnerability by intracoronary imaging, to consider subsequent non-invasive testing or alternatively repeat FFR at a later date. Further studies are required to stablish the ideal timing to perform FFR after AMI, in order to minimize the impact of any microvascular disturbance. The role of FFR in the assessment of vulnerable plaques *per se* also requires additional evaluation in clinical trials.

Consent

Written informed consent was obtained from the patient for publication of this case report and any accompanying images. A copy of the written consent is available for review by the Editor of this journal.

Abbreviations

ACS: Acute coronary syndrome; AMI: Acute myocardial infarction; FFR: Fractional flow reserve; IMR: Index of microcirculatory resistance; IVUS: Intravascular ultra-sound; LAD: Left anterior descending artery; MACE: Major adverse cardiac events; MVD: Multi-vessel disease; PCI: Percutaneous coronary intervention; Pd/Pa: Distal coronary pressure to aortic pressure ratio; STEMI: ST-segment elevation myocardial infarction; TCFA: Thin-cap fibroatheromas; VH: Virtual histology.

Competing interests

The authors declare that they have no competing interests.

Authors' contributions

LL, conception and design, analysis and interpretation of data, manuscript writing. JSM, VM and JC, attending physician, acquisition and analysis of data, revising it critically for important intellectual content. JMF, EJ, JG and MP, interpretation of data, revising it critically for important intellectual content. All authors read and approved the final manuscript.

Authors' information

Not applicable.

Acknowledgements

I do not have any specific acknowledge to make.

References

1. Hasdai D, Behar S, Wallentin L, Danchin N, Gitt AK, Boersma E, et al. A prospective survey of the characteristics, treatments and outcomes of patients with acute coronary syndromes in Europe and the Mediterranean basin; the Euro Heart Survey of Acute Coronary Syndromes (Euro Heart Survey ACS). Eur Heart J. 2002;23:1190–201.
2. Sorajja P, Gersh BJ, Cox DA, McLaughlin MG, Zimetbaum P, Costantini C, et al. Impact of multivessel disease on reperfusion success and clinical outcomes in patients undergoing primary percutaneous coronary intervention for acute myocardial infarction. Eur Heart J. 2007;28:1709–16.
3. Windecker S, Kolh P, Alfonso F, Collet J-P, Cremer J, Falk V, et al. 2014 ESC/EACTS Guidelines on myocardial revascularization: The Task Force on Myocardial Revascularization of the European Society of Cardiology (ESC) and the European Association for Cardio-Thoracic Surgery (EACTS). Eur Heart J. 2014;35:2541–619.
4. Steg PG, James SK, Atar D, Badano LP, Blömstrom-Lundqvist C, Borger MA, et al. ESC Guidelines for the management of acute myocardial infarction in patients presenting with ST-segment elevation. Eur Heart J. 2012;33:2569–619.
5. Pijls NHJ, van Schaardenburgh P, Manoharan G, Boersma E, Bech J-W, van' t Veer M, et al. Percutaneous coronary intervention of functionally nonsignificant stenosis: 5-year follow-up of the DEFER Study. J Am Coll Cardiol. 2007;49:2105–11.
6. Tonino PAL, De Bruyne B, Pijls NHJ, Siebert U, Ikeno F, Van' t Veer M, et al. Fractional flow reserve versus angiography for guiding percutaneous coronary intervention. N Engl J Med. 2009;360:213–24.
7. Pijls NHJ, Fearon WF, Tonino PAL, Siebert U, Ikeno F, Bornschein B, et al. Fractional flow reserve versus angiography for guiding percutaneous coronary intervention in patients with multivessel coronary artery disease: 2-year follow-up of the FAME (Fractional Flow Reserve Versus Angiography for Multivessel Evaluation) study. J Am Coll Cardiol. 2010;56:177–84.
8. De Bruyne B, Pijls NHJ, Kalesan B, Barbato E, Tonino PAL, Piroth Z, et al. Fractional flow reserve-guided PCI versus medical therapy in stable coronary disease. N Engl J Med. 2012;367:991–1001.
9. Hennigan B, Layland J, Fearon WF, Oldroyd KG. Fractional flow reserve and the index of microvascular resistance in patients with acute coronary syndromes. EuroIntervention. 2014;10 Suppl T:T55–63.
10. Claeys MJ, Bosmans JM, Hendrix J, Vrints CJ. Reliability of fractional flow reserve measurements in patients with associated microvascular dysfunction: importance of flow on translesional pressure gradient. Catheter Cardiovasc Interv. 2001;54:427–34.
11. Hamm CW, Bassand J-P, Agewall S, Bax J, Boersma E, Bueno H, et al. ESC Guidelines for the management of acute coronary syndromes in patients presenting without persistent ST-segment elevation: The Task Force for the management of acute coronary syndromes (ACS) in patients presenting without persistent ST-segment elevatio. Eur Heart J. 2011;32:2999–3054.
12. Ntalianis A, Sels J-W, Davidavicius G, Tanaka N, Muller O, Trana C, et al. Fractional flow reserve for the assessment of nonculprit coronary artery stenoses in patients with acute myocardial infarction. JACC Cardiovasc Interv. 2010;3:1274–81.
13. Cuculi F, De Maria GL, Meier P, Dall'Armellina E, de Caterina AR, Channon KM, et al. Impact of microvascular obstruction on the assessment of coronary

flow reserve, index of microcirculatory resistance, and fractional flow reserve after ST-segment elevation myocardial infarction. J Am Coll Cardiol. 2014;64:1894–904.

14. Fearon WF, Balsam LB, Farouque HMO, Robbins RC, Fitzgerald PJ, Yock PG, et al. Novel index for invasively assessing the coronary microcirculation. Circulation. 2003;107:3129–32.
15. Fearon WF, Shah M, Ng M, Brinton T, Wilson A, Tremmel JA, et al. Predictive value of the index of microcirculatory resistance in patients with ST-segment elevation myocardial infarction. J Am Coll Cardiol. 2008;51:560–5.
16. Stone GW, Maehara A, Lansky AJ, de Bruyne B, Cristea E, Mintz GS, et al. A prospective natural-history study of coronary atherosclerosis. N Engl J Med. 2011;364:226–35.
17. Bourantas CV, Garcia-Garcia HM, Farooq V, Maehara A, Xu K, Généreux P, et al. Clinical and angiographic characteristics of patients likely to have vulnerable plaques: analysis from the PROSPECT study. JACC Cardiovasc Imaging. 2013;6:1263–72.
18. Yun KH, Mintz GS, Farhat N, Marso SP, Taglieri N, Verheye S, et al. Relation between angiographic lesion severity, vulnerable plaque morphology and future adverse cardiac events (from the Providing Regional Observations to Study Predictors of Events in the Coronary Tree study). Am J Cardiol. 2012;110:471–7.
19. Versteeg D, Hoefer IE, Schoneveld AH, de Kleijn DPV, Busser E, Strijder C, et al. Monocyte toll-like receptor 2 and 4 responses and expression following percutaneous coronary intervention: association with lesion stenosis and fractional flow reserve. Heart. 2008;94:770–6.
20. Waksman R, Legutko J, Singh J, Orlando Q, Marso S, Schloss T, et al. FIRST: Fractional Flow Reserve and Intravascular Ultrasound Relationship Study. J Am Coll Cardiol. 2013;61:917–23.
21. Hüseyinova G, Aslanger E, Çakır O, Atıcı A, Panç C, Demirkıran A, et al. Potential contribution of virtual histology plaque composition to hemodynamic-morphologic dissociation in patients with non-ST elevation acute coronary syndrome. Int J Cardiol. 2015;187:33–8.
22. Smits PC, Vlachojannis GJ, Lunde K, Omerovic E, Schotborgh CE, Richardt G, et al. TCT-328 FFR-guided complete revascularization during primary PCI: Preliminary data from the COMPARE ACUTE trial. J Am Coll Cardiol. 2014;64:11_S.

6

Usefulness of the heart-rate variability complex for predicting cardiac mortality after acute myocardial infarction

Tao Song[1], Xiu Fen Qu[1*], Ying Tao Zhang[2], Wei Cao[1], Bai He Han[1], Yang Li[1], Jing Yan Piao[1], Lei Lei Yin[1] and Heng Da Cheng[3]

Abstract

Background: Previous studies indicate that decreased heart-rate variability (HRV) is related to the risk of death in patients after acute myocardial infarction (AMI). However, the conventional indices of HRV have poor predictive value for mortality. Our aim was to develop novel predictive models based on support vector machine (SVM) to study the integrated features of HRV for improving risk stratification after AMI.

Methods: A series of heart-rate dynamic parameters from 208 patients were analyzed after a mean follow-up time of 28 months. Patient electrocardiographic data were classified as either survivals or cardiac deaths. SVM models were established based on different combinations of heart-rate dynamic variables and compared to left ventricular ejection fraction (LVEF), standard deviation of normal-to-normal intervals (SDNN) and deceleration capacity (DC) of heart rate. We tested the accuracy of predictors by assessing the area under the receiver-operator characteristics curve (AUC).

Results: We evaluated a SVM algorithm that integrated various electrocardiographic features based on three models: (A) HRV complex; (B) 6 dimension vector; and (C) 8 dimension vector. Mean AUC of HRV complex was 0.8902, 0.8880 for 6 dimension vector and 0.8579 for 8 dimension vector, compared with 0.7424 for LVEF, 0.7932 for SDNN and 0.7399 for DC.

Conclusions: HRV complex yielded the largest AUC and is the best classifier for predicting cardiac death after AMI.

Keywords: Acute myocardial infarction, Cardiac death, Support vector machine, Heart-rate variability, Machine learning

Background

Risk stratification of survival after acute myocardial infarction (AMI) could be very useful in guiding post-AMI care, such as implantation of a cardioverter-defibrillator or other optimal medical therapy [1-3]. The degree of left-ventricular ejection fraction (LVEF) impairment is generally used to predict the risk for AMI; however, because most patients exhibit preserved left-ventricular contractile function when acute revascularization procedures are performed after AMI, the ability to stratify risk based on LVEF is reduced. Several previous studies have indicated that decreased heart-rate variability (HRV), a marker of cardiac autonomic nervous system dysfunction, is associated with a high risk for severe ventricular arrhythmias and mortality in the post-AMI population [4]. However, conventional methods to analyze HRV, such as standard time and frequency domain measures, have relatively poor accuracy for predicting outcomes with current treatment strategies [5-7]. Recent Holter-based predictive variables, such as heart-rate turbulence and deceleration capacity (DC) of heart rate, have demonstrated greater prognostic power in post-AMI patients; however, the clinical usefulness is not well established. HRV methods can capture several aspects of autonomic heart rate modulation, but individual HRV indices do not reflect global effects of autonomic nervous system dysfunction on the disease. This may be the cause

* Correspondence: xiufenq@sina.cn
[1]Department of Cardiology, the First Affiliated Hospital of Harbin Medical University, No.23 Youzheng Street, Nangang District, Harbin City 150001, Heilongjiang Province, China
Full list of author information is available at the end of the article

of the limited predictive capacity of HRV approaches. Therefore, a comprehensive method to quantify the global effects of the autonomic nervous system on heart rate modulation and to provide individualized risk stratification in the post-AMI population is desperately needed. In this study, we developed a support vector machine (SVM) algorithm based on heart-rate dynamics that measures the relationship between autonomic nervous dysfunction and AMI mortality. We used this novel analytical tool to more accurately classify high-risk AMI patients. We postulate that the integrated features of HRV are better than individual measures of HRV and DC at predicting mortality risk in the post-AMI human population.

Methods

Participants

For this study, 226 patients aged from 18 to 80 years who were admitted for AMI to the Cardiology Department of the 1st hospital of the Harbin Medical University in Harbin, China from January 2009 to December 2009 were enrolled. AMI was diagnosed at the time of admission by at least 2 of the following findings: chest pain for ≥20 min; creatine kinase-MB more than double the upper normal limit of our laboratory; ST-segment elevation ≥0.1 mv in at least two limb leads or ≥0.2 mv in at least two contiguous precordial leads; and primary motion abnormality of the left ventricular regional wall in the echocardiography or MRI examination. We excluded patients if they: (1) had severe valvular, pulmonary, hepatic, renal or other severe concomitant noncardiovascular disease; (2) were logistically unable to participate; (3) exhibited sinus rhythm for <80% of the total 24-hour Holter recording; (4) had atrial flutter, atrial fibrillation or pacemaker rhythm; (5) had inadequately analyzable electrocardiographic data; and/or (6) had inadequate follow-up data. Furthermore, all of patients underwent routine cardiac medication and AMI treatment according to the contemporary guidelines [8].

The analysis of electrocardiographic data and the monitoring of patients were approved by the Institutional Ethics Committee for human research of the Harbin Medical University. Since the data collection was noninvasive and did not affect routine clinical management of the patients, the Ethics Committee deemed oral informed consent to be sufficient for patient participation.

Procedures

Holter electrocardiograms were recorded for 24 hours during the second week after infarction (average 8–14 days) for patients that were stable during this period. The recordings were digitized at 128 Hz, automatically processed with a GE Holter system (GE medical, USA), and scanned with GE Holter analysis software following standard procedures as specified by the manufacturer. Manual verification of uncorrected QRS classifications and reduction of noise was conducted as needed. Meanwhile, we assessed LVEF by single-plane echocardiography one week after index infarction, with <0.35 predefined as seriously abnormal. Other risk predictors included age, history of myocardial infarction, diabetes mellitus, hypertension, and medical treatments, which were determined by the physician using a standardized protocol.

Automatic feature extraction

Machine learning algorithms require data to be represented by features, such as the indices that occur in an electrocardiographic recording. In this study, a total of 10 indices were extracted from every Holter recording. The electrocardiographic features of the patients are shown in Table 1 and include the following: indices of HRV; heart-rate turbulence; mean heart beat; DC; and acceleration capacity of heart rate. As proposed by the Task Force of the European Society of Cardiology and the North American Society of Pacing and Electrophysiology [9], we calculated the following conventional risk predictors from time domain measures of HRV in the 24-hour Holter recordings. Time domain measures of the R-R time series were used to quantify the variability of the R-R intervals, including standard deviation of all normal-to-normal intervals [SDNN (ms)], average standard deviation of all normal-to-normal intervals (ms), standard deviation of average normal-to-normal intervals (ms), mean normal-to-normal intervals (ms), and triangle index of geometric figure parameter of the R-R time series. The spectral measures of HRV were analyzed using the methods recommended by the Task Force, and the cut-off values of reduced spectral indexes were also predefined. These traditional indices of HRV have a proven ability to predict mortality [10] and are easy to calculate.

Table 1 Electrocardiographic features of heart-rate dynamics extracted from Holter recordings

Methods	Features
Time domain of HRV	Standard deviation of all normal-to-normal intervals
	Average standard deviation of all normal-to-normal intervals
	Standard deviation of average normal-to-normal intervals
	Mean normal-to-normal intervals
	Triangle index of a geometric figure
Counting of R-R series	Mean heart rates per hour
Heart rate turbulence	Turbulence onset
	Turbulence slope
Phase rectified signal averaging	Heart rate deceleration capacity
	Heart rate acceleration capacity

High resting heart rate has been associated with cardiac death [11]. In this study, mean heart rate was calculated as heart beat number per hour. We assessed other newer risk predictors of heart-rate dynamics as well. Heart-rate turbulence indices, including turbulence onset and turbulence slope (ms), reflect the baroreflex mediated short-term oscillation of cardiac cycle lengths after spontaneous ventricular premature complexes. These were calculated in the instances when ventricular premature beats were found in the Holter recordings [12]. Turbulence slope was defined as the maximum slope of the regression line assessed over any sequence within five subsequent sinus R-R intervals during the first fifteen sinus heart beats following an ectopic ventricular beat. A decreased heart rate turbulence is related to autonomic dysfunction and has a powerful ability to predict sudden cardiac death [13]. Two newer Holter-based risk variables, which are developed by a phase rectified signal averaging technique—namely, DC (ms) and acceleration capacity (ms) of heart rate—were calculated to provide a separate assessment of autonomic modulation of the heart rate. DC reflects the regulation of the vagus nerve on heart rate. This is of clinical importance because vagus withdraw has been regarded as an important mechanism of sudden death [14]. Furthermore, these features are all thought to reflect functional changes of the autonomic nervous system.

SVM algorithm

In machine learning, SVM are supervised learning models with associated learning algorithms that analyze data and recognize patterns. SVMs are used for classification and regression analyses, and the classification strongly depends on the available feature set and the tuning of hyper-parameters [15]. We used SVMs to analyze the predictive power of the combined indices from every Holter recording. In this study, SVM was developed to maximize the margin of the hyper-plane dividing electrocardiographic data into two classes, survivals and cardiac deaths, by finding the best hyper-plane that separates clusters of features represented in an n-dimensional space. A hyper-plane can be written as the set of points X satisfying $W^TX + b = 0$, where W^T is a normal vector perpendicular to the hyper-plane, X is the vector of electrocardiographic features, and b is bias or offset of the hyper-plane from the origin. Inputs of SVM are mapped onto a high dimensional feature space via kernel functions, and the optimal hyper-planes are constructed to separate samples into two classes [16]. SVMs were trained and tested using the leave-one-out and cross-validation methods, which were applied to evaluate the accuracy of classification. At every step, one electrocardiographic data subset was left out from the total training dataset and treated as undefined data. The classification model was constructed with the remaining data and the algorithm classified the "left-out" electrocardiographic data. The same procedure was applied to the training dataset. The results of SVM were normalized in the range from 0 to 1. We prospectively defined a cut-off point as >0.5 indicated higher probabilities of death, while <0.5 indicated higher probability of survival. Through training and testing, we finished feature selection and searched for the optimal vector that had the greatest predictive power.

At the same time, comparisons were made with LVEF, SDNN and DC using the identical dataset. The SDNN measured from the 24-hour R-R intervals was chosen as a conventional index of HRV, with a value <70 ms predefined as abnormal [10]. Meanwhile, DC measured from the 24-hour recording was chosen as a novel index of heart-rate dynamics, with a value <4.5 ms predefined as abnormal [14].

Follow-up and endpoints

Patients with AMI underwent physical examination 6 months after discharge and annually thereafter by telephone assessment. The patients were followed for a mean of 28 months after AMI. In cases of death, the causes were verified from the hospital records, death certificates, autopsy records and telephone interviews with either the primary physicians or those who had witnessed the death. An independent endpoint committee determined the cause of death according to the available data from the aforementioned sources. Witnessed deaths due to cardiac diseases including myocardial infarction, heart failure, severe malignant arrhythmia and those occurring after attempted resuscitation by defibrillator were all classified as cardiac death. Unwitnessed deaths occurring in a previously asymptomatic patient with no other life-threatening diseases was classified as cardiac death as well. Based on these determinations, the electrocardiographic data were then classified as survivals or cardiac deaths. To avoid bias, the computer center received only electrocardiographic data and classification results without other clinical information of patients.

Statistical analysis

We calculated receiver-operator characteristic curves to evaluate prediction accuracy of SVM models, LVEF, and conventional risk indices of HRV and DC. We quantified receiver-operator characteristic curves by taking the integrals of the curves (area under the curve; AUC), with the continuous variable being set to a plurality of different critical values, to calculate a series of sensitivity and specificity thresholds. The sensitivity was used as the ordinate and negative positive rate (1- specific) as the abscissa to plot the curves. The AUC of a method was prospectively defined as the statistical measure of the predictive power. The accuracy, sensitivity, specificity, positive predictive value and negative predictive value of each variable were taken into account [17]. The difference between two receiver-operator characteristic curves was compared by non-parametric test, with a P value less than 0.05 considered statistically significant.

Results

Based on initial evaluation with the GE analysis software, 6 electrocardiograms were excluded because of non-cardiac death and 12 electrocardiograms were excluded because of unacceptable deviations in the recordings or otherwise inadequately analyzable data. Thus, a total of 208 patient dynamic electrocardiograms were included in the subsequent analyses. Among these data, 196 (94.2%) recordings were classified as survivals and 12 (5.8%) recordings were classified as cardiac deaths, including 7 sudden cardiac deaths and 5non-sudden cardiac deaths. Among these patients, 207 of the 208 patients were used as the "training" subjects and the remaining patient was used as a "test" subject. Repeating the dataset from the test subject 208 times, the classification accuracy was then calculated by the number of correctly classified patients divided by the total number of patients. The clinical characteristics of the patients are shown in Table 2. For the treatment, 112 patients (53.8%) underwent PTCA, and thrombolysis was performed in 45 patients (21.6%). In addition, other treatments such as β-blockers, ACE inhibition or ARBs were used in more than 75% patients, and aspirin or statins were used in more than 97% patients. Therefore, most patients in this study received modern standard of care for AMI.

Table 2 Patient baseline characteristics and treatment

Clinical features	Survivals (n = 196)	Cardiac deaths (n = 12)
Study characteristics		
Follow-up (months)	27.99 ± 6.02	11.17 ± 10.85
Patient characteristics		
Age (years)	60.19 ± 11.39	71.83 ± 7.29*
Sex (female)	52 (27%)	6 (50%)*
LVEF	54.86 ± 11.18	46.00 ± 11.15*
LVEF < 0.35	9 (4.6%)	3 (25%)*
Smoking (ex or current)	110 (56%)	4 (33%)*
Diabetes mellitus	42 (21%)	8 (67%)*
Previous myocardial infarction	25 (13%)	2 (17%)
Hypertension	95 (48%)	11 (92%)*
Treatment		
PTCA	117 (60%)	7 (58%)
Thrombolysis	44 (22%)	2 (17%)
No acute revascularization	35 (18%)	3 (25%)
Aspirin or clopidogrel	194 (99%)	12 (100%)
β-blockers	158 (81%)	10 (83%)
Statins	192 (98%)	10 (83%)*
ACEI/ARB	150 (77%)	9 (75%)
Diuretic	134 (68%)	7 (58%)

Data are number (%) unless otherwise stated. *P < 0.05.

Among the established 10 electrocardiographic features we evaluated, heart-rate turbulence indices depended on the existence of ventricular premature beats. However, a ventricular premature beat might not have existed in every recording, a total of 83 recordings have no ventricular premature in this cohort. Inherent to the procedures of machine learning, a missing feature in the dataset was difficult to accommodate in the analyses. To avoid biases according to this consideration, the features with possible missing data points were not employed. As a result, heart-rate turbulence could not be used as a classifier in this study. Ultimately, 8 features of extracted heart-rate dynamics indices were used to construct SVM models. The electrocardiographic features of the patients after feature selection and the differences between the two classes are shown in Table 3.

Linear predictive models are in most cases ineffective in solving death prediction problems. To circumvent this challenge, we searched for the kernel's parameters that could be optimized to obtain the best classification accuracy. This optimized first employed training and testing the technique to check each combination of parameter choices. Then, the parameters that resulted in the best accuracy were selected. Next, the final models were trained on the whole training set using the chosen parameters. The result was a 5 dimension HRV feature vector, which is called a HRV complex. In this study, we constructed 3 SVMs using different combinations of the features that performed better than other combinations tested: (A) HRV complex (5 time domain measures of HRV); (B) 6 dimension vector (HRV + DC + acceleration capacity, with mean normal-to-normal intervals removed); and (C) 8 dimension vector (HRV + DC + acceleration capacity + mean heart rate). The results of accuracy, sensitivity, specificity, positive predictive value and negative predictive value of SVMs are shown in Table 4. Although SVMs had an accuracy rate of only 0.80, they had greater sensitivities and better negative predictive values. Among the SVMs, the sensitivities of HRV complex and 6 dimension vector both reached 0.91, whereas SDNN had sensitivity of only 0. 58. The results of sensitivity, specificity, positive predictive value and negative predictive value of the HRV complex, SDNN and DC in subgroup with LVEF > 0.35 are shown in Table 5. The HRV complex had better sensitivity, positive predictive value and negative predictive value as compared with SDNN and DC in these patients.

Receiver-operator characteristic curves for predictions of SVM models are shown in Figure 1. The mean AUCs

Table 3 Electrocardiographic characteristics of the patients, after feature selection, that were used to construct SVM predictive models

Variables	Survivals (n = 196)	Cardiac deaths (n = 12)	P value
Standard deviation of all normal-to-normal intervals	96.22 ± 27.86	64.52 ± 14.65	<0.001
Standard deviation of average normal-to-normal intervals	83.66 ± 26.65	58.47 ± 15.68	0.001
Average standard deviation of all normal-to-normal intervals	43.40 ± 13.67	25.74 ± 6.84	<0.001
Mean normal-to-normal intervals	893.54 ± 115.46	826.85 ± 84.21	0.051
Triangle index (number%)	27.48 ± 8.81	16.80 ± 4.20	<0.001
Heart rate deceleration capacity	6.31 ± 1.91	4.21 ± 1.44	<0.001
Heart rate acceleration capacity	-6.27 ± 1.98	-4.12 ± 1.42	<0.001
Mean heart rates per hour (number)	68.36 ± 9.00	73.50 ± 7.70	0.054

Data are ms unless otherwise specified.

of receiver-operator characteristic curves are shown in Table 6. In SVM models, AUC of the HRV complex (0.8902) was larger than that of the 6 dimension vector (0.8880) and the 8 dimension vector (0.8579). Compared to traditional indices, the AUCs of the SVM models were significantly larger than those of LVEF (0.7424, $p < 0.01$), SDNN (0.7932, $p < 0.05$) and DC (0.7399, $p < 0.01$). Hence, SVM predictive models based on heart-rate dynamics variables yield larger AUCs than LVEF, SDNN and DC.

Discussion

In this study, we used noninvasive heart-rate dynamics indices extracted from electrocardiographic datasets from patients following AMI to develop a computer-aided predictive tool that improves risk stratification. By combining the predictive power of multiple heart-rate dynamics variables, SVM models are an effective approach to quantify the risk of cardiac death and are capable of prospectively identifying high-risk patients in the post-AMI population. The HRV complex we describe in this study provides a novel analysis method to evaluate the effect of autonomic nervous system dysfunction on cardiac death following AMI. Moreover, this new predictive strategy has an enhanced discriminating threshold for AMI as compared to current electrocardiographic and echocardiographic methods (i.e. LVEF, SDNN and DC).

Autonomic nervous system dysfunction has a significant adverse effect on outcomes in post-AMI patients. Therefore, quantitative assessment of autonomic dysfunction could enhance the predictability of cardiac death [18,19]. The effects of autonomic modulators on the heart can be quantified by noninvasive HRV methods, and conventional indices of HRV developed by simple calculation of R-R series have demonstrated prognostic value for mortality [20]. Nevertheless, individual HRV indices do not reflect the combined effects of the autonomic nervous system on heart rate, and therefore these traditional measures have only a partial predictive capability. In this study, to advance our ability to predict outcomes in AMI patients, individual HRV indices were regarded as the features of high-risk of cardiac death, and a SVM was used to combine the predictive power of multiple HRV indices. As a result, we developed a novel HRV analysis method, termed HRV complex, which was effective at predicting cardiac death after AMI. Whether our method will be effective to quantify entire autonomic nervous system dysfunction will require additional studies. Nevertheless, our results clearly show that the HRV complex has a better prognostic capacity compared with SDNN or DC of heart rate. The HRV complex also outperforms the combination of HRV indices and DC. In this sense, the HRV complex is a better prognostic tool than individual HRV indices, and the

Table 4 Accuracy, sensitivity, specificity, positive predictive value and negative predictive value of HRV complex, 6 dimension, 8 dimension, LVEF, SDNN and DC (%)

Methods		Accuracy	Sensitivity	Specificity	Positive predictive value	Negative predictive value
	HRV complex	79.81	91.67	79.08	21.15	99.36
SVM	6 dimension	79.33	91.67	78.57	20.75	99.35
	8 dimension	79.33	83.33	79.08	19.61	98.73
	LVEF	91.83	25.00	95.41	25.00	95.41
	SDNN	83.65	58.33	85.20	19.44	97.09
	DC	80.77	50.00	82.65	15.00	96.43

Table 5 Sensitivity, specificity, positive predictive value and negative predictive value of HRV complex, SDNN and DC in patients with LVEF > 0.35 (%)

Methods	Sensitivity	Specificity	Positive predictive value	Negative predictive value
HRV complex	88.89	80.21	17.78	99.34
SDNN	55.56	86.63	16.67	97.59
DC	55.56	82.89	13.51	97.48

classifiers that incorporate the combined effects of vagal and sympathetic modulators are better than a single nerve modulator.

An ideal risk stratification tool needs to be accurate, cost effective and have the capacity to reduce the risk of death across different patient populations [21,22]. In this study, the specificity of LVEF is higher than other methods; however, the sensitivity is quite low. Due to the fact that the number of survivals and cardiac deaths are unbalanced, the higher specificity does not reflect the capacity of classification. This leads to a lower predictive value than a tool based on LVEF. To overcome this limitation, machine-learning approaches, which utilize "training" and "testing" exercises with a well-characterized dataset, were used. SVM is a good learning method that is well suited for small samples, and it does not involve probability measures. Thus, SVM is different from the existing statistical methods and not easily susceptible to overfitting. SVM uses insights from training samples to forecast probabilities and greatly simplifies the classification and regression problems. In this study, we used the leave-one-out and cross-validation method to carry out "training" and "testing." this method achieves most of the benefits of machine learning [23]. In the subgroup of patients with LVEF > 0.35, the sensitivity of HRV complex is about 0.89, meaning that the HRV complex could recognize ~89% of high risk patients which were otherwise identified as low risk by LVEF.

To verify the HRV complex's usefulness for the discrimination of patients likely to benefit from post-AMI therapy, the SVM model was designed to test the ability of HRV variables to stratify an AMI patient population. In the present study, we used cardiac death, which may arise clinically as the result of an autonomic disorder after severe cardiovascular damage (e.g. a fall in blood pressure eliciting a surge in sympathetic outflow), as the main endpoint. The HRV complex has several potential advantages over a single stratification tool. First, it combines predictive variables and is therefore more accurate. Through "training" and "testing", the SVM predictive

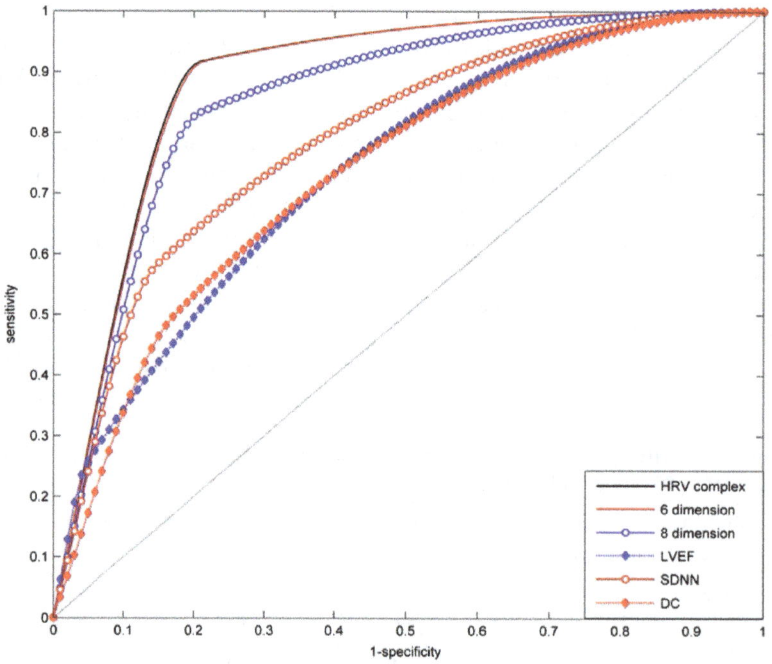

Figure 1 Receiver-operator characteristic curves for predicting cardiac deaths by HRV complex, 6 dimension, 8 dimension, LVEF, SDNN and DC. Sensitivity is determined from the proportion of cardiac deaths identified as high risk; specificity is determined from the proportion of survivors identified as low risk.

Table 6 Average AUCs of ROC of HRV complex, 6 dimension, 8 dimension, LVEF, SDNN and DC

Methods	AUC	P value
SVM		
HRV complex	0.8902	-
6 dimension	0.8880	>0.05
8 dimension	0.8579	>0.05
LVEF	0.7424	<0.01
SDNN	0.7932	<0.05
DC	0.7399	<0.01

model combines the prognostic power of several established stratification tools. Second, the HRV complex provides a digital risk estimate rather than a binary distinction of just "high" or "low" risk. This quantified risk assessment can aid clinicians in determining optimal cost-effective preventive strategies. Finally, the HRV complex reflects the underlying mechanism of cardiac death after AMI, and as a result will better predict outcomes as compared with current methods. We suspect that autonomic dysfunction as the trigger of cardiac death could be determined by our method. Thus, this stratification tool could improve the discrimination of patients eligible for cardioverter-defibrillator implantation [24].

We assessed the accuracy of prediction by our model by calculating the AUCs of the receiver-operator characteristic curves. This method accounts for dependency of specificity on sensitivity and is independent of specific cut-off values. Classifiers with AUCs > 0.80 are considered good in classification [25]. AUCs of methods A, B, and C in our study of SVMs were all higher than 0.80, demonstrating their strong predictive abilities. The HRV complex yielded the largest AUC (0.8902), exhibiting the largest prognostic capability, which was slightly larger than the 6 or 8 dimension vector models (0.8880 and 0.8579, respectively). This is likely because some features, such as mean heart rate, mean N-N intervals or acceleration capacity of heart rate, have relatively small effects on the distinction between high and low-risk populations. In the present population studied, the largest separation of receiver-operator characteristic curves between HRV complex and SDNN or DC had a sensitivity level of about 90%. The HRV complex-based risk assessment was especially suitable for accurate identification of high-risk patients who would benefit from further interventions or device implantation. Impaired DC of heart rate has been reported as a powerful predictor of all-cause mortality after AMI [14]. However, it did not play an important role in this study. This may be due to the sample size in the present study and/or because DC is not suitable to specifically predict cardiac (as opposed to all-cause) death after AMI. The accuracy of SVMs was quite good, but the size of the training dataset was small and the number of deaths was small. Hence, it is necessary to evaluate how a larger training set affects the predictive accuracy of SVMs in future studies.

There are several limitations to this study. First, we only use traditional established risk predictors of HRV to construct predictive models without including other strong risk markers, such as some nonlinear measurements of heart rate dynamics and T wave alterations [26,27]. The addition of these markers may provide incremental predictive power. Second, we employed HRV indices from 24-hour Holter recordings and did not determine the difference of risk classification by the HRV complex during daytime versus nighttime. We only obtained a single Holter recording in the second week after AMI; it is possible that serial or more frequent measurements would reveal differential risk amongst these patients. Third, whether the proposed SVM models can perform well using other datasets remains unknown. Therefore, this novel predictive algorithm should be studied in a larger number of patients. Fourth, we used cardiac death as the main endpoint. Although sudden cardiac death includes a subset of patients who succumb to lethal arrhythmias and who would therefore benefit from prophylactic interventions, no universally accepted definition for sudden cardiac death is available. Thus, we could not estimate how many of the patients in our study would be candidates for device therapy to prevent/respond to arrhythmias. In this study, we showed that the HRV complex was a useful risk predictor following AMI. However, we have no data to show whether specific treatments in response to such a predictor will improve patient outcomes. This goal will be pursued in a future study.

Conclusions

This study identifies a novel risk predictor that we have termed the HRV complex, which improves stratification of post-AMI patients. The predictive accuracy of HRV complex is better than LVEF, individual established indices of HRV and DC of heart rate. The performance suggests that the HRV complex is an accurate, non-invasive, quantitative screening metric for improving risk stratification of the post-AMI population. It has great potential to provide a framework to aid clinical decision-making in the prediction of cardiac deaths.

Competing interests

The authors declare that they have no competing interests.

Authors' contributions

TS, XQ, YL and HC have substantial contributions to conception and design. TS, YZ, WC, BH, JP and LY have participated in acquisition of data, or analysis and interpretation of data. TS, XQ, YZ, YL and HC have been involved in drafting the manuscript and revising it. All authors read and approved the final manuscript.

Acknowledgments
We would like to thank our colleagues at the First Affiliated Hospital of Harbin Medical University and Harbin Institute of Technology.

Funding
The project was supported in part by Scientific Research Fund of Heilongjiang Provincial Education Department, China (no. 12511295) and Scientific Research Fund of Heilongjiang Provincial Science and Technology Department, China (no. GC13C203).

Author details
[1]Department of Cardiology, the First Affiliated Hospital of Harbin Medical University, No.23 Youzheng Street, Nangang District, Harbin City 150001, Heilongjiang Province, China. [2]School of Computer Science and Technology, Harbin Institute of Technology, Harbin, China. [3]Department of Computer Science, Utah State University, Salt Lake City, UT, USA.

References

1. Bardy GH, Lee KL, Mark DB, Poole JE, Packer DL, Boineau R, Domanski M, Troutman C, Anderson J, Johnson G: **Amiodarone or an implantable cardioverter–defibrillator for congestive heart failure.** *N Engl J Med* 2005, **352**(3):225–237.
2. Kusmirek SL, Gold MR: **Sudden cardiac death: the role of risk stratification.** *Am Heart J* 2007, **153**(4):25–33.
3. Moss AJ, Zareba W, Hall WJ, Klein H, Wilber DJ, Cannom DS, Daubert JP, Higgins SL, Brown MW, Andrews ML: **Prophylactic implantation of a defibrillator in patients with myocardial infarction and reduced ejection fraction.** *N Engl J Med* 2002, **346**(12):877–883.
4. Kurths J, Voss A, Saparin P, Witt A, Kleiner H, Wessel N: **Quantitative analysis of heart rate variability.** *CHAOS* 1995, **5**(1):88–94.
5. Huikuri HV, Tapanainen JM, Lindgren K, Raatikainen P, Mäkikallio TH, Airaksinen KJ, Myerburg RJ: **Prediction of sudden cardiac death after myocardial infarction in the beta-blocking era.** *J Am Coll Cardiol* 2003, **42**(4):652–658.
6. Mäkikallio TH, Barthel P, Schneider R, Bauer A, Tapanainen JM, Tulppo MP, Schmidt G, Huikuri HV: **Prediction of sudden cardiac death after acute myocardial infarction: role of Holter monitoring in the modern treatment era.** *Eur Heart J* 2005, **26**(8):762–769.
7. Priori SG, Aliot E, Blomstrom-Lundqvist C, Bossaert L, Breithardt G, Brugada P, Camm AJ, Cappato R, Cobbe SM, Di Mario C: **Task force on sudden cardiac death of the European Society of Cardiology.** *Eur Heart J* 2001, **22**(16):1374–1450.
8. Antman EM, Anbe DT, Armstrong PW, Bates ER, Green LA, Hand M, Hochman JS, Krumholz HM, Kushner FG, Lamas GA: **ACC/AHA guidelines for the management of patients with ST-elevation myocardial infarction: a report of the American College of Cardiology/American Heart Association Task Force on Practice Guidelines (Committee to Revise the 1999 Guidelines for the Management of Patients with Acute Myocardial Infarction).** *J Am Coll Cardiol* 2004, **44**(3):E1–E211.
9. Camm A, Malik M, Bigger J, Breithardt G, Cerutti S, Cohen R, Coumel P, Fallen E, Kennedy H, Kleiger R: **Heart rate variability: standards of measurement, physiological interpretation and clinical use. Task Force of the European Society of Cardiology and the North American Society of Pacing and Electrophysiology.** *Circulation* 1996, **93**(5):1043–1065.
10. Buccelletti E, Gilardi E, Scaini E, Galiuto L, Persiani R, Biondi A, Basile F, Silveri NG: **Heart rate variability and myocardial infarction: systematic literature review and metanalysis.** *Eur Rev Med Pharmacol Sci* 2009, **13**(4):299–307.
11. Soliman EZ, Elsalam MA, Li Y: **The relationship between high resting heart rate and ventricular arrhythmogenesis in patients referred to ambulatory 24 h electrocardiographic recording.** *Europace* 2010, **12**(2):261–265.
12. Schmidt G, Malik M, Barthel P, Schneider R, Ulm K, Rolnitzky L, Camm AJ, Bigger JT Jr, Schömig A: **Heart-rate turbulence after ventricular premature beats as a predictor of mortality after acute myocardial infarction.** *Lancet* 1999, **353**(9162):1390–1396.
13. Bauer A, Malik M, Schmidt G, Barthel P, Bonnemeier H, Cygankiewicz I, Guzik P, Lombardi F, Müller A, Oto A: **Heart rate turbulence: standards of measurement, physiological interpretation, and clinical use: International Society for Holter and Noninvasive Electrophysiology Consensus.** *J Am Coll Cardiol* 2008, **52**(17):1353–1365.
14. Bauer A, Kantelhardt JW, Barthel P, Schneider R, Mäkikallio T, Ulm K, Hnatkova K, Schömig A, Huikuri H, Bunde A: **Deceleration capacity of heart rate as a predictor of mortality after myocardial infarction: cohort study.** *Lancet* 2006, **367**(9523):1674–1681.
15. Gaspar P, Carbonell J, Oliveira JL: **On the parameter optimization of Support Vector Machines for binary classification.** *J Integr Bioinform* 2012, **9**(3):201.
16. Huang S, Shen Q, Duong TQ: **Quantitative prediction of acute ischemic tissue fate using support vector machine.** *Brain Res* 2011, **1405**:77–84.
17. Vihinen M: **How to evaluate performance of prediction methods? Measures and their interpretation in variation effect analysis.** *BMC Genomics* 2012, **13**(Suppl 4):S2.
18. Schwartz P, La Rovere M, Vanoli E: **Autonomic nervous system and sudden cardiac death. Experimental basis and clinical observations for post-myocardial infarction risk stratification.** *Circulation* 1992, **85**(1 Suppl):I77.
19. Chen LS, Zhou S, Fishbein MC, CHEN PS: **New perspectives on the role of autonomic nervous system in the genesis of arrhythmias.** *J Cardiovasc Electrophysiol* 2007, **18**(1):123–127.
20. La Rovere MT, Bigger JT Jr, Marcus FI, Mortara A, Schwartz PJ: **Baroreflex sensitivity and heart-rate variability in prediction of total cardiac mortality after myocardial infarction. ATRAMI (Autonomic Tone and Reflexes After Myocardial Infarction) Investigators.** *Lancet* 1998, **351**(9101):478–484.
21. Kim HK, Jeong MH, Ahn Y, Kim JH, Chae SC, Kim YJ, Hur SH, Seong IW, Hong TJ, Choi DH: **Hospital discharge risk score system for the assessment of clinical outcomes in patients with acute myocardial infarction (Korea Acute Myocardial Infarction Registry [KAMIR] score).** *Am J Cardiol* 2011, **107**(7):965–971. e961.
22. Atwater BD, Thompson VP, Vest RN, Shaw LK, Mazzei WR, Al-Khatib SM, Hranitzky PM, Bahnson TD, Velazquez EJ, Califf RM: **Usefulness of the Duke Sudden Cardiac Death risk score for predicting sudden cardiac death in patients with angiographic (>75% narrowing) coronary artery disease.** *Am J Cardiol* 2009, **104**(12):1624–1630.
23. Ebrahimpour M, Putniņš TJ, Berryman MJ, Allison A, Ng BW-H, Abbott D: **Automated authorship attribution using advanced signal classification techniques.** *PLoS One* 2013, **8**(2):e54998.
24. Secemsky EA, Verrier RL, Cooke G, Ghossein C, Subacius H, Manuchehry A, Herzog CA, Passman R: **High prevalence of cardiac autonomic dysfunction and T-wave alternans in dialysis patients.** *Heart Rhythm* 2011, **8**(4):592–598.
25. Alonzo T, Pepe M: **Development and evaluation of classifiers.** *Methods Mol Biol* 2007, **404**:89.
26. Vandeput S, Verheyden B, Aubert A, Van Huffel S: **Nonlinear heart rate dynamics: circadian profile and influence of age and gender.** *Med Eng Phys* 2012, **34**(1):108–117.
27. Monasterio V, Laguna P, Cygankiewicz I, Vázquez R, Bayés-Genís A, Bayés de Luna A, Martínez JP: **Average T-wave alternans activity in ambulatory ECG records predicts sudden cardiac death in patients with chronic heart failure.** *Heart Rhythm* 2012, **9**(3):383–389.

7

Pre-hospital delay in patients with first time myocardial infarction

Gunnar Nilsson[1*], Thomas Mooe[2], Lars Söderström[3] and Eva Samuelsson[2]

Abstract

Background: In myocardial infarction (MI), pre-hospital delay is associated with increased mortality and decreased possibility of revascularisation. We assessed pre-hospital delay in patients with first time MI in a northern Swedish population and identified determinants of a pre-hospital delay ≥ 2 h.

Methods: A total of 89 women (mean age 72.6 years) and 176 men (mean age 65.8 years) from a secondary prevention study were enrolled in an observational study after first time MI between November 2009 and March 2012. Total pre-hospital delay was defined as the time from the onset of symptoms suggestive of MI to admission to the hospital. Decision time was defined as the time from the onset of symptoms until the call to Emergency Medical Services (EMS). The time of symptom onset was assessed during the episode of care, and the time of call to EMS and admission to the hospital was based on recorded data. The first medical contact was determined from a mailed questionnaire. Determinants associated with pre-hospital delay ≥ 2 h were identified by multivariable logistic regression.

Results: The median total pre-hospital delay was 5.1 h (IQR 18.1), decision time 3.1 h (IQR 10.4), and transport time 1.2 h (IQR 1.0). The first medical contact was to primary care in 52.3 % of cases (22.3 % as a visit to a general practitioner and 30 % by telephone counselling), 37.3 % called the EMS, and 10.4 % self-referred to the hospital. Determinants of a pre-hospital delay ≥ 2 h were a visit to a general practitioner (OR 10.77, 95 % CI 2.39–48.59), call to primary care telephone counselling (OR 3.82, 95 % CI 1.68–8.68), chest pain as the predominant presenting symptom (OR 0.24, 95 % CI 0.08–0.77), and distance from the hospital (OR 1.03, 95 % CI 1.02–1.04). Among patients with primary care as the first medical contact, 67.0 % had a decision time ≥ 2 h, compared to 44.7 % of patients who called EMS or self-referred ($p = 0.002$).

Conclusions: Pre-hospital delay in patients with first time MI is prolonged considerably, particularly when primary care is the first medical contact. Actions to shorten decision time and increase the use of EMS are still necessary.

Keywords: Myocardial infarction, Observational study, Pre-hospital delay, Primary care

Background

Pre-hospital delay in myocardial infarction (MI) is associated with increased mortality [1, 2] and decreased possibility of revascularisation [3, 4]. Delay times exceeding 2.0 h are still commonly reported [5–8]. A cut-off time for pre-hospital delay is arbitrary, as mortality increases with time to reperfusion therapy [1, 9]. However, a 2-h cut-off is often applied because MI patients treated within 2 h receive the most clinical benefit from reperfusion therapy [3, 10].

Total pre-hospital delay can be divided into decision time (time from the onset of symptoms suggestive of MI until the call for medical help) and transport time (time from the call for medical help to hospital admission), also called "home-to-hospital delay" [11], with the decision time as the major part [12–15]. The scientific terminology for pre-hospital delay is not consistent; "time-to-treatment" and "treatment-seeking delay"

* Correspondence: gunnar.nilsson@regionjh.se
[1]Department of Public Health and Clinical Medicine, Unit of Research, Education and Development - Östersund, Umeå University, Umeå, Sweden
Full list of author information is available at the end of the article

are alternative terms, making comparisons between studies difficult [16].

Several determinants are associated with pre-hospital delay, including low socio-economic status, female gender, co-morbidities (e.g., diabetes and coronary disease), the patient's cognitive and emotional status, and determinants related to the healthcare provider [17, 18]. In some reports, patients with primary care as the first medical contact (FMC) have an increased pre-hospital delay [7, 19–21], often with less severe cardiac events than other patients [22]. Primary care clinics and telephone counselling services are frequently the FMC for patients with a suspected MI [7, 21], as symptoms related to MI often are not identified as cardiac [23]. Symptoms of MI may also be vague or atypical, leading to delayed care [24–27]. The impact of a previous MI on pre-hospital delay has varied in different studies. Results have shown shorter [28–31], longer [2, 32], or even neutral [21, 33] pre-hospital delays in association with a previous MI.

Pre-hospital delay in MI is related to the context [22, 27], and research on this issue should be based on data-sets that include relevant socio-demographic and healthcare-related data. The northern Swedish setting is characterised by long distances to the hospital, an aged population, and low to average education level. Traditionally, primary care has been the FMC for both acute and chronic diseases. By combining data from three different sources, we provide a more detailed picture of the pre-hospital delay issue compared to studies using a narrower data catch. Our aim was to assess the pre-hospital delay in men and women in a northern Swedish population with first time MI, and to identify determinants of a prolonged pre-hospital delay ≥ 2 h.

Methods

Participants

Participants in this observational study were recruited from the population of Region Jämtland Härjedalen, northern Sweden (in 2012: population 126 201, 53 % living in rural communities and 47 % in the capital community) [34]. The capital community of the region, Östersund, is the location of the regional hospital with clinics for cardiology and emergency medical services (EMS). The distance from participants' place of residence to the hospital ranged from 0.4 to 234 km. A referral from a GP was not required for patients to access emergency care or ambulance transport to a hospital in cases of chest pain suggestive of myocardial infarction. The primary care clinics were run by the regional healthcare authorities or contracted to provide primary care on the same taxation system and with the same patient charges. Participating patients were hospitalised with MI type 1, according to the universal definition [35], between November 26, 2009 and March 26, 2012. Eligible participants were identified from a population-based secondary prevention study that recruited patients after acute coronary syndromes (ACS) and stroke, within the Region Jämtland Härjedalen [36]. For patients living in rural communities, ambulance services and primary care clinics were accessible locally. Medical telephone counselling was available from primary care clinics 08:00 a.m. - 17:00 p.m. on weekdays and from Swedish Healthcare Direct (SHD) at all hours, with the possibility of directing patients to the Emergency Medical Services (EMS) or a primary care clinic as appropriate. The SHD, a part of the primary care organisation of the region, provided medical telephone counselling by nursing staff as a complementary service to the primary care clinics. The EMS alarm number was also accessible for calls from the public on a 24-h basis. The EMS with ambulance-based pre-hospital care, including thrombolytic therapy, was organised by the Emergency Care Centre, Östersund Hospital. Visits to primary care, emergency care, and ambulance transport were subject to patient charges of approximately 15–27 € during the study period. Deceased patients and patients declining consent or with insufficient data on pre-hospital delay were excluded from the present study.

Data sources and measurements

We used three different data sources. First, to acquire demographic and medical baseline data, a structured interview was carried out during the initial hospitalisation by nursing staff engaged in the secondary prevention study. The outline of the secondary prevention study of patients with ACS was published previously [36]. Second, previous chest pain symptoms, expectations of medical care, pre-hospital events, and FMC before admission to the hospital were recorded from a postal questionnaire sent to patients within 3–6 months after MI. Two reminders were sent to ensure participation. Third, for patients transported by ambulance, the symptoms reported by the patient at triage, the time of call to the EMS, and the time of admission to the hospital were recorded from ambulance records. For patients with private transport to the hospital, triage data and time of admission to the hospital were recorded from prospective records at the Emergency Care Centre.

Time of onset of symptoms suggestive of MI was determined during the episode of care, by nursing staff engaged in the secondary care study. Uncertainty in the time of symptom onset was estimated in hours, more or less, relative to the recorded onset time. The definitions of time intervals are explained in Fig. 1. For patients with private transport, only total pre-hospital delay was possible to calculate because the time to call to the EMS was unavailable.

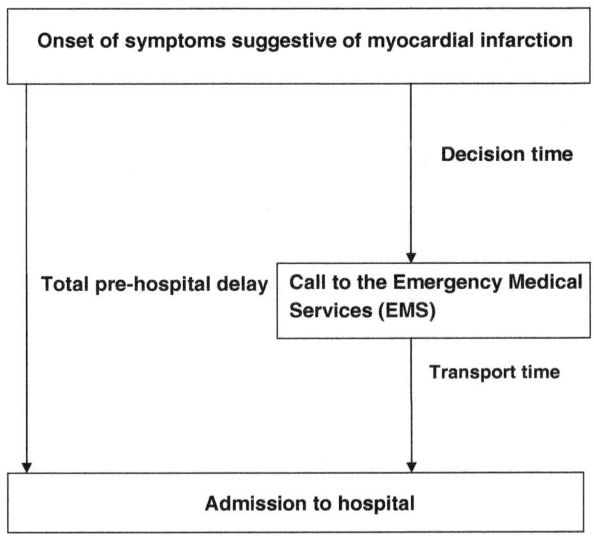

Fig. 1 Pre-hospital delay and definition of time intervals

Patients' expectations for medical care the day of admission to the hospital was assessed on a visual analogue scale from 0–100. The pain intensity at triage was assessed on a visual analogue scale from 0–10. If several assessments of pain were recorded during triage, the highest value was chosen. If a statement of no pain was recorded, the value was recorded as 0.

The distance from the patient's residence to the hospital was computed by Google Maps. Socio-economic classification was based on the Swedish Socioeconomic Classification (SEI) [37]. Marital status was determined from hospital records.

Three questions on previous chest pain symptoms were originally used in the "Rose angina questionnaire" [38–40] and the Swedish translation for primary care patients assessed for coronary disease [41]. Questions on the sequence of events before admission to the hospital were presented with fixed alternatives. The question "In your own opinion, did you suspect a myocardial infarction the day you fell ill?" was asked with yes and no as potential answers. A question on FMC before admission was presented with fixed alternatives, with the possibility of providing additional information, for classification into the following categories: "Personal visit to a GP before referral"; "Referral by call to a primary care centre/Swedish Healthcare Direct"; "Called the Emergency Medical Services;" and "Self-referred to hospital". Ambulance transport of patients was confirmed by ambulance records stating the location, date, time, medical actions, and condition of the patient at triage. For patients with private transport, the same triaging procedure was carried out at the emergency department. Presenting symptoms were classified as: "Predominantly chest pain symptoms", e.g., pain, ache, burn, or pressure in the chest; "Predominantly other pain symptoms", e.g., predominance of pain in the abdomen, arm, shoulder, or neck; and "Predominance of symptoms other than pain", e.g., severe fatigue, syncope, or circulatory shock.

MIs were diagnosed in accordance with the universal definition of MI type 1 [35]. The type of MI, ST elevation MI (STEMI) or non-ST elevation MI (NSTEMI), was not treated as a determinant of pre-hospital delay because it is an outcome measurement from the pre-hospital perspective.

Delay caused by medical misjudgement

All medical records were scrutinised for patients who were sent home from clinics or kept waiting to detect cases in which medical misjudgement contributed to a pre-hospital delay ≥ 2 h.

Statistical analysis

Patient characteristics are presented as proportions, means, or medians. The median and inter quartile range (IQR) were used for highly skewed distributions. To compare proportions, we used the chi-squared test or Fisher's exact test as appropriate. To compare means or medians, we used the Student's t-test (two sided) or the Mann–Whitney U-test as appropriate. We used univariate logistic regression to identify determinants of pre-hospital delay and $p < 0.25$ for determinants to be included in the multivariable logistic model. We reduced the model stepwise by excluding the least significant variable manually until only significant variables remained. The level of significance was set at $p < 0.05$. To assess the discriminatory power of the multivariable model, we used receiver operating characteristic (ROC) curves and calculated the area under the curve (AUC) [42, 43]. Statistical analyses were performed in the software IBM SPSS version 22.

Results

Descriptive data

We recruited 265 consenting patients, 89 of which were women, to take part in this study (Fig. 2). The mean patient age was 68.1 years; the mean age of participating women was 72.6 years. "Manual workers" was the predominant socio-economic group (62.7 %). The receiving hospital for 258 patients was the central hospital in Östersund; the other seven patients were admitted to other Swedish hospitals due to temporary visits outside their normal place of residence. The FMC was primary care in 52.3 % of all cases (22.3 % as a visit to a general practitioner (GP) and 30 % by telephone counselling), 37.3 % called the EMS, and 10.4 % self-referred to the hospital. A majority of patients (76.6 %) used ambulance transport (198 by road and 5 by air ambulance). Patients visiting a GP, calling a primary care clinic/SHD, or

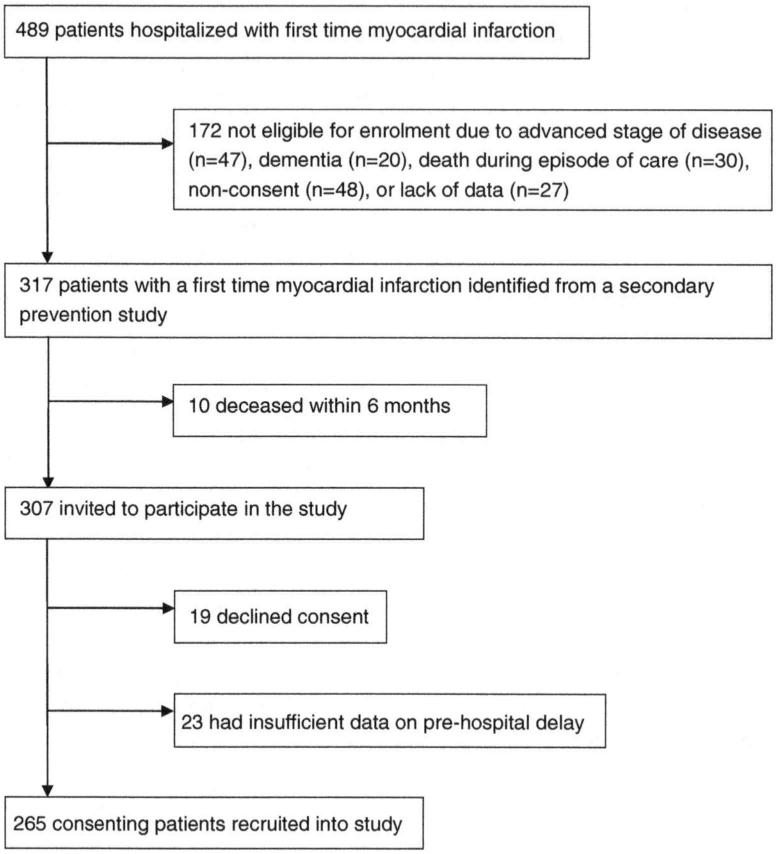

Fig. 2 Participant recruitment

calling the EMS as the FMC were transported by ambulance in 72.4, 79.5, and 99 % of cases, respectively. Finally, 97 patients (36.6 %) were diagnosed as STEMI (21 women and 76 men), and the others as NSTEMI.

Main results

The median total pre-hospital delay was 5.1 (IQR 18.1) hours, with a median decision time of 3.1 (IQR 10.4) hours and median transport time of 1.2 (IQR 1.0) hours. No differences were found between men and women (Table 1). The median transport time was 0.78 (IQR 0.5) hours in the central community and 1.65 (IQR 1.1) hours in the rural communities (p <0.001). No significant differences were found in the decision time or total pre-hospital delay between the central and rural communities. The uncertainty of the time of symptom onset was a median 0.0 h (IQR 1.0), with the 80th percentile at 2.0 h.

A highly skewed distribution in total pre-hospital delay and decision time was observed with wide IQRs among both men and women (Table 1 and Additional file 1). Patients with a total pre-hospital delay ≥2 h lived farther from the hospital and were more likely to have consulted a GP before admission to the hospital, to be diabetic, and to report recurrent angina symptoms than those with a total pre-hospital delay <2 h. Patients with a total pre-hospital delay <2 h were more likely to have called the EMS or self-referred to the hospital, and they were

Table 1 Total pre-hospital delay, decision time, and transport time for patients with first time myocardial infarction

Characteristic	Total n = 265	Men n = 176 (66.4 %)	Women n = 89 (33.6 %)	*P*-value, Mann–Whitney *U* Test
Total pre-hospital delay, median (IQR)	5.1 (18.1)	5.9 (17.4)	4.1 (19.3)	0.436
Decision time, median (IQR)[a]	3.1 (10.4)	3.7 (10.1)	2.0 (11.8)	0.411
Transport time, median (IQR)[a]	1.2 (1.0)	1.3 (1.0)	1.2 (1.0)	0.052

All data are given in hours. Total pre-hospital delay is the time between onset of symptoms suggestive of myocardial infarction and admission to the hospital. Decision time is the time between onset of symptoms suggestive of myocardial infarction and the call to Emergency Medical Services. Transport time is the time between the call to Emergency Medical Services and admission to the hospital. [a]Calculated for 200/203 patients transported to the hospital by ambulance

more likely to report chest pain as the predominant symptom at triage than those with a total pre-hospital delay ≥2 h (Table 2).

Characteristics associated with a total pre-hospital delay ≥ 2 h in the adjusted model were: visit to a GP before referral (OR 10.77, 95 % CI 2.39–48.59), referral by a call to a primary care centre/SHD (OR 3.82, 95 % CI 1.68–8.68), chest pain as the predominant symptom at triage (negative association; OR 0.24, 95 % CI 0.08–0.77), and distance (km) to hospital (OR 1.03, 95 % CI 1.02–1.04) (Table 3). Patients in contact with primary care, as a GP visit or by telephone counselling, also had a prolonged decision time (Table 3). Chest pain as the predominant symptom at triage was associated with a shorter decision time (Table 3). We examined the characteristics of the regression model for interaction with gender, but none of the findings were significant. Age, gender, and levels of scholarship did not contribute to significant improvement of the multivariable model. The discriminatory ability of the multivariable model (Table 3) was evaluated by ROC curves; the AUC was 0.84 (95 % CI 0.79–0.90, p <0.001) for total pre-hospital delay and 0.68 (95 % CI 0.60–0.76, p <0.001) for decision time.

Among patients with primary care as the FMC, 67.0 % had a decision time ≥ 2 h, compared to 44.7 % of patients calling the EMS or self-referring to the hospital (p = 0.002). Compared to patients who self-referred or called the EMS before admission to the hospital, primary care patients were younger (mean age 66.3 years (SD 12.0) vs. 69.7 (SD 10.9) years, p = 0.016) and lived a greater distance from the hospital (median distance 37.5 km (IQR 10.0–99.5) vs. 21.0 km (IQR 4.0–68.5), p = 0.012). Patients with a FMC to primary care more often reported recurrent angina symptoms preceding the MI (34.6 % vs. 21.8 %, p = 0.022), a lower pain intensity at triage (5.1 (SD 3.1) vs. 6.3 (SD 2.9), p = 0.030), and less frequently asked a friend/next of kin for help before admission to the hospital (20.5 % vs. 38.8 %, p = 0.001) than patients who self-referred or called the EMS. Patients with a FMC to primary care were less frequently diagnosed with STEMI than patients who self-referred or called the EMS as the FMC (25.7 % vs. 49.2 %, p < 0.001). Among primary care patients with private transport to the hospital and lived in rural communities, the total pre-hospital delay time increased stepwise compared to the total population (Table 4).

Delay caused by medical misjudgement

We identified three patients with delayed care ≥ 2 h due to medical misjudgement; two were sent home from primary care clinics but returned within 12 to 24 h, and one patient was delayed for 2 h at a primary care centre before referral.

Non-participants

Non-participating patients did not differ significantly with respect to age, gender, or distance from the hospital compared to participants.

Discussion

Key findings

The median total pre-hospital delay was 5.1 h, with decision time as the major contributor. The FMC was to primary care (as a GP visit or by telephone counselling) in approximately half of all patients. Visiting a GP or calling primary care for telephone counselling prior to hospital admission were both associated with a total pre-hospital delay and decision time ≥ 2 h. Chest pain as the predominant symptom at triage was associated with shorter total pre-hospital delay and decision time.

Interpretation of findings

The pre-hospital delay among our study participants exceeded that reported in several previous studies on ACS and MI. Pre-hospital delay in the European patients' study arm of the Global Registry of Acute Coronary Events (GRACE) study was a median 2.3–2.7 h for STEMI and 2.7–3.1 h for NSTEMI cases between 2000 and 2006 (lowest value in 2006) [28]. In the Northern Sweden MONICA Study, a delay time ≥ 2 h was found in 64 % of patients with diabetes and 58 % of non-diabetics [44]. In a cohort of Norwegian patients with first time MI, 52 % of women and 51 % of men had a total pre-hospital delay exceeding 2 h [19]. A pre-hospital delay similar to our data was reported in an Irish setting in 2013; the median pre-hospital delay for STEMI patients was 2.7 h and for NSTEMI patients 4.5 h [7].

There are several possible explanations for the prolonged delay in our study. First, unlike the MONICA cohort and the Norwegian multicentre study by Lovlien et al [19, 44], we did not apply an upper age limit, and we recruited a somewhat higher proportion of female participants. Second, the prolonged pre-hospital delay among our study patients is likely related to the context of medical care, as primary care as the FMC is recommended for patients and the EMS is the second choice in most circumstances [7, 19–22]. In our study, primary care as the FMC was associated with both prolonged pre-hospital delay and decision time. Pre-hospital delay attributable to healthcare provider contact was described previously [22, 30, 45] but remains to be addressed because such provider-related delay may account for more loss in total delay time compared to patient delay [46–48]. This problem is even more important if patients believe that calling primary care, and not EMS, is always the appropriate action [49]. This could explain the association between primary care as the FMC and pre-hospital delay that we observed.

Table 2 Characteristics of first time myocardial infarction patients according to total pre-hospital delay ($n = 265$)

Characteristic	<2 h	≥2 h	*P*-value
	n = 52 (19.6 %)	*n* = 213 (80.4 %)	
Mean age, years (SD)	67.5 (11.3)	68.2 (11.7)	0.668
Female sex	19/52 (36.5 %)	70/213 (32.9 %)	0.615
Married or cohabiting	23/32 (71.9 %)	106/172 (61.6 %)	0.270
Distance to hospital in km, median (IQR)	7.0 (27.5)	49.8 (87.4)	<0.001
University or college degree	7/51 (13.7 %)	31/213 (14.6 %)	0.880
Manual worker	33/51 (66.0 %)	132/212 (61.9 %)	0.746
Medical history			
Previous revascularisation	2/52 (3.8 %)	7/213 (3.3 %)	0.691
Previous stroke or TIA	3/52 (5.8 %)	10/213 (4.7 %)	0.742
Angina pectoris, current diagnosis	2/52 (3.8 %)	20/213 (9.4 %)	0.267
Hypertension, current diagnosis	25/52 48.1 %)	104/213 (48.8 %)	0.923
Diabetes mellitus, medication for	5/52 (9.6 %)	46/213 (21.6 %)	0.049
Dyslipidaemia, medication for	6/52 (11.5 %)	44/213 (20.7 %)	0.132
Previous chest pain symptoms			
Ever have chest pain or discomfort in the chest	21/52 (40.4 %)	63/203 (31.0 %)	0.201
Chest pain walking at an ordinary pace on the level	3/51 (5.9 %)	23/198 (11.6 %)	0.232
Chest pain walking uphill or in a hurry	14/51 (27.5 %)	68/202 (33.7 %)	0.397
On the day of admission to hospital			
Myocardial infarction suspected by patient	23/52 (44.2 %)	71/210 (33.8 %)	0.161
"I decided by myself to seek medical care"	23/49 (46.9 %)	99/209 (47.47.4 %)	0.957
"I took advice from a next of kin/friend"	9/49 (18.4 %)	50/209 (23.9 %)	0.405
"A next of kin/friend contacted medical care"	17/49 (34.7 %)	60/209 (28.7 %)	0.410
Expectations of medical care, mean (SD)[a]	80.2 (15.0)	76.2 (21.4)	0.208
First medical contact before admission to hospital			
Personal visit to a GP before referral	2/52 (3.8 %)	56/208 (26.9 %)	<0.001
Referred by call to a primary care centre/Swedish Healthcare Direct	10/52 (19.2 %)	68/208 (32.7 %)	0.058
Called the Emergency Medical Services	27/52 (51.9 %)	70/208 (33.7 %)	0.015
Self-referred to hospital	13/52 (25.0 %)	14/208 (6.7 %)	<0.001
Ambulance transport to hospital	36/52 (69.2 %)	167/213 (78.4 %)	0.161
Symptoms reported by patient at triage			
Predominantly chest pain	48/52 (92.3 %)	170/211 (80.6 %)	0.044
Predominantly other pain	3/52 (5.8 %)	27/211 (12.8 %)	0.153
Symptoms other than pain predominated	1/52 (1.9 %)	14/211 (6.6 %)	0.189
Symptom onset related to physical strain	10/52 (19.2 %)	37/210 (17.6 %)	0.786
Recurrent angina within 2 weeks before admission	9/52 (17.3 %)	69/213 (32.4 %)	0.032
Pain intensity, mean (SD)[b]	6.7 (2.7)	5.5 (3.1)	0.099

TIA transitory ischaemic attack
[a]Visual analogue scale from 0 to 100 where 0 is lowest and 100 is highest possible expectations; five patients with missing values
[b]Visual analogue scale from 0 to 10 where 0 is no pain and 10 is worst possible pain; assessed at triage in 115/265 patients

Furthermore, many of our study participants lived far from the hospital, with consequences on transport time. However, 76.6 % used an ambulance for transportation to the hospital, which is a greater proportion of patients than in previous reports from Ireland, Australia, and Sweden (40–50 % of ACS patients with ambulance transport) [50–52]. Among our patients, 37.3 % primarily called the EMS, 99 % of which were transported by ambulance, compared to 72.4 % of patients who visited a GP as the FMC. GP visits before hospital admission may

Table 3 Characteristics associated with prolonged pre-hospital delay in patients with first time myocardial infarction

Characteristic	Total prehospital delay ≥ 2 h		Decision time ≥ 2 h	
	Adjusted OR (95 % CI)	*P*-value	Adjusted OR (95 % CI)	*P*-value
Personal visit to a GP before referral	10.77 (2.39–48.59)	0.002	3.85 (1.66–8.90)	0.002
Referred by call to a primary care centre/Swedish Healthcare Direct	3.82 (1.68–8.68)	0.001	2.00 (1.03–3.87)	0.041
Chest pain predominating symptom at triage	0.24 (0.08–0.77)	0.016	0.34 (0.12–0.90)	0.031
Distance to hospital, km	1.03 (1.02–1.04)	<0.001	1.00 (1.00–1.01)	0.586

Total pre-hospital delay is the time between onset of symptoms suggestive of myocardial infarction and admission to the hospital. Decision time is the time between onset of symptoms suggestive of myocardial infarction and the call to Emergency Medical Services

have resulted in delayed transport and fewer patients transported by ambulance, as recently reported in an Irish setting [51]. Ambulance stations with access to thrombolytic therapy were located in all rural communities, and a shortage of ambulance resources is unlikely to have contributed to delayed care among our patients.

In our study, the average education level was low and a majority of participants were manual workers, but these were not determinants of pre-hospital delay. Previous research has demonstrated a relationship between low socio-economic level and pre-hospital delay [18, 53, 54], but definitions of socio-economic status and cut-offs for pre-hospital delay differ, making comparisons difficult.

Future aspects

The association between the patient's choice of FMC and pre-hospital delay force us to rethink the kind of assessment of chest pain that is most appropriate in primary care. Clinical prediction rules to rule out coronary disease in low-risk patients has been proposed as one possibility for selecting patients with chest pain for cardiologic care [55, 56]; point-of-care troponin T testing is another possibility [57], but such measures are unlikely to decrease pre-hospital delay related to health care providers. As proposed previously, medical telephone counselling should be the focus of an epidemiological study to further develop the management of ACS calls [22]. Our findings support patients with new onset chest pain being encouraged to call the EMS and not primary care telephone counselling. As public campaigns to reduce pre-hospital delay have yielded negative results [58], future efforts should target high-risk patients, preferably by individualised patient education, which has been reported to reduce pre-hospital time in patients with recurrent ACS episodes [15]. A high-risk approach is further supported by the increasing delay-time among certain subgroups in our study, such as primary care patients with private transport to the hospital and rural residency (Table 4). The discriminatory ability of the multivariable model supports the core determinants of pre-hospital delay being related to a patient's decision-making process and choice of health care provider [22, 46].

Table 4 Total pre-hospital delay according to first medical contact (FMC), transport mode, and residency

Characteristic	Number of patients	Total pre-hospital delay in hours, median (IQR)
Total	265	5.1 (18.1)
Primary care as FMC	136	8.7 (33.3)
Primary care as FMC and private transport to hospital	32	20.9 (69.1)
Primary care as FMC, private transport to hospital, and rural residency	12	74.0 (140.8)

Primary care as FMC: Visit to a GP, call to a primary care centre or Swedish Healthcare Direct

Strengths and limitations

We used different data sources to provide detailed information on each study participant. A high participation rate (86.3 %) and the population-based study approach strengthened the external validity. Data on symptom presentation at triage were recorded from ambulance and emergency care records, reflecting conditions at the time of care as closely as possible. Previous medical history, socio-economic status, and time of symptom onset were assessed by trained nursing staff during the episode of care. The exact time of the onset of symptoms indicating MI can be hard to establish and is a common problem in studies reporting on pre-hospital delay [16]. An estimation of the uncertainty in the time of symptom onset was included in our study plan.

The subdivision of total pre-hospital delay into decision time and transport time was not possible to calculate in patients with private transport to the hospital, which limits our analysis of decision time and transport time to patients with ambulance transport. Delay due to medical misjudgement was determined from retrospective data, which may have been insufficient. We recruited patients from a population-based secondary prevention program after MI and ACS, meaning that the generalisability of our findings is limited to surviving patients eligible for a prevention programme. The rural context, with many patients living distantly from hospital but with access to primary care and ambulance services, is another limitation for the overall generalisability of our findings. The postal questionnaire covering previous chest pain symptoms, sequence of events, and FMC prior to hospitalisation was delivered within 3-6 months after the MI, and recall bias cannot be ruled out.

Comparisons across different studies are complicated by different definitions of pre-hospital delay [16]. We applied a bivariate approach with a 2-h cut-off to identify determinants associated with pre-hospital delay. This time limit was chosen from a theoretical point of view [3] and to allow comparisons with other studies using the same cut-off [14, 19, 28, 44, 59].

Conclusions

In this study of patients in a northern Swedish population with first time MI, the total pre-hospital delay was considerably prolonged (median 5.1 h), with decision time as the major contributor (median 3.1 h). Primary care patients had a longer pre-hospital delay, mainly due to a longer decision time. Actions to shorten decision time and increase the use of EMS are still necessary.

Abbreviations

ACS: Acute coronary syndrome; AUC: Area under the curve; ECG: Electrocardiogram; EMS: Emergency medical services; FMC: First medical contact; GP: General Practitioner; MI: Myocardial infarction; NSTEMI: Non-ST elevation myocardial infarction; ROC: Receiver operating characteristic; SHD: Swedish Healthcare Direct; STEMI: ST elevation myocardial infarction.

Competing interests

The authors declare that they have no competing interests.

Authors' contributions

GN designed the study, performed the statistical analyses, and drafted the manuscript. ES supervised the study design, participated in data analysis, and helped draft the manuscript. TM supervised the study design, participated in data analysis, and helped draft the manuscript. LS gave advice on the statistical analyses, participated in data analysis, and helped draft the manuscript. All authors read and approved the final manuscript.

Authors' information

GN: GP, doctoral student, Department of Public Health and Clinical Medicine, Unit of Research, Education and Development - Östersund, Umeå University, Sweden.
ES: GP, Associate Professor, Family Medicine, Department of Public Health and Clinical Medicine, Umeå University, Sweden.
TM: Consultant in cardiology, Östersund Hospital, Associate Professor of Medicine, Department of Public Health and Clinical Medicine, Umeå University, Sweden.
LS: Master of Science, Unit of Research, Education and Development - Östersund Hospital, Östersund, Sweden.

Acknowledgements

The authors wish to express their sincere gratitude to all study participants and the staff engaged in the Nailed ACS Risk Factor Trial.

Funding

This study was funded by grants from the Unit of Research, Education and Development, Östersund Hospital, Region Jämtland Härjedalen, Sweden (Dnr-JLL- 370941, 368631 and 467081). The funders had no role in the study design, data collection, data analysis, or in writing of the report.

Author details

[1]Department of Public Health and Clinical Medicine, Unit of Research, Education and Development - Östersund, Umeå University, Umeå, Sweden. [2]Department of Public Health and Clinical Medicine, Umeå University, Umeå, Sweden. [3]Unit of Research, Education and Development, Östersund Hospital, Region Jämtland Härjedalen, Östersund, Sweden.

References

1. De Luca G, Suryapranata H, Ottervanger JP, Antman EM. Time delay to treatment and mortality in primary angioplasty for acute myocardial infarction: every minute of delay counts. Circulation. 2004;109(10):1223–5.
2. Newby LK, Rutsch WR, Califf RM, Simoons ML, Aylward PE, Armstrong PW, et al. Time from symptom onset to treatment and outcomes after thrombolytic therapy. GUSTO-1 Investigators. J Am Coll Cardiol. 1996;27(7): 1646–55.
3. Goldberg RJ, Mooradd M, Gurwitz JH, Rogers WJ, French WJ, Barron HV, et al. Impact of time to treatment with tissue plasminogen activator on morbidity and mortality following acute myocardial infarction (The second National Registry of Myocardial Infarction). Am J Cardiol. 1998;82(3):259–64.
4. Kushner FG, Hand M, Smith Jr SC, King III SB, Anderson JL, Antman EM, et al. focused updates: ACC/AHA guidelines for the management of patients with ST-elevation myocardial infarction (updating the 2004 guideline and 2007 focused update) and ACC/AHA/SCAI guidelines on percutaneous coronary intervention (updating the 2005 guideline and 2007 focused update) a report of the American College of Cardiology Foundation/American Heart Association Task Force on Practice Guidelines. J Am Coll Cardiol. 2009; 54(23):2205–41.
5. Goldberg RJ, Steg PG, Sadiq I, Granger CB, Jackson EA, Budaj A, et al. Extent of, and factors associated with, delay to hospital presentation in patients with acute coronary disease (the GRACE registry). American J Cardiol. 2002; 89(7):791–6.
6. Isaksson RM, Holmgren L, Lundblad D, Brulin C, Eliasson M. Time trends in symptoms and prehospital delay time in women vs. men with myocardial infarction over a 15-year period. The Northern Sweden MONICA Study. Eur J Cardiovasc Nurs. 2008;7(2):152–8.
7. McKee G, Mooney M, O'Donnell S, O'Brien F, Biddle MJ, Moser DK. Multivariate analysis of predictors of pre-hospital delay in acute coronary syndrome. Int J Cardiol. 2013;168(3):2706–13.
8. Saczynski JS, Yarzebski J, Lessard D, Spencer FA, Gurwitz JH, Gore JM, et al. Trends in prehospital delay in patients with acute myocardial infarction (from the Worcester Heart Attack Study). Am J Cardiol. 2008;102(12):1589–94.
9. Estevez-Loureiro R, Lopez-Sainz A, Perez de Prado A, Cuellas C, Calvino Santos R, Alonso-Orcajo N, et al. Timely reperfusion for ST-segment elevation myocardial infarction: Effect of direct transfer to primary angioplasty on time delays and clinical outcomes. World J Cardiol. 2014;6(6):424–33.
10. Chareonthaitawee P, Gibbons RJ, Roberts RS, Christian TF, Burns R, Yusuf S. The impact of time to thrombolytic treatment on outcome in patients with acute myocardial infarction. For the CORE investigators (Collaborative Organisation for RheothRx Evaluation). Heart. 2000;84(2):142–8.
11. Perkins-Porras L, Whitehead DL, Strike PC, Steptoe A. Pre-hospital delay in patients with acute coronary syndrome: factors associated with patient decision time and home-to-hospital delay. Eur J Cardiovasc Nurs. 2009;8(1):26–33.
12. Moss AJ, Goldstein S. The pre-hospital phase of acute myocadial infarction. Circulation. 1970;41(5):737–42.
13. Ottesen MM, Dixen U, Torp-Pedersen C, Kober L. Prehospital delay in acute coronary syndrome–an analysis of the components of delay. Int J Cardiol. 2004;96(1):97–103.
14. Rasmussen CH, Munck A, Kragstrup J, Haghfelt T. Patient delay from onset of chest pain suggesting acute coronary syndrome to hospital admission. Scand Cardiovasc J. 2003;37(4):183–6.
15. Mooney M, McKee G, Fealy G, O' Brien F, O'Donnell S, Moser D. A randomized controlled trial to reduce prehospital delay time in patients with acute coronary syndrome (ACS). J Emerg Med. 2014;46(4):495–506.
16. Mackay MH, Ratner PA, Nguyen M, Percy M, Galdas P, Grunau G. Inconsistent measurement of acute coronary syndrome patients' pre-hospital delay in research: a review of the literature. Eur J Cardiovasc Nurs. 2014;13(6):483–93.
17. Khraim FM, Carey MG. Predictors of pre-hospital delay among patients with acute myocardial infarction. Patient Educ Couns. 2009;75(2):155–61.
18. Moser DK, Kimble LP, Alberts MJ, Alonzo A, Croft JB, Dracup K, et al. Reducing delay in seeking treatment by patients with acute coronary syndrome and

stroke: a scientific statement from the American Heart Association Council on cardiovascular nursing and stroke council. Circulation. 2006;114(2):168–82.

19. Lovlien M, Schei B, Hole T. Prehospital delay, contributing aspects and responses to symptoms among Norwegian women and men with first time acute myocardial infarction. Eur J Cardiovasc Nurs. 2007;6(4):308–13.
20. O'Donnell S, Condell S, Begley C, Fitzgerald T. Prehospital care pathway delays: gender and myocardial infarction. J Adv Nurs. 2006;53(3):268–76.
21. Johansson I, Stromberg A, Swahn E. Factors related to delay times in patients with suspected acute myocardial infarction. Heart Lung. 2004; 33(5):291–300.
22. Alonzo AA. The effect of health care provider consultation on acute coronary syndrome care-seeking delay. Heart Lung. 2007;36(5):307–18.
23. Tummala SR, Farshid A. Patients' understanding of their heart attack and the impact of exposure to a media campaign on pre-hospital time. Heart Lung Circ. 2015;24(1):4–10.
24. Isaksson RM, Brulin C, Eliasson M, Naslund U, Zingmark K. Prehospital experiences of older men with a first myocardial infarction: a qualitative analysis within the Northern Sweden MONICA Study. Scand J Caring Sci. 2011;25(4):787–97.
25. Isaksson RM, Brulin C, Eliasson M, Naslund U, Zingmark K. Older women's prehospital experiences of their first myocardial infarction. J Cardiovasc Nurs. 2013;28(4):360–9.
26. Kirchberger I, Heier M, Wende R, von Scheidt W, Meisinger C. The patient's interpretation of myocardial infarction symptoms and its role in the decision process to seek treatment: the MONICA/KORA Myocardial Infarction Registry. Clin Res Cardiol. 2012;101(11):909–16.
27. Pattenden J, Watt I, Lewin RJ, Stanford N. Decision making processes in people with symptoms of acute myocardial infarction: qualitative study. BMJ. 2002;324(7344):1006–9.
28. Goldberg RJ, Spencer FA, Fox KA, Brieger D, Steg PG, Gurfinkel E, et al. Prehospital Delay in Patients With Acute Coronary Syndromes (from the Global Registry of Acute Coronary Events [GRACE]). Am J Cardiol. 2009; 103(5):598–603.
29. Meischke H, Larsen MP, Eisenberg MS. Gender differences in reported symptoms for acute myocardial infarction: impact on prehospital delay time interval. Am J Emerg Med. 1998;16(4):363–6.
30. Sheifer SE, Rathore SS, Gersh BJ, Weinfurt KP, Oetgen WJ, Breall JA, et al. Time to presentation with acute myocardial infarction in the elderly: associations with race, sex, and socioeconomic characteristics. Circulation. 2000;102(14):1651–6.
31. Leizorovicz A, Haugh MC, Mercier C, Boissel JP. Pre-hospital and hospital time delays in thrombolytic treatment in patients with suspected acute myocardial infarction. Analysis of data from the EMIP study. European Myocardial Infarction Project. Eur Heart J. 1997;18(2):248–53.
32. Yarzebski J, Goldberg RJ, Gore JM, Alpert JS. Temporal trends and factors associated with extent of delay to hospital arrival in patients with acute myocardial infarction: the Worcester Heart Attack Study. Am Heart J. 1994; 128(2):255–63.
33. Dracup K, Moser DK, Eisenberg M, Meischke H, Alonzo AA, Braslow A. Causes of delay in seeking treatment for heart attack symptoms. Soc Sci Med. 1995;40(3):379–92.
34. Statistical database. Statistics Sweden. 2015. http://www.statistikdatabasen.scb.se/. Accessed 25 Aug 2015.
35. Thygesen K, Alpert JS, White HD. Universal definition of myocardial infarction. Eur Heart J. 2007;28(20):2525–38.
36. Mooe T, Bjorklund F, Graipe A, Huber D, Jakobsson S, Kajermo U, et al. The Nurse-Based Age Independent Intervention to Limit Evolution of Disease After Acute Coronary Syndrome (NAILED ACS) Risk Factor Trial: Protocol for a Randomized Controlled Trial. JMIR Res Protoc. 2014;3(3):e42.
37. Statistics Sweden. Swedish socio-economic classification (SEI). In: Reports on Statistical Co-ordination 1982:4. http://www.scb.se/Grupp/Hitta_statistik/Forsta_Statistik/Klassifikationer/_Dokument/SEI-AGG_Eng.pdf. Accessed 25 Aug 2015.
38. Lawlor DA, Adamson J, Ebrahim S. Performance of the WHO Rose angina questionnaire in post-menopausal women: are all of the questions necessary? J Epidemiol Community Health. 2003;57(7):538–41.
39. Rose G, McCartney P, Reid DD. Self-administration of a questionnaire on chest pain and intermittent claudication. Br J Prev Soc Med. 1977;31(1):42–8.
40. Rose GA. The diagnosis of ischaemic heart pain and intermittent claudication in field surveys. Bull World Health Organ. 1962;27:645–58.
41. Nilsson G, Mooe T, Stenlund H, Samuelsson E. Diagnostic characteristics and prognoses of primary-care patients referred for clinical exercise testing: a prospective observational study. BMC Fam Pract. 2014;15:71.
42. Fan J, Upadhye S, Worster A. Understanding receiver operating characteristic (ROC) curves. CJEM. 2006;8(1):19–20.
43. Faraggi D, Reiser B. Estimation of the area under the ROC curve. Stat Med. 2002;21(20):3093–106.
44. Angerud KH, Brulin C, Naslund U, Eliasson M. Longer pre-hospital delay in first myocardial infarction among patients with diabetes: an analysis of 4266 patients in the northern Sweden MONICA Study. BMC Cardiovasc Disord. 2013;13:6.
45. GISSI–Avoidable Delay Study Group. Epidemiology of avoidable delay in the care of patients with acute myocardial infarction in Italy. A GISSI-generated study. Arch Intern Med. 1995;155(14):1481–8.
46. Alonzo AA. The impact of physician consultation on care-seeking during acute episodes of coronary heart disease. Med Care. 1977;15(1):34–50.
47. Bouma J, Broer J, Bleeker J, van Sonderen E, Meyboom-de Jong B, DeJongste MJ. Longer pre-hospital delay in acute myocardial infarction in women because of longer doctor decision time. J Epidemiol Community Health. 1999;53(8):459–64.
48. Broer J, Bleeker JK, Bouma J, de Jongste MJ, Erdman RA, Meyboom-de JB. Regional differences in prehospital time delay for patients with acute myocardial infarction; Rotterdam and Groningen, 1990-1995. Ned Tijdschr Geneeskd. 2000;144(2):78–83.
49. Leslie WS, Urie A, Hooper J, Morrison CE. Delay in calling for help during myocardial infarction: reasons for the delay and subsequent pattern of accessing care. Heart. 2000;84(2):137–41.
50. Kerr D, Holden D, Smith J, Kelly AM, Bunker S. Predictors of ambulance use in patients with acute myocardial infarction in Australia. Emerg Med J. 2006; 23(12):948–52.
51. Mooney M, O'Brien F, McKee G, O'Donnell S, Moser D. Ambulance use in acute coronary syndrome in Ireland: a cross-sectional study. Eur J Cardiovasc Nurs. 2015; doi:10.1177/1474515115579134.
52. Thuresson M, Jarlov MB, Lindahl B, Svensson L, Zedigh C, Herlitz J. Factors that influence the use of ambulance in acute coronary syndrome. Am Heart J. 2008;156(1):170–6.
53. Lovlien M, Schei B, Hole T. Myocardial infarction: psychosocial aspects, gender differences and impact on pre-hospital delay. J Advanc Nurs. 2008; 63(2):148–54.
54. Park YH, Kang GH, Song BG, Chun WJ, Lee JH, Hwang SY, et al. Factors related to prehospital time delay in acute ST-segment elevation myocardial infarction. J Korean Med Sci. 2012;27(8):864–9.
55. Bosner S, Becker A, Abu Hani M, Keller H, Sonnichsen AC, Haasenritter J, et al. Accuracy of symptoms and signs for coronary heart disease assessed in primary care. Br J Gen Pract. 2010;60(575):e246–57.
56. Gencer B, Vaucher P, Herzig L, Verdon F, Ruffieux C, Bosner S, et al. Ruling out coronary heart disease in primary care patients with chest pain: a clinical prediction score. BMC Med. 2010;8:9.
57. Nilsson S, Andersson PO, Borgquist L, Grodzinsky E, Janzon M, Kvick M, et al. Point-of-Care Troponin T Testing in the Management of Patients with Chest Pain in the Swedish Primary Care. Int J Family Med. 2013;2013:532093.
58. Dracup K, McKinley S, Riegel B, Moser DK, Meischke H, Doering LV, et al. A randomized clinical trial to reduce patient prehospital delay to treatment in acute coronary syndrome. Circ Cardiovasc Qual Outcomes. 2009;2(6):524–32.
59. Ting HH, Bradley EH, Wang Y, Lichtman JH, Nallamothu BK, Sullivan MD, et al. Factors associated with longer time from symptom onset to hospital presentation for patients with ST-elevation myocardial infarction. Arch Intern Med. 2008;168(9):959–68.

8

TSC-22 up-regulates collagen *3a1* gene expression in the rat heart

Annina Kelloniemi[1], Jani Aro[1], Juha Näpänkangas[2], Elina Koivisto[1], Erja Mustonen[1], Heikki Ruskoaho[1,3] and Jaana Rysä[1,4*]

Abstract

Background: The transforming growth factor (TGF)-β is one of the key mediators in cardiac remodelling occurring after myocardial infarction (MI) and in hypertensive heart disease. The TGF-β-stimulated clone 22 (TSC-22) is a leucine zipper protein expressed in many tissues and possessing various transcription-modulating activities. However, its function in the heart remains unknown.

Methods: The aim of the present study was to characterize cardiac TSC-22 expression *in vivo* in cardiac remodelling and in myocytes *in vitro*. In addition, we used TSC-22 gene transfer in order to examine the effects of TSC-22 on cardiac gene expression and function.

Results: We found that TSC-22 is rapidly up-regulated by multiple hypertrophic stimuli, and in post-MI remodelling both TSC-22 mRNA and protein levels were up-regulated (4.1-fold, $P<0.001$ and 3.0-fold, $P<0.05$, respectively) already on day 1. We observed that both losartan and metoprolol treatments reduced left ventricular TSC-22 gene expression. Finally, TSC-22 overexpression by local intramyocardial adenovirus-mediated gene delivery showed that TSC-22 appears to have a role in regulating collagen *type IIIa1* gene expression in the heart.

Conclusions: These results demonstrate that TSC-22 expression is induced in response to cardiac overload. Moreover, our data suggests that, by regulating collagen expression in the heart *in vivo*, TSC-22 could be a potential target for fibrosis-preventing therapies.

Keywords: Cardiac hypertrophy, Heart failure, Pressure overload, Myocardial infarction

Background

Various stimuli such as increased mechanical stress, neurohumoral activation or myocardial injury initiate pathological alterations in the heart, referred to as cardiac remodelling [1]. Common features of pathological cardiac remodelling include alterations in cardiomyocyte size, modulation of the extracellular matrix (ECM), inflammation, and microvascular perturbations [1]. Cardiac remodelling leads to further deterioration of cardiac function, and eventually to heart failure, one of the leading causes of mortality and morbidity worldwide [1, 2].

At molecular level, cardiac remodelling is the result of altered gene expression that is regulated by the activation of numerous transcription factors including GATA-4, myocyte enhancer factor-2, Nkx2.5, serum response factor and SMADs [3]. Transcription factors are, in turn, regulated by several signalling pathways such as mitogen-activated kinases (MAPKs) p38, extracellular signal-regulated kinase (ERK) and c-Jun N-terminal kinase (JNK) [4, 5]. One of the key mediators involved in the pathological remodelling in cardiac hypertrophy and after myocardial infarction is the transforming growth factor beta (TGF-beta) [6], which regulates cardiomyocyte hypertrophy, fibroblast proliferation, inflammatory response and extracellular matrix metabolism through direct and indirect mechanisms [7, 8]. TGF-β also regulates several cardiac transcription factors including Smad 4, Smad 6/7 and cAMP response element-binding protein (CREB1) [6, 9]. Although it has been studied extensively, the role of transcriptional regulation of pathological cardiac remodelling is not yet fully understood.

* Correspondence: jaana.rysa@uef.fi
[1]Research Unit of Biomedicine (Pharmacology & Toxicology), University of Oulu, Oulu, Finland
[4]School of Pharmacy, Faculty of Health Sciences, University of Eastern Finland, Kuopio, Finland
Full list of author information is available at the end of the article

TSC-22 (TGF-β stimulated clone 22) is a member of leucine zipper proteins, first isolated as TGF-β responsive gene form mouse osteoblastic cells [10]. Although the DNA binding surface of TSC-22 differs from that of the other basic leucine zipper proteins, it can homodimerize and heterodimerize with other transcription factors such as SMADs [11–14], and it has transcriptional repression activity [11]. Several physiological roles for TSC-22 have been identified: TSC-22 is thought to be a tumour suppressor in several cancer cell lines and tumour tissue [15–21], regulating developmental processes in *Xenopus laevis* during gastrulation and in oogenesis of *Drosophila melanogaster* [14, 22], apoptosis [17, 21], and systemic cholesterol metabolism [23] as well as promoting cardiac myofibroblast differentiation and fibrosis [13]. TSC-22 is up-regulated by many stimuli, including different cytokines, fibroblast growth factor 2 (FGF2), and epidermal growth factor (EGF) [24]. In addition, elevated TSC-22 mRNA-levels have been reported in an experimental model of essential hypertension, in spontaneously hypertensive rats (SHRs) [25], and after experimental myocardial infarction in rats [26]. Thus, TSC-22 may have an important role in controlling the transcriptional response of cardiac remodelling.

Here we assessed TSC-22 expression levels in the heart and used adenovirus-mediated gene delivery in the normal rat heart in order to investigate the effects of TSC-22 on cardiac gene expression and function. In addition, we analysed the effect of TSC-22 overexpression on hypertrophic gene response in cultured neonatal rat ventricular myocytes (NRVMs). We demonstrated that multiple hypertrophic stimuli and post-MI remodelling regulate TSC-22 expression in the heart. Our data shows that TSC-22 has a role in regulating collagen *Col3a1* gene expression in the heart *in vivo*, suggesting it may be involved in the development of cardiac ECM remodelling.

Methods

Expression and purification of TSC-22 for antibody production

For TSC-22 (also known as TSC-22D1) protein production, the cDNA coding for rat TSC-22 (GeneBank accession number L25785) was subcloned into the *Nde*I-*Bam*HI site of pET-15b expression vector (Novagen/Merck, Darmstadt, Germany) containing an amino terminal $(His)_6$-tag. The construct was transformed into the *E. coli* BL21(DE3) cells and grown in LB-medium in the presence of ampicillin (100 μg/ml) at +37 °C. Protein expression was induced by 1 mM isopropyl b-D-thiogalactoside (IPTG) for 3 h, after which the cells were harvested, suspended in a lysis buffer (100 mM NaH_2PO_4, 10 mM Tris–HCl, 8 M urea, pH 8.0) and stored at −70 °C. The cells were melted and sonicated 10 times for 10 s (200–300 V). The soluble protein fraction was obtained by centrifuging at 10 000 × *g* for 30 min at +4 °C.

Recombinant protein containing a His-tag at the amino terminus was purified on a Ni-NTA-agarose (Qiagen, Venlo, Netherlands) according to the manufacturer's instructions. Briefly, the agarose was stirred with the soluble fraction of the *E. coli* supernatant for 2 h. The matrix was washed in the buffer (100 mM NaH_2PO_4, 10 mM Tris–HCl, 8 M urea, pH 6.3). Proteins were first eluted in the buffers containing 100 mM NaH_2PO_4, 10 mM Tris–HCl, 8 M urea, pH 5.9 and pH 4.5, respectively and continued in the buffer containing 100 mM NaH_2PO_4, 10 mM Tris–HCl, 8 M urea, 250 mM imidazole, pH 3.5.

Eluted proteins were concentrated with a Centricon Centrifugal Filter device (Millipore, Billerica, MA, USA) and separated with preparative SDS-PAGE. The gel was stained by 0.25 mM KCl [27] and TSC-22 was cut from the gel and eluted in a 3 ml buffer containing 20 mM Tris–HCl pH 8.0, 0.01 % SDS, 1 mM $CaCl_2$ at +37 °C overnight, after which the buffer was changed into phosphate-buffered saline (PBS) by PD-10 column (GE Healthcare, Little Chalfont, United Kingdom). The antibody against TSC-22 was produced in rabbits by Davids Biotechnology (Regensburg, Germany). TSC-22 protein was injected three different times for immunization, and rabbit serum antibody was purified by precipitation and affinity purification. The specificity of the TSC-22 antibody was tested with the pure TSC-22 protein used as an antigen.

Animals

Newborn, 2- to 4-day-old Sprague–Dawley rats of both sexes and male 2- to 3-month-old SD rats weighing from 250 to 300 g as well as 12-to-20-month-old spontaneously hypertensive rats (SHR) of the Okamoto-Aoki strain and age-matched Wistar-Kyoto (WKY) rats from the colony of the Centre of Experimental Animals at the University of Oulu, Finland, were used. The SHR strain was originally obtained from Møllegaards Avslaboratorium, Skensved, Denmark. All rats were kept in plastic cages with free access to tap water and regular rat chow in a room with a controlled 40 % humidity and a temperature of 22 °C. A 12 h light and 12 h dark environmental light cycle was maintained. All experimental protocols were approved by the Animal Use and Care Committee of the University of Oulu and the Provincial Government of Western Finland Department of Social Affairs and Health. The study conforms to the Guide for the Care and Use of Laboratory Animals published by the US National Institutes of Health.

Experimental design in conscious normotensive and hypertensive rats

The Sprague Dawley rats were anesthetized with 0.26 mg/kg fentanyl citrate, 8.25 mg/kg fluanisone and 4.1 mg/kg midazolam i.p., and instrumented for vehicle and drug infusions as previously described [25]. The experiments were started in conscious animals by measuring mean arterial pressure (MAP) and heart rate for 30 min before baseline hemodynamic measurements were made. Then arginine vasopressin (AVP) (Peninsula Laboratories Europe) at a dose of 0.05 mg/kg per minute or vehicle (0.9 % NaCl) was infused i.v. at 37.5 ml/min for 30 min and 4 h.

Angiotensin II (Sigma Chemicals) (33 μg/kg/h) or vehicle (0.9 % NaCl) was administered through subcutaneously implanted osmotic minipumps (Alzet, Durect Corporation, Cupertino, CA, USA) in conscious rats for 6, 12 and 72 h, and 2 weeks as described previously [25]. In a separate series of experiments, vehicle (0.9 % NaCl), Ang II (33 μg/kg/h), losartan (400 μg/kg/h) [25] (a generous gift from Merck), or Ang II in combination with losartan was administered for 6 h.

In addition, osmotic minipumps (Alzet) releasing metoprolol (Sigma-Aldrich, St. Louis, MO, USA) (1.5 mg/kg/h) or losartan (400 μg/kg/h) were placed subcutaneously in WKY and SHRs, as described above. At the end of experiments, the rats were decapitated, the thoracic cavity was opened, and the heart was removed, left ventricular samples were blotted dry, weighed, frozen in liquid nitrogen and stored at −70 °C for further analysis.

Experimental myocardial infarction

Myocardial infarction was produced by ligation of the left anterior descending coronary artery (LAD) [28]. The male Sprague–Dawley rats were anesthetized, a left thoracotomy and pericardial incision was made, and the LAD was ligated as previously described [29], producing left ventricular dilation, thinning of the anterior wall and hypertrophy of the posterior wall [29]. In a separate series of experiments, osmotic minipumps (Alzet) releasing metoprolol (Sigma-Aldrich) 1.5 mg/kg/h or losartan (400 μg/kg/h) were placed subcutaneously. The sham operated rats underwent the same surgical procedure without osmotic minipumps or ligation of LAD.

Recombinant adenovirus vectors and adenoviral gene transfer *in vivo*

The recombinant adenoviruses containing the coding regions of the constitutively active MKK3b (RAdMKK3bE) and wild-type (WT) p38α (RAdp38α) genes driven by the cytomegalovirus immediate early promoter were generated as described [30]. Recombinant replication-deficient adenovirus RAd*lacZ*, which contains the *Escherichia coli* β-galactosidase (*LacZ*) gene, was used as a control virus. The recombinant adenovirus AxCAmTSC-22 (deposited by Kazunari Yokoyama) and AxCALacZ (deposited by Izumu Saito) were provided by the DNA Bank, RIKEN BioResource Center (Tsukuba, Japan) with the support of National Bio-Resources Project of Ministry of Education, Culture, Sports, Science and Technology Japan (MEXT). The recombinant adenovirus harbouring mouse TSC-22 (TGF beta 1-inducible gene) cDNA AxCAmTSC-22 (hereinafter referred to as TSC-22) and AxCALacZ (hereinafter referred to as LacZ) expressing beta-galactosidase, used as a control virus, were under the control of a CAG promoter [31].

Adenovirus-mediated gene transfer into the left ventricle was performed as a local intramyocardial injection, as previously described [32]. Male Sprague–Dawley rats weighing 250–300 g were anesthetized with medetomidine hydrochloride (Domitor 250 μg/kg, i.p.) and ketamine hydrochloride (Ketamine 50 mg/kg, i.p.). A left thoracotomy and pericardial incision was made. Recombinant TSC-22 adenovirus with a dose of 7×10^9 pfu in a 100-μL volume was injected using a Hamilton precision syringe directly into the anterior wall of the left ventricle; the heart was then repositioned in the chest and the incision was closed. After the operation, the anaesthesia was partially antagonized with atipamezole hydrochloride (Antisedan 1.5 mg/kg, i.p.) and the rats were given buprenorphine hydrochloride (Temgesic, 0.05-0.2 mg/kg s.c.) for analgesia.

Echocardiography

Transthoracic echocardiography was performed using a commercially available Acuson Ultrasound System (SequoiaTM 512) and a 15-MHz linear transducer (15 L8) (Acuson, Mountain View, CA, USA) as previously described [29, 33]. Echocardiographic measurements were performed by a skilled sonographer blinded to the treatments. After echocardiography, the animals were sacrificed, their hearts were weighed and the tissue samples were immersed in liquid nitrogen and stored at −70 °C for later analysis.

Cell culture

Cell cultures of cardiac ventricular cells were isolated from 2-to-4 day old Sprague–Dawley rats as described [34]. The animals were killed by cervical dislocation and the ventricles were excised and cut into small pieces, and thereafter incubated 1–2 h at +37 °C in a solution containing 100 mM NaCl, 10 mM KCl, 1.2 mM KH_2PO_4, 4.0 mM $MgSO_4$, 50 mM taurine, 20 mM glucose, 10 mM Hepes, 2 mg/ml collagenase type 2 (Worthington, Lakewood, NJ, USA), 2 mg/ml pancreatin (Sigma-Aldrich, St Louis, MO, USA) and 1 % penicillin–streptomycin (PS). The detached cells were collected after incubation by centrifuging at 900 rpm for 5 min. The bottom layer of the pellet containing undamaged isolated cardiomyocytes was plated on 35 mm dishes at a density of $1.4 \times 10^5/cm^2$. The cells were cultured overnight in Dulbecco's modified Eagle's medium nutrient mixture F-12 ham with

L-glutamine (DMEM/F12) containing 10 % foetal bovine serum (FBS) and 1 % PS. Thereafter the cells were cultured in complete serum free medium (CSFM) containing DMEM/F12, 2.5 mg/ml bovine serum albumin, 1 μM insulin, 5.64 μg/ml transferrin, 32 nM selenium, 2.8 mM Na-pyruvate, 0.1 nM T_3 and 1 % PS. The cells were infected with adenoviruses 24 h after the cells were plated at the virus concentration of 2, 4 or 8 MOI (multiplicity of infection). Fresh CSFM was changed 24 h after the infection and cells were cultured in all 72 h before being washed twice with ice-cold PBS and stored at −70 °C. Endothelin-1 (ET-1) treatment was performed as described before [35, 36].

Isolation and analysis of RNA

Total RNA from tissue samples was isolated by the guanidine thiocyanate-CsCl method and from cultured cardiomyocytes with TRIzol Reagent according to the manufacturer's protocol (Invitrogen, CA, USA) by using the Phase Lock Gel system (Eppendorf AG, Hamburg, Germany) as previously described [37]. For Northern Blot analyses, 20 μg samples of RNA from LV tissue were separated on agarose–formaldehyde gel electrophoresis and transferred to nylon membranes (Osmonics Inc.). PCR-amplified Northern probes corresponding following genes: rat TSC-22 and 18S were random primer-labelled with [α^{32}P]dCTP, and the membranes were hybridized and washed as described previously [25]. The hybridization signals were normalized to 18S RNA quantified from the same samples.

Rat TSC-22, Atrial natriuretic peptide (ANP), B-type natriuretic peptide (BNP), interleukin-6 (IL-6), connective tissue growth factor (CTGF), plasminogen activator inhibitor-1 (PAI-1), fibronectin-1 (Fn-1), collagen type Iα1 (Col1a1) and type IIIα1 (col3a1), Bcl-2-associated X protein (Bax2), B-cell lymphoma 2A (Bcl2A) and 18S mRNA levels were measured by real time quantitative PCR using TaqMan chemistry on an ABI 7300 Sequence Detection System (Applied Biosystems, Foster City, CA, USA) as described previously [37]. The sequences of the forward and reverse primers and fluorogenic probes for RNA are given in Table 1. The results were normalized to 18S RNA quantified from the same samples.

Protein extraction

The tissue was broken in liquid nitrogen, and homogenized in a lysis buffer consisting of 20 mmol/L Tris (pH 7.5), 10 mmol/L NaCl, 0.1 mmol/L EDTA, 0.1 mmol/L EGTA, 1 mmol/L β-glycerophosphate, 1 mmol/L Na_3VO_4, 2 mmol/L benzamidine, 1 mmol/L PMSF, 50 mmol/L NaF, 1 mmol/L DTT and 10 μg/mL of each leupeptin, pepstatin and aprotinin as previously described [32, 37]. The tissue homogenates were centrifuged at 2000 rpm in +4 °C for 1 min. To separate the total protein fraction, 5× NEB was added to the tissue homogenate, following by centrifugation at 12,500 rpm for 20 min. The supernatant was stored in −70 °C until assayed.

Table 1 Sequences of primers and fluorogenic probes used in real time quantitative RT-qPCR analysis (sequences 5′ to 3′)

Gene	Forward Primer	Reverse Primer	Fluorogenic Probe
TSC-22	GCAGGAGAACAATC	TGCAGCTGGG	CCAGTCCGGAG
	TGTTGAAGAC	CCTGAAAC	CAGCTCGCC
ANP	GAAAAGCAAACTG	CCTACCCCCG	TCGCTGGCCCT
	AGGGCTCTG	AAGCAGCT	CGGAGCCT
BNP	TGGGCAGAAGATAG	ACAACCTCAG	CGGCGCAGTCA
	ACCGGA	CCCGTCACAG	GTCGCTTGG
IL-6	ATATGTTCTCAGGG	TGCATCATCGC	CAGAATTGCCATTGCA
	AGATCTTGGAA	TGTTCATACAA	CAACTCTTTTCTCA
CTGF	CGCCAACCGCAAGA	CACGGACCCA	CACTGCCAAAGA
	TTG	CCGAAGAC	TGGTGCACCCTG
PAI-1	GCTGACCACAGCAG	GTGCCCCTCTCA	CCCGGCAGCAGAT
	GGAAA	CTGATATTGAA	CCAAGATGCTAT
col1a1	CCCCTTGGTCTTGG	GCACGGAAAC	CTTTGCTTCCCAGATGT
	AGGAA	TCCAGCTGAT	CCTATGGCTATGATG
Fn-1	GCGAGGCAGGATC	CCAATCTTGTA	ACCATTGCAAAT
	AGCTG	GGACTGACCCC	CGCTGCCATGAA
Bax2	TCCCCCCGAGAGG	CCCAGTTGAAG	CCGGGTGGCAGCT
	TCTTCT	TTGCCATCA	GACATGTTTG
Bcl2A	GGAACTATATGG	AGGCTGAGCA	CGACCTCTGTTTG
	CCCCAGCAT	GGGTCTTCAG	ATTTCTCCTGGCTGTC
col3a1	AGCTGGCCTTCCTC	GCTGTTTTTGCAG	TTCCAGCCGG
	AGACTTC	TGGTATGTAATG	GCCTCCCAG
18S	TGGTTGCAAAGCT	AGTCAAATTA	CCTGGTGGTGC
	GAAACTTAAAG	AGCCGCAGGC	CCTTCCGTCA

TSC-22 transforming growth factor beta-stimulated clone 22; *ANP* atrial natriuretic peptide; *BNP* B-type natriuretic peptide; *IL-6* interleukin-6; *CTGF* connective tissue growth factor; *PAI-1* plasminogen activator inhibitor-1; *col1a1* collagen type Iα1; *Fn-1* fibronectin-1; *Bax2* Bcl-2-associated X protein; *Bcl2A* B-cell lymphoma 2A; *col3a1* collagen type IIIα1

To extract total protein from cultured cardiomyocytes, the cells were scraped in 100–150 μl of 1× NEB buffer containing protease-inhibitor cocktail (1:100 volume), phosphatase-inhibitor cocktail (1:100 volume) and 1 mM dithiothreitol (DTT) (1:1000 volume). Cells were vortexed for 20 s and centrifuged 12,500 rpm for 20 min at +4 °C. The supernatant was collected as the total protein fragment. The entire procedure was carried out at +4 °C. The supernatant was stored in −70 °C until assayed. Protein concentrations were determined by colorimetric assay (Bio-Rad Laboratories, Hercules, CA, USA).

Western blotting

Western blots were performed as previously described [35]. Briefly, 15–60 μg of protein was loaded onto a

SDS-PAGE gel and transferred to nitrocellulose filters. The membranes were blocked in 5 % non-fat milk and incubated with anti-TSC-22 polyclonal antibody (dilution 1:500 in 0.5 % milk-TBS-Tween) overnight. After incubation with secondary anti-rabbit antibody (Cell Signaling Technology, Danvers, MA, USA) at the dilution of 1:2000, the protein amount was detected by ECL Plus (GE Healthcare Life Sciences). For Odyssey detection, the membranes were blocked in Odyssey Blocking Buffer – TBS (1:1) and incubated with anti-TSC-22 polyclonal antibody or anti-GAPDH (glyceraldehyde-3-phosphate dehydrogenase) (Millipore, MA, USA) overnight. After incubation with secondary Alexa Fluor anti-rabbit or anti-mouse antibody (Invitrogen), the protein levels were detected using Odyssey Infrared Detection.

Histological analysis

For immunohistochemical analysis, the hearts were fixed in 10 % buffered formalin solution. Transverse sections of the left ventricle were embedded in paraffin, and 5-μm-thick sections were cut from the midsection of the heart, at the level of the papillary muscles. Sections were deparaffinised in xylene and dehydrated in graded ethanol, and to identify cellular localization of TSC-22, incubated with specific anti-TSC-22 polyclonal antibody at a dilution of 1:500. The primary antibody was detected by a peroxidase conjugated Dako REAL™ EnVision™ Detection System, Peroxidase/DAB kit (Dako, Glostrup, Denmark) according to the manufacturer's instructions, and the samples were counterstained with hematoxylin and eosin. All measurements were performed by persons blinded to the treatments.

Human LV tissue samples

LV samples were obtained from explanted human hearts from 4 patients with cardiomyopathy (2 dilated, 1 idiopathic, 1 hypertrophic) undergoing heart transplantation. Non-diseased donor hearts unsuitable for transplant were used to obtain control myocardial tissue ($n = 2$). All tissues were obtained with signed informed consent of the subjects. The project was approved by the local Ethics Committee (Ethical permission number: 5012-0/2011-EKU142/PI/11–Semmelweis University, Hungary) and conducted in accordance with the guidelines of the Declaration of Helsinki.

Statistics

Statistical analysis was performed by unpaired Student's *t*-test or One-way Analysis of variance (ANOVA) followed by a least significant difference (LSD) post hoc test for multiple comparisons. A value of $P<0.05$ was considered to be statistically significant. The results are expressed as mean ± standard error of the mean (SEM).

Results

Cardiac remodelling in chronic hypertension and after experimental myocardial infarction modulates TSC-22 gene expression

DNA-microarray studies have previously shown that TSC-22 mRNA levels are elevated both in old SHRs [33] and after experimental MI in rats [26]. First, we examined TSC-22 protein levels, which were higher in 12-to-20-month-old SHR (1.6-fold, $P<0.05$) compared with age-matched normotensive WKY rats (Fig. 1a). Then we investigated the induction of TSC-22 in the heart more carefully after MI. Similarly to gene expression profiles of Stanton et al. [26], LV TSC-22 mRNA levels were up-regulated 4 weeks after MI (Fig. 1b). In addition, a significant increase in mRNA levels was seen already on day 1 following MI when compared to sham-operated animals (4.1-fold, $P<0.001$), indicating that TSC-22 induction in the post-infarction cardiac remodelling process is rapid and persistent. Similar profiles to mRNA, in the degree and the time course of the induction, were seen in the protein up-regulation, as assessed by Western blot analysis (Fig. 1c). TSC-22 mRNA and proteins were also found to be expressed in the left ventricle of control human hearts and in patients with cardiomyopathy, but there were no changes in the expression levels between failing and control hearts (data not shown).

TSC-22 gene expression is induced in the adult heart with acute pressure overload

Next, we studied the effect of acute and chronic pressure overload on LV TSC-22 expression. Ang II increased TSC-22 mRNA levels from 6 h to 2 weeks, the greatest increase (12.0-fold, $P<0.001$) being observed after 6 h of Ang II infusion (Fig. 2a). Accordingly, *in vivo* administration of AVP induced a small, but significant increase in TSC-22 already after 1 h, and at 4 h, TSC-22 mRNA levels were markedly elevated (5.5-fold, $P<0.001$) (Fig. 2b). Moreover, the Ang II type 1-receptor antagonist losartan completely abolished the changes in TSC-22 gene expression induced by Ang II in the left ventricle (Fig. 2c).

The effect of long-term treatment of heart failure with metoprolol and hypertension with metoprolol or losartan on TSC-22 expression

Next, we aimed to characterize whether TSC-22 expression changes in response to a treatment with a beta-blocker metoprolol or losartan in left ventricular hypertrophy or heart failure. First, we characterized the LV TSC-22 gene expression in rats treated with metoprolol during the remodelling in post-MI [38]. Post-infarction treatment with metoprolol improved LV systolic and diastolic function and attenuated LV remodelling as previously described [38]. After MI, LV TSC-22 mRNA levels were increased 2.8-fold ($P < 0.001$) (Fig. 3a). Metoprolol

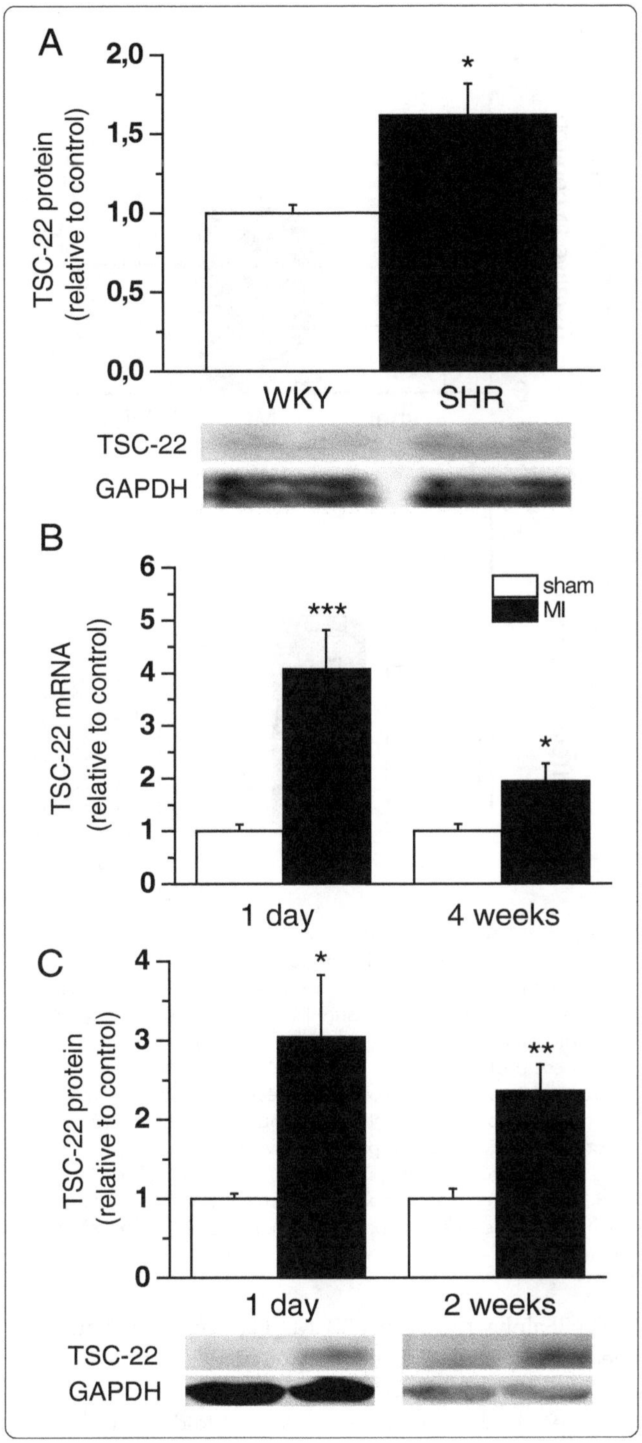

Fig. 1 Effects of cardiac remodelling on chronic hypertension and, after experimental myocardial infarction (MI), on transforming growth factor beta-stimulated clone 22 (TSC-22) expression. **a** Left ventricular (LV) tissue TSC-22 total protein levels were analysed by Western blot from 12 and 20 months old Wistar Kyoto (WKY) and spontaneously hypertensive rat (SHR) hearts ($n = 5$). Open bars represent WKY and solid bars SHR *$P<0.05$ versus WKY (Student's *t*-test). The effect of MI on LV tissue TSC-22 mRNA levels (**b**) measured by Northern blot or RT-PCR and TSC-22 protein levels (**c**) analysed by Western blot ($n = 6–8$). Open bars represent sham and solid bars MI *$P<0.05$, **$P<0.01$, ***$P<0.001$ versus sham (Student's *t*-test). The results are expressed as mean ± SEM. Representative Western blots are shown

administration for 2 weeks via osmotic minipumps reduced LV TSC-22 mRNA levels by 32 % ($P<0.05$). Next, we infused metoprolol for two weeks in 12-month-old SHRs. Metoprolol treatment lowered the heart beat and reduced enlargement of LV end-diastolic dimension (7.7 ± 0.1 in SHR vs. 8.5 ± 0.1 in SHR treated with metoprolol; $P<0.001$). Again, metoprolol reduced significantly the TSC-22 mRNA levels in metoprolol-treated SHRs when compared with untreated SHRs (Fig. 3b). A similar decrease in TSC-22 gene expression was also seen after 2 weeks of losartan infusion in SHRs (Fig. 3b), when reduced thickness of the LV wall was seen in losartan-treated SHRs compared to untreated SHRs (interventricular septal thickness −15.4 %, $P<0.001$ and left ventricular posterior wall thickness in diastole −18.2 %, $P<0.05$).

Signalling pathways regulating TSC-22 gene expression

We determined the cellular mechanisms involved in the regulation of TSC-22 gene expression by testing the effect of hypertrophic agonist ET-1 on TSC-22 mRNA levels in neonatal rat ventricular myocytes (NRVMs). ET-1 (100 nM) significantly increased TSC-22 gene expression with maximal mRNA levels at 12 h (2.7–fold, $P<0.001$) (Fig. 4a) and protein levels at 24 h (4.7-fold, $P<0.001$) (Fig. 4b). Next, we investigated intracellular signalling pathways mediating ET-1 induced TSC-22 gene expression by focusing on MAPKs, since all MAPK pathways are key signalling routes known to be activated in the heart in response to hypertrophic stimuli including ET-1 [4]. The neonatal rat ventricular myocytes were exposed to kinase inhibitors SB203580 (10 μM) or PD98059 (10 μM), and the cells were treated with 100 nM ET-1 for 1 h. Neither PD98059 (Fig. 4c) nor SB203580 (Fig. 4d) had significant effect on ET-1 –induced increase in TSC-22 mRNA levels in NRVMs. However, the p38α and p38β MAPK inhibitor SB203580 significantly increased TSC-22 mRNA levels in NRVMs (Fig. 4d).

Finally, in order to determine whether p38 MAPKs regulate cardiac TSC-22 gene expression *in vivo*, adenoviruses expressing constitutively active MKK3bE and

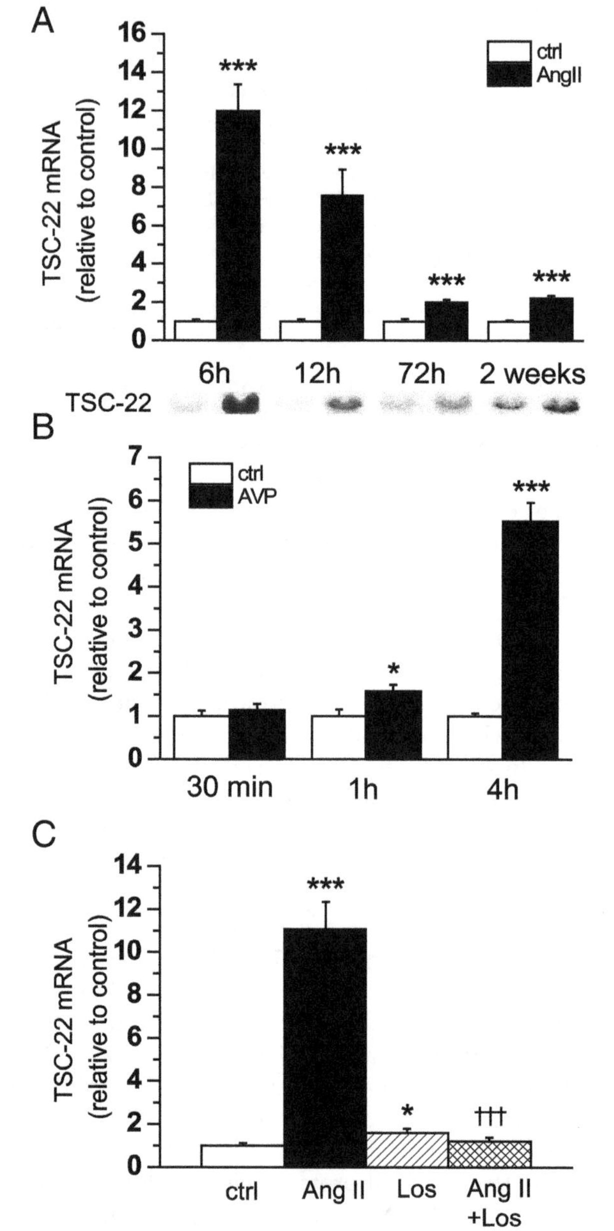

Fig. 2 The effect of acute and chronic pressure overload on transforming growth factor beta-stimulated clone 22 (TSC-22) gene expression. **a** The effect of angiotensin II (Ang II) administration (33 μg/kg/h) on left ventricular (LV) TSC-22 mRNA levels assessed by Northern blot analysis in rats (n = 6–8). Open bars represent control and black bars Ang II ***P <0.001 versus control (Student's t-test). **b** TSC-22 mRNA levels after arginine vasopressin (AVP) infusion (n = 9). Open bars represent control and solid bars AVP *P <0.05, ***P <0.001 versus control (Student's t-test). **c** The effect of Ang II and AT_1-receptor antagonist losartan (Los) on LV TSC-22 mRNA levels at 6 h (n = 5–8). *P <0.05, ***P <0.001 versus control. †††P <0.001 versus Ang II (one-way ANOVA followed by least significance difference post hoc test). The results are expressed as mean ± SEM. Representative Northern blots are shown

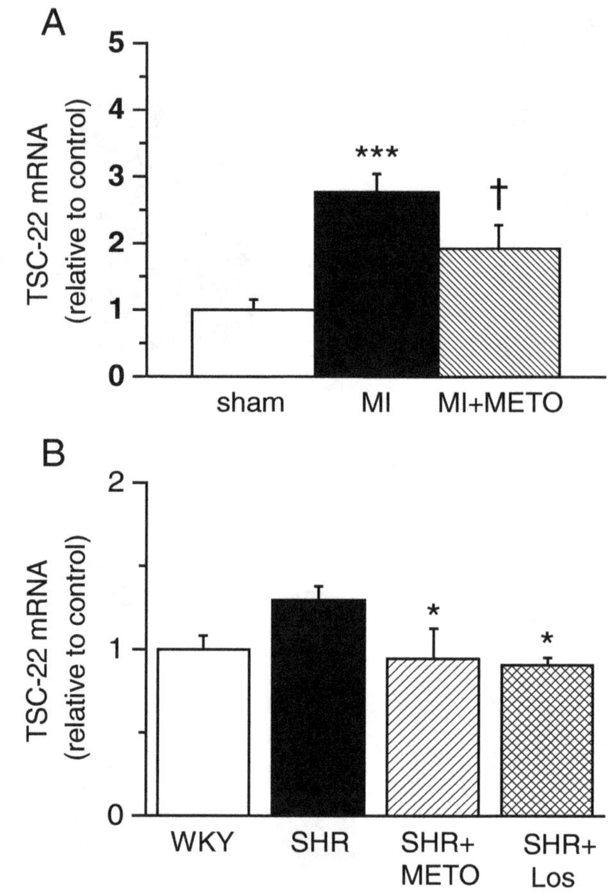

Fig. 3 The effect of long-term treatment of heart failure and hypertension with metoprolol on transforming growth factor beta-stimulated clone 22 (TSC-22) expression. **a** Left ventricular (LV) TSC-22 mRNA levels measured by RT-PCR from rats 2 weeks after myocardial infarction (MI) and after metoprolol (METO) treatment post-MI (n = 7-8). ***P <0.001 versus sham. †P <0.001 versus MI (one-way ANOVA followed by least significance difference post hoc test). **b** LV TSC-22 mRNA levels from 12-month-old Wistar Kyoto (WKY) rats, untreated spontaneously hypertensive rats (SHR) and SHRs treated with metoprolol (METO) or losartan (Los) for 14 days (n = 5-6). *P <0.05 versus untreated SHR (one-way ANOVA followed by least significance difference post hoc test). The results are expressed as mean ± SEM

WT p38alpha to cause p38 MAPK-overexpression were injected into the LV free wall of adult Sprague–Dawley rats. Adenoviral p38 MAPK overexpression significantly increased both TSC-22 mRNA (1.8-fold, P<0.01) and protein levels (4.1-fold, P<0.01) at day 3 following gene transfer (Fig. 4e-f).

The role of TSC-22 in regulating cardiac gene expression

In order to study the direct myocardial effects of TSC-22 in regulating cardiac gene expression, we established an *in vivo* gene transfer protocol to locally increase TSC-22 levels in the adult rat heart. First, the efficiency and functionality of the adenovirus gene transfer was

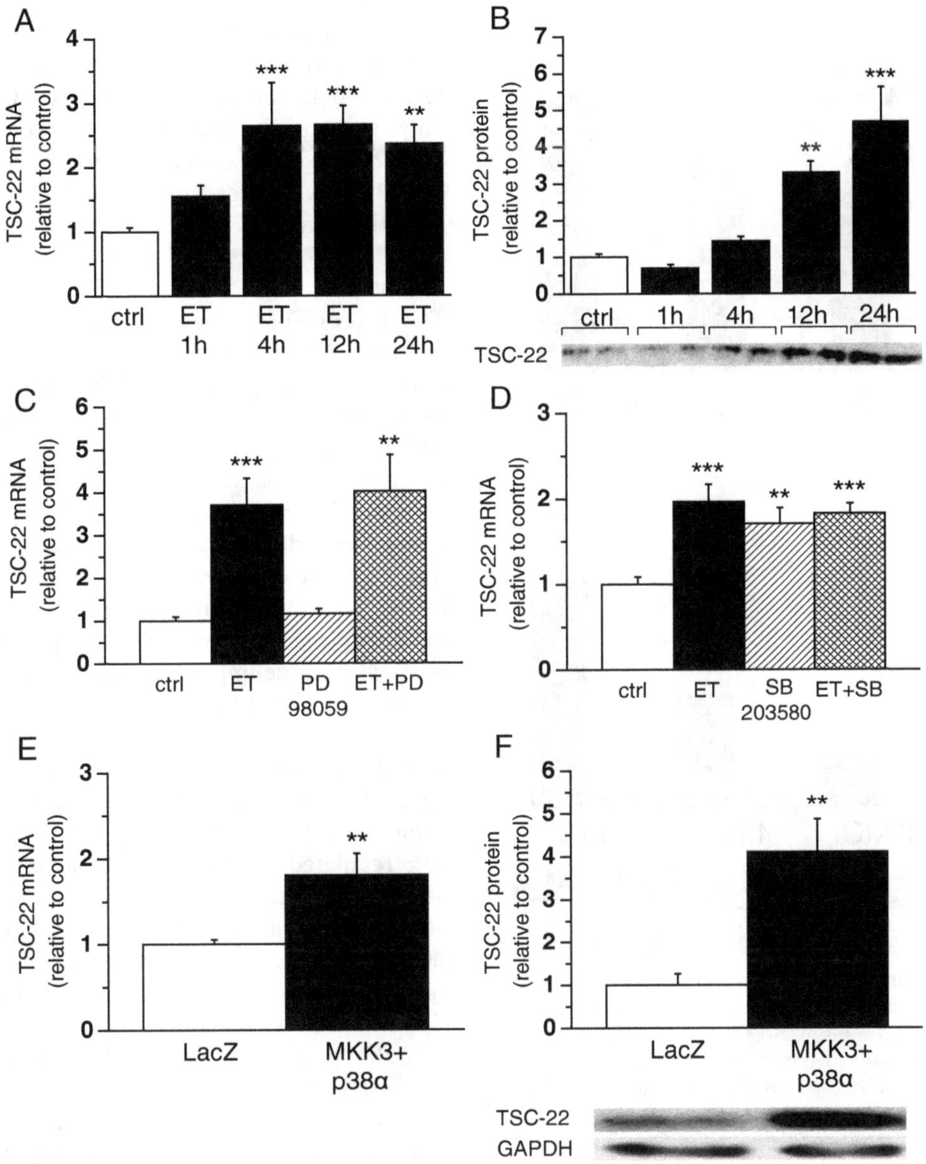

Fig. 4 Signalling pathways regulating transforming growth factor beta-stimulated clone 22 (TSC-22) gene expression. Cultured neonatal rat ventricular myocytes (NRVMs) were treated with endothelin-1 (ET, 100 nM) for 1, 4, 12 and 24 h. **a** TSC-22 mRNA levels were measured by RT-PCR ($n = 9–12$ from three independent experiments) **b**) and TSC-22 total protein levels were determined by Western blot ($n = 4$). Open bars represent control and solid bars ET **$P < 0.01$, ***$P < 0.001$ versus control (one-way ANOVA followed by least significance difference post hoc test). TSC-22 mRNA levels in NRVMs exposed to kinase inhibitor (**c**) PD98059 (10 μM) or **d**) SB203580 (10 μM), and treated with 100 nM ET for 1 h ($n = 8–9$, from three independent experiments). **$P < 0.01$, ***$P < 0.001$ versus control (Student's *t*-test). TSC-22 **e**) mRNA levels measured by Northern blot and **f**) total protein levels analysed by Western blot in left ventricle (LV) of Sprague–Dawley (SD)-rats after adenovirus induced MKK3bE and WT p38alpha overexpression at day 3 ($n = 7–10$). Open bars represent LacZ and solid bars MKK3bE and WT p38alpha **$P < 0.01$ versus LacZ (Student's *t*-test). The results are expressed as mean ± SEM. Representative Western blots are shown

studied by transducing the cardiomyocyte cell cultures with TSC-22 adenovirus. Adenovirus transduction markedly increased both TSC-22 mRNA and protein levels at the virus amounts of 2, 4 and 8 MOI in a dose-dependent manner (Fig. 5a, b).

Next, the effect of TSC-22 gene delivery on cardiac function was studied *in vivo* [32]. TSC-22 mRNA levels were increased in response to adenoviral TSC-22 overexpression at three days up to 2 weeks (7.7-fold, $P < 0.001$ and 1.7-fold, $P < 0.01$, respectively) following injections (Fig. 6a). Similarly, the induction in TSC-22 protein levels was seen 3 days after TSC-22 gene transfer (Fig. 6b). TSC-22 gene transfer had no significant effect on LV dimensions or cardiac function as assessed by echocardiography (Table 2).

To evaluate the localization of TSC-22, we performed immunohistochemical studies of TSC-22 overexpressing

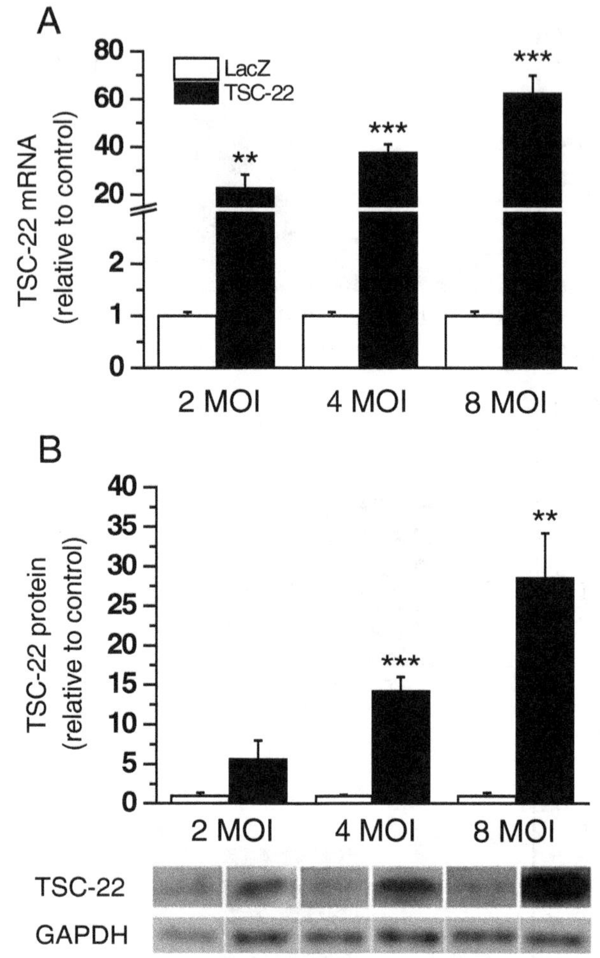

Fig. 5 Effects of transforming growth factor beta-stimulated clone 22 (TSC-22) overexpression in cultured neonatal rat ventricular myocytes (NRVMs). TSC-22 **a**) mRNA levels measured by RT-PCR ($n = 8–12$) or **b**) total protein levels determined by Western blot analysis ($n = 4$) from cultured NRVMs transduced with TSC-22 or LacZ adenovirus for 48 h at the virus amount of 2 MOI, 4 MOI and 8 MOI. $^{**}P < 0.01$, $^{***}P < 0.001$ versus LacZ (Student's *t*-test). The results are expressed as mean ± SEM. Representative Western blots are shown

hearts and LacZ injected control hearts. At 3 days, TSC-22 immunohistochemistry showed a very strong cytoplasmic staining that localized to the endothelium of myocardial capillaries at the injection site (Fig. 6c). In addition, some myocytes in the inflammation area of TSC-22 overexpressing hearts displayed cytoplasmic and nuclear positivity in TSC-22 immunostaining. In control hearts, there was also some positivity in the myocytes of inflammation areas, but this was weaker than in TSC-22 overexpressing hearts, and no remarkable endothelial positivity could be seen.

Next, we determined the influence of TSC-22 gene transfer on expression of several well-established markers of cardiac hypertrophy, fibrosis and apoptosis. TSC-22 gene delivery did not have an influence on expression levels of natriuretic peptides (ANP and BNP), inflammatory and ECM modulatory factors (IL-6, CTGF, PAI-1, Fn-1, col1a1) or apoptosis (Bax2, Bcl2A). The only statistically significant difference between the TSC-22 and LacZ-treated groups was in increased col3a1 gene expression levels 2 weeks after TSC-22 gene delivery (Fig. 6d).

Discussion

TGF-β is one of the key mediators both in the embryonic development of the heart and a number of cardiac diseases such as post-MI remodelling and pressure overload hypertrophy [7, 8]. TGF-β activates transcription factors such as SMAD proteins, and TSC-22. TSC-22 is suggested to have functions in controlling tumorigenesis, apoptosis, cholesterol homeostasis, cardiac fibrosis as well as development and differentiation processes [14–23]. Overall in this study, we extended knowledge of the role of TSC-22 in the heart. We found that TSC-22 gene expression is rapidly up-regulated by multiple hypertrophic stimuli and post-MI remodelling in the heart. We showed that both losartan and metoprolol treatments reduced left ventricular TSC-22 gene expression levels. We also observed that growth-promoting factor ET-1, activated TSC-22 mRNA and protein expression in cultured neonatal ventricular myocytes, and that p38MAPK signalling regulated cardiac TSC-22 expression *in vivo*. By using local intramyocardial adenovirus-mediated gene delivery, we evaluated the effect of TSC-22 overexpression on cardiac gene expression, showing that TSC-22 appears to have a role in regulating *col3a1* gene expression in the heart.

In the present study, we showed that TSC-22 gene expression was rapidly up-regulated in response to AVP- and Ang II-infused pressure overload, mimicking the expression patterns of immediate-early genes such as *Egr-1, c-jun* and *c-fos* in response to hemodynamic stress [39]. Elevated mRNA levels have previously been described by chronic pressure overload in the left ventricle of 20-month-old SHRs and at 2 to 16 weeks after experimental myocardial infarction in the rat [26, 33]. Altogether, the data implies that TSC-22 is up-regulated throughout the time course of cardiac remodelling suggesting it has a constitutive role in activating cardiac remodelling-related gene expression. However, although TSC-22 was expressed in the human heart both at mRNA and protein level, it was not up-regulated in patients with end-stage heart failure. Even though we cannot rule out the species difference (human vs. rodent), one possibility is that elevated amounts of TSC-22 are needed for controlling the transcriptional response of the active remodelling process and in the functional deterioration but no longer at the failing stage.

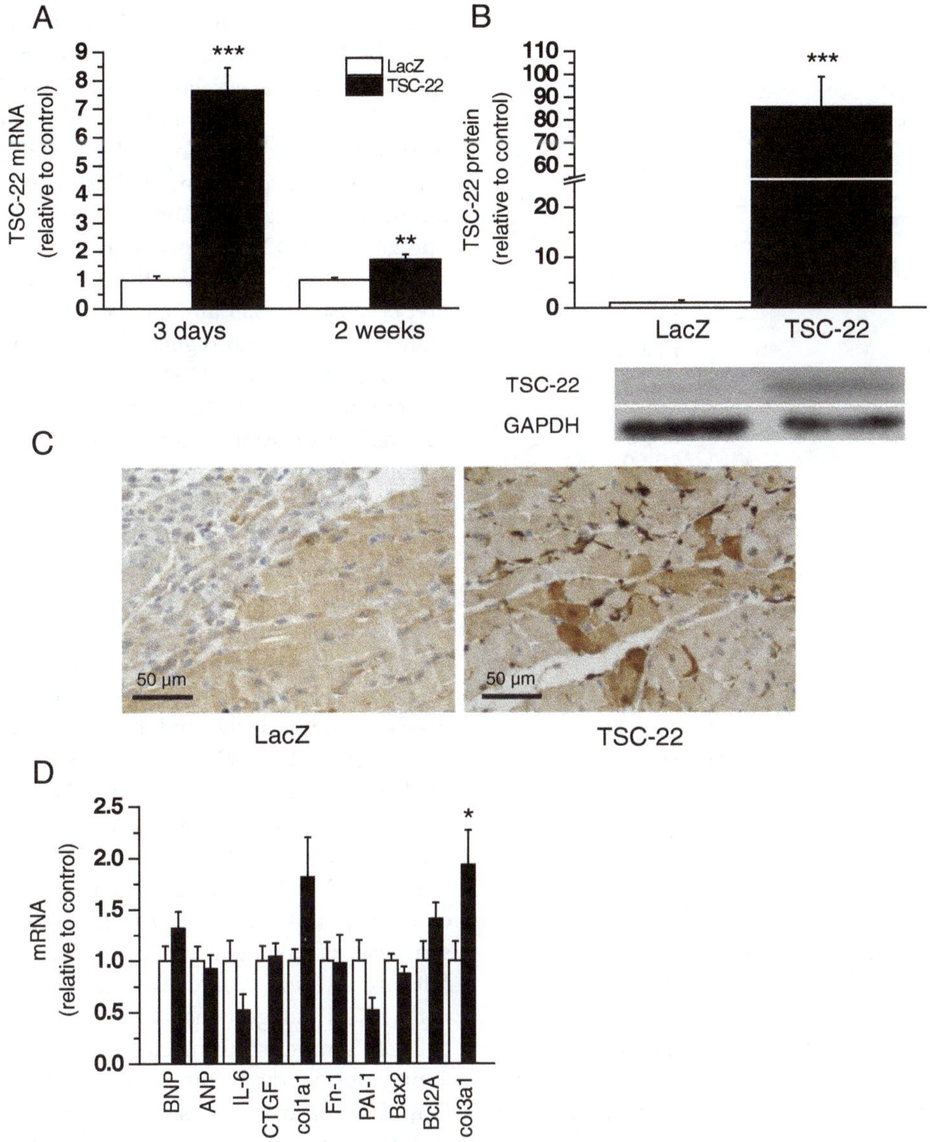

Fig. 6 Effects of adenovirus-mediated transforming growth factor beta-stimulated clone 22 (TSC-22) gene delivery in normal rat hearts. TSC-22 **a** mRNA levels measured by RT-PCR 3 days or 2 weeks ($n = 5$–8) and **b** total protein levels analysed by Western blot ($n = 8$) 3 days after gene delivery in left ventricular (LV) tissue samples of Sprague–Dawley (SD)-rat hearts. **c** Localization of TSC-22 at cellular level was studied by immunohistochemical staining against TSC-22 at day 3 after gene transfer. **d** mRNA levels of B-type natriuretic peptide (BNP), atrial natriuretic peptide (ANP), interleukin-6 (IL-6), connective tissue growth factor (CTGF), collagen type Iα1 (col1a1), fibronectin-1 (Fn-1), plasminogen activator inhibitor-1 (PAI-1), Bcl-2-associated X protein (Bax2), B-cell lymphoma 2A (Bcl2A) and collagen type IIIα1(col3a1) measured by RT-PCR from LV of SD-rat hearts 2 weeks after gene delivery ($n = 5$). *$P < 0.05$, **$P < 0.01$, ***$P < 0.001$ versus LacZ (Student's t-test). The results are expressed as mean ± SEM. Representative Western blots are shown

Cardiac remodelling after myocardial infarction and in hypertensive hypertrophy is an important target for drug treatment. In our study, both beta-blocker and ATR-antagonist treatment reduced left ventricular TSC-22 gene expression levels. Several studies suggest that there is an association between TGF-β1 and both the renin-angiotensin-aldosterone and the beta-adrenergic systems [7, 8, 40]. Ang II induces TGF-β1 expression in cardiac myocytes and fibroblasts *in vitro* [7, 8, 40]. TGF-β1 is implicated in AngII-induced cardiac hypertrophy and beta-adrenergic signalling in the heart *in vivo* [41–43]. Furthermore, TGF-β1 has been shown to modulate beta-adrenergic receptors in various cell types [8, 44]. However, in TGF-β1 transgenic mice chronic β-adrenoceptor blockade was able to reverse the structural and functional changes of the heart, but treatment with the AT1-receptor antagonist losartan was not [45]. In our study, using the rat chronic pressure overload model, both

Table 2 Effect of intramyocardial TSC-22 gene delivery on cardiac function in the normal adult rat heart

Variable	Group	TSC-22 3 days	TSC-22 2 weeks
Interventricular septum diastole (mm)	LacZ	1.9 ± 0.1	2.0 ± 0.1
	TSC-22	2.1 ± 0.1	2.0 ± 0.1
Interventricular septum systole (mm)	LacZ	2.6 ± 0.1	2.5 ± 0.2
	TSC-22	2.7 ± 0.2	2.8 ± 0.2
Left ventricle diastole (mm)	LacZ	7.6 ± 0.3	8.6 ± 0.1
	TSC-22	7.2 ± 0.3	8.7 ± 0.2
Left ventricle systole (mm)	LacZ	5.1 ± 0.3	6.1 ± 0.3
	TSC-22	4.7 ± 0.3	6.1 ± 0.3
Posterior wall distole (mm)	LacZ	2.3 ± 0.2	1.6 ± 0.1
	TSC-22	2.0 ± 0.3	1.5 ± 0.1
Posterior wall systole (mm)	LacZ	2.1 ± 0.2	2.3 ± 0.2
	TSC-22	2.1 ± 0.1	2.3 ± 0.1
Ejection fraction (%)	LacZ	66.7 ± 2.3	58.2 ± 4.5
	TSC-22	69.1 ± 3.0	62.8 ± 3.0
Fractional shortening (%)	LacZ	32.8 ± 1.7	27.4 ± 2.7
	TSC-22	34.7 ± 2.5	30.3 ± 2.0
IVRT	LacZ	no data	24.8 ± 2.2
	TSC-22	no data	25.0 ± 1.6
E/A-ratio	LacZ	no data	5.1 ± 0.8
	TSC-22	no data	2.7 ± 0.6*
		$n = 7–8$	$n = 5$

Adenoviral gene construct expressing TSC-22 or LacZ were injected into LV free wall and echocardiographic measurements were performed at 3 days and 2 weeks after gene transfer. The results are expressed as mean ± SEM. *$P < 0.05$ versus LacZ (Student's *t*-test). IVRT, isovolumic relaxation time

betablocker metoprolol and AT1R antagonist losartan caused a reduction of TSC-22 gene expression, which could be due to the beneficial effects of these drugs on the development of cardiac fibrosis [46–48]. In SHR ventricular remodelling, cardiac hypertrophy is associated with an increase in fibrosis [49, 50], and it has been shown that endogenous AngII, mediated by AT1 receptors, plays a role in the formation of fibrosis e.g. by stimulating of TGF-β1-synthesis [7, 8, 40]. The effect of the AT1 receptor antagonist on TSC-22 gene expression was also observed in response to acute pressure overload, which can also be due to the inhibition of an Ang II-induced increase in blood pressure. So, it is likely that the effects of losartan on TSC-22 expression are explained by multiple mechanisms.

Almost nothing is known about the mechanisms and signalling pathways that regulate cardiac TSC-22 gene expression. We observed that ET-1 activated TSC-22 mRNA and protein expression in cultured neonatal ventricular myocytes. In our study, no ERK inhibitor PD98059 or p38 inhibitor SB203580 had an effect on ET-1-mediated activation of TSC-22 gene expression in cardiac myocytes. In fact, SB203580 alone was able to increase TSC-22 levels significantly. In addition, the role of p38 MAPK as a regulator of TSC-22 expression was studied in the adult heart *in vivo*. Since adenovirus-mediated overexpression of p38 MAPK *in vivo* increased TSC-22 gene expression, our results suggest that cardiac remodelling after MI and in hypertensive hypertrophy upregulates TSC-22 expression in the heart via the p38 MAPK pathway. However, the results are difficult to interpret because the p38 inhibitor SB203580 did not alter ET-1 induced TSC-22 up-regulation *in vitro*, which might be due to the fact that SB203580 by itself at the dose used in cell culture was able to increase TSC-22 gene expression. Although expression information alone is not sufficient to establish firm functional associations, the increased expression in the p38 MAPK overexpressed hearts exhibiting fibrosis and infiltration of inflammatory cells [32] supports previous findings that the TSC-22 may contribute to the development of cardiac fibrosis [13].

A key finding of our present study is that TSC-22 gene delivery in the adult rat heart regulates collagen synthesis. TSC-22 overexpression *in vivo* increased *col3a1* gene expression significantly, and there was a similar trend in col1a1 mRNA levels. In previous studies, lentivirus-mediated overexpression of TSC-22 enhanced the TGFβ -induced expression of a- collagen I in cultured rat fibroblasts [13] and in kidney cells, TSC-22 was shown to regulate col1a2 [51]. Collagens type I and III are major constituents of cardiac ECM [52], and in fibrosis e.g. the synthesis of collagen and degradation of collagen scaffold are altered. Our data together with previous findings [13, 51] suggest that TSC-22 has a role in regulating collagen synthesis during cardiac remodelling. Contrary to a previous study using neonatal rat cardiac fibroblasts [13], TSC-22 overexpression did not have any effect on PAI-1 or fibronectin, which may due to the cell type specific differences in the regulation of gene expression. Similarly to a previous study [53], TSC-22 was located in both nuclear and cytoplasmic regions, indicating that TSC-22 might have an effect on cardiac structure by regulating ECM-modulating genes at transcriptional level.

To summarize, we studied the TSC-22 expression during cardiac modelling in post-MI and hypertensive hypertrophy. We noticed that TSC-22 expression is rapidly increased in response to pressure overload and myocardial injury, and elevated expression levels are sustained until the failing phase of heart failure. Our analysis provides new insights into the transcriptional regulation of cardiac remodelling by showing that TSC-22 appears to have a role in regulating collagen 3a1 expression in the heart *in vivo*. In accordance with previous findings, our data suggests that TSC-22 could be a target for preventing the formation of cardiac fibrosis.

Conclusions

In conclusion, TSC-22 expression in the rat heart is regulated by multiple hypertrophic stimuli and post-MI remodelling. Our data suggests that TSC-22 might regulate collagen synthesis in the heart *in vivo* and could be a potential target for fibrosis-preventing therapies.

Abbreviations

AngII: Angiotensin II; col: Collagen; ET-1: Endothelin-1; LV: Left ventricle; MAPK: Mitogen activated kinase; MI: Myocardial infarction; NRVM: Neonatal rat ventricular myocytes; SHR: Spontaneously hypertensive rat; TGF-β: Transforming growth factor –β; TSC-22: TGF-β-stimulated clone 22; WKY: Wistar Kyoto.

Competing interests

The authors declare that they have no competing interests.

Authors' contributions

Conceived and designed the experiments: AK, JA, HR, JR; Performed the experiments: AK, JA, EK, JR. Analysed the data: AK, JA, JN, EM, EK, HR, JR. Contributed to the writing of the manuscript: AK, HR, JR. All authors read and approved the final manuscript.

Acknowledgements

We thank Dr J. Miyazaki at Osaka University, Japan for the CAG promoter. This work was supported by grants from the Academy of Finland (JR, grant number 276747; HR, grant number 266661), Aarne Koskelo Foundation, Finnish Cultural Foundation, the Finnish Foundation for Cardiovascular Research and the Sigfrid Jusélius Foundation. We thank Marja Arbelius, Pirjo Korpi, Kati Lampinen, Kaisa Penttilä and Sirpa Rutanen for their expert technical assistance.

Author details

[1]Research Unit of Biomedicine (Pharmacology & Toxicology), University of Oulu, Oulu, Finland. [2]Department of Pathology, Institute of Diagnostics, Oulu University Hospital, University of Oulu, Oulu, Finland. [3]Division of Pharmacology and Pharmacotherapy, Faculty of Pharmacy, University of Helsinki, Helsinki, Finland. [4]School of Pharmacy, Faculty of Health Sciences, University of Eastern Finland, Kuopio, Finland.

References

1. Mann DL, Barger PM, Burkhoff D. Myocardial recovery and the failing heart: myth, magic, or molecular target? J Am Coll Cardiol. 2012;60:2465–72.
2. Go AS, Mozaffarian D, Roger VL, Benjamin EJ, Berry JD, Blaha MJ, et al. Heart disease and stroke statistics–2014 update: a report from the American Heart Association. Circulation. 2014;129:e28–292.
3. Oka T, Xu J, Molkentin JD. Re-employment of developmental transcription factors in adult heart disease. Semin Cell Dev Biol. 2007;18:117–31.
4. Rose BA, Force T, Wang Y. Mitogen-activated protein kinase signaling in the heart: angels versus demons in a heart-breaking tale. Physiol Rev. 2010;90:1507–46.
5. Akazawa H, Komuro I. Roles of cardiac transcription factors in cardiac hypertrophy. Circ Res. 2003;92:1079–88.
6. Dobaczewski M, Chen W, Frangogiannis NG. Transforming growth factor (TGF)-beta signaling in cardiac remodeling. J Mol Cell Cardiol. 2011;51:600–6.
7. Bujak M, Frangogiannis NG. The role of TGF-beta signaling in myocardial infarction and cardiac remodeling. Cardiovasc Res. 2007;74:184–95.
8. Rosenkranz S. TGF-beta1 and angiotensin networking in cardiac remodeling. Cardiovasc Res. 2004;63:423–32.
9. Liu G, Ding W, Neiman J, Mulder KM. Requirement of Smad3 and CREB-1 in mediating transforming growth factor-beta (TGF beta) induction of TGF beta 3 secretion. J Biol Chem. 2006;281:29479–90.
10. Shibanuma M, Kuroki T, Nose K. Isolation of a gene encoding a putative leucine zipper structure that is induced by transforming growth factor beta 1 and other growth factors. J Biol Chem. 1992;267:10219–24.
11. Kester HA, Blanchetot C, Hertog J, Van der Saag PT, Van der Burg B. Transforming growth factor- beta -stimulated clone-22 is a member of a family of leucine zipper proteins that can homo- and heterodimerize and has transcriptional repressor activity. J Biol Chem. 1999;274:27439–47.
12. Choi SJ, Moon JH, Ahn YW, Ahn JH, Kim DU, Han TH. Tsc-22 enhances TGF-beta signaling by associating with Smad4 and induces erythroid cell differentiation. Mol Cell Biochem. 2005;271:23–8.
13. Yan X. TSC-22 promotes transforming growth factor beta-mediated cardiac myofibroblast differentiation by antagonizing Smad7 activity. Mol Cell Biol. 2011;31:3700–9.
14. Dobens LL, Hsu T, Twombly V, Gelbart WM, Raftery LA, Kafatos FC. The Drosophila bunched gene is a homologue of the growth factor stimulated mammalian TSC-22 sequence and is required during oogenesis. Mech Dev. 1997;65:197–208.
15. Kawamata H, Nakashiro K, Uchida D, Hino S, Omotehara F, Yoshida H, et al. Induction of TSC-22 by treatment with a new anti-cancer drug, vesnarinone, in a human salivary gland cancer cell. Br J Cancer. 1998;77:71–8.
16. Kawamata H, Fujimori T, Imai Y. TSC-22 (TGF-beta stimulated clone-22): a novel molecular target for differentiation-inducing therapy in salivary gland cancer. Curr Cancer Drug Targets. 2004;4:521–9.
17. Ohta S, Yanagihara K, Nagata K. Mechanism of apoptotic cell death of human gastric carcinoma cells mediated by transforming growth factor beta. Biochem J. 1997;324(Pt 3):777–82.
18. Shostak KO, Dmitrenko VV, Vudmaska MI, Naidenov VG, Beletskii AV, Malisheva TA, et al. Patterns of expression of TSC-22 protein in astrocytic gliomas. Exp Oncol. 2005;27:314–8.
19. Iida M, Anna CH, Gaskin ND, Walker NJ, Devereux TR. The putative tumor suppressor Tsc-22 is downregulated early in chemically induced hepatocarcinogenesis and may be a suppressor of Gadd45b. Toxicol Sci. 2007;99:43–50.
20. Yu J, Ershler M, Yu L, Wei M, Hackanson B, Yokohama A, et al. TSC-22 contributes to hematopoietic precursor cell proliferation and repopulation and is epigenetically silenced in large granular lymphocyte leukemia. Blood. 2009;113:5558–67.
21. Yoon CH, Rho SB, Kim ST, Kho S, Park J, Jang IS, et al. Crucial role of TSC-22 in preventing the proteasomal degradation of p53 in cervical cancer. PLoS One. 2012;7:e42006.
22. Hashiguchi A, Okabayashi K, Asashima M. Role of TSC-22 during early embryogenesis in Xenopus laevis. Dev Growth Differ. 2004;46:535–44.
23. Jager J, Greiner V, Strzoda D, Seibert O, Niopek K, Sijmonsma TP, et al. Hepatic transforming growth factor-beta 1 stimulated clone-22 D1 controls systemic cholesterol metabolism. Mol Metab. 2014;3:155–66.
24. Dohrmann CE, Noramly S, Raftery LA, Morgan BA. Opposing effects on TSC-22 expression by BMP and receptor tyrosine kinase signals in the developing feather tract. Dev Dyn. 2002;223:85–95.
25. Rysa J, Aro J, Ruskoaho H. Early left ventricular gene expression profile in response to increase in blood pressure. Blood Press. 2006;15:375–83.
26. Stanton LW, Garrard LJ, Damm D, Garrick BL, Lam A, Kapoun AM, et al. Altered patterns of gene expression in response to myocardial infarction. Circ Res. 2000;86:939–45.
27. Prussak CE, Almazan MT, Tseng BY. Peptide production from proteins separated by sodium dodecyl-sulfate polyacrylamide gel electrophoresis. Anal Biochem. 1989;178:233–8.
28. Pfeffer MA, Pfeffer JM, Fishbein MC, Fletcher PJ, Spadaro J, Kloner RA, et al. Myocardial infarct size and ventricular function in rats. Circ Res. 1979;44:503–12.
29. Tenhunen O, Soini Y, Ilves M, Rysa J, Tuukkanen J, Serpi R, et al. p38 Kinase rescues failing myocardium after myocardial infarction: evidence for angiogenic and anti-apoptotic mechanisms. FASEB J. 2006;20:1907–9.
30. Wang Y, Huang S, Sah VP, Ross Jr J, Brown JH, Han J, et al. Cardiac muscle cell hypertrophy and apoptosis induced by distinct members of the p38 mitogen-activated protein kinase family. J Biol Chem. 1998;273:2161–8.
31. Niwa H, Yamamura K, Miyazaki J. Efficient selection for high-expression transfectants with a novel eukaryotic vector. Gene. 1991;108:193–9.
32. Tenhunen O, Rysa J, Ilves M, Soini Y, Ruskoaho H, Leskinen H. Identification of cell cycle regulatory and inflammatory genes as predominant targets of p38 mitogen-activated protein kinase in the heart. Circ Res. 2006;99:485–93.
33. Rysa J, Leskinen H, Ilves M, Ruskoaho H. Distinct upregulation of extracellular matrix genes in transition from hypertrophy to hypertensive heart failure. Hypertension. 2005;45:927–33.
34. Ronkainen VP, Ronkainen JJ, Hanninen SL, Leskinen H, Ruas JL, Pereira T, et al. Hypoxia inducible factor regulates the cardiac expression and secretion of apelin. FASEB J. 2007;21:1821–30.

35. Aro J, Tokola H, Ronkainen VP, Koivisto E, Tenhunen O, Ilves M, et al. Regulation of cardiac melusin gene expression by hypertrophic stimuli in the rat. Acta Physiol (Oxf). 2013;207:470–84.
36. Koivisto E, Karkkola L, Majalahti T, Aro J, Tokola H, Kerkela R, et al. M-CAT element mediates mechanical stretch-activated transcription of B-type natriuretic peptide via ERK activation. Can J Physiol Pharmacol. 2011;89:539–50.
37. Luosujarvi H, Aro J, Tokola H, Leskinen H, Tenhunen O, Skoumal R, et al. A novel p38 MAPK target dyxin is rapidly induced by mechanical load in the heart. Blood Press. 2010;19:54–63.
38. Mustonen E, Leskinen H, Aro J, Luodonpää M, Vuolteenaho O, Ruskoaho H, et al. Metoprolol treatment lowers thrombospondin-4 expression in rats with myocardial infarction and left ventricular hypertrophy. Basic Clin Pharmacol Toxicol. 2010;107:709–17.
39. Hoshijima M, Chien KR. Mixed signals in heart failure: cancer rules. J Clin Invest. 2002;109:849–55.
40. Brand T, Schneider MD. The TGF beta superfamily in myocardium: ligands, receptors, transduction, and function. J Mol Cell Cardiol. 1995;27:5–18.
41. Rosenkranz S, Flesch M, Amann K, Haeuseler C, Kilter H, Seeland U, et al. Alterations of beta-adrenergic signaling and cardiac hypertrophy in transgenic mice overexpressing TGF-beta(1). Am J Physiol Circ Physiol. 2002;283:H1253–62.
42. Schultz Jel J, Witt SA, Glascock BJ, Nieman ML, Reiser PJ, Nix SL, et al. TGF-beta1 mediates the hypertrophic cardiomyocyte growth induced by angiotensin II. J Clin Invest. 2002;109:787–96.
43. Schluter KD, Frischkopf K, Flesch M, Rosenkranz S, Taimor G, Piper HM. Central role for ornithine decarboxylase in beta-adrenoceptor mediated hypertrophy. Cardiovasc Res. 2000;45:410–7.
44. Schluter KD, Zhou XJ, Piper HM. Induction of hypertrophic responsiveness to isoproterenol by TGF-beta in adult rat cardiomyocytes. Am J Physiol. 1995;269(5 Pt 1):C1311–6.
45. Huntgeburth M, Tiemann K, Shahverdyan R, Schluter KD, Schreckenberg R, Gross ML, et al. Transforming growth factor beta(1) oppositely regulates the hypertrophic and contractile response to beta-adrenergic stimulation in the heart. PLoS One. 2011;6:e26628.
46. Brouri F, Hanoun N, Mediani O, Saurini F, Hamon M, Vanhoutte PM, et al. Blockade of β1- and desensitization of β 2-adrenoceptors reduce isoprenaline-induced cardiac fibrosis. Eur J Pharmacol. 2004;485:227–34.
47. De Carvalho FC, Sun Y, Weber KT. Angiotensin II receptor blockade and myocardial fibrosis of the infarcted rat heart. J Lab Clin Med. 1997;129:439–46.
48. Schieffer B, Wirger A, Meybrunn M, Seitz S, Holtz J, Riede UN, et al. Comparative effects of chronic angiotensin-converting enzyme inhibition and angiotensin II type 1 receptor blockade on cardiac remodeling after myocardial infarction in the rat. Circulation. 1994;89:2273–82.
49. Boluyt MO, Robinson KG, Meredith AL, Sen S, Lakatta EG, Crow MT, et al. Heart failure after long-term supravalvular aortic constriction in rats. Am J Hypertens. 2005;18(2 Pt 1):202–12.
50. Kuoppala A, Shiota N, Lindstedt KA, Rysä J, Leskinen HK, Luodonpää M, et al. Expression of bradykinin receptors in the left ventricles of rats with pressure overload hypertrophy and heart failure. J Hypertens. 2003;21:1729–36.
51. Kato M, Wang L, Putta S, Wang M, Yuan H, Sun G, et al. Post-transcriptional up-regulation of Tsc-22 by Ybx1, a target of miR-216a, mediates TGF-{beta}-induced collagen expression in kidney cells. J Biol Chem. 2010;285:34004–15.
52. Jane-Lise S, Corda S, Chassagne C, Rappaport L. The extracellular matrix and the cytoskeleton in heart hypertrophy and failure. Heart Fail Rev. 2000;5:239–50.
53. Hino S, Kawamata H, Uchida D, Omotehara F, Miwa Y, Begum NM, et al. Nuclear translocation of TSC-22 (TGF-beta-stimulated clone-22) concomitant with apoptosis: TSC-22 as a putative transcriptional regulator. Biochem Biophys Res Commun. 2000;278:659–64.

Initiation of and long-term adherence to secondary preventive drugs after acute myocardial infarction

Sigrun Halvorsen[1*], Jarle Jortveit[2], Pål Hasvold[3], Marcus Thuresson[4] and Erik Øie[5]

Abstract

Background: Secondary preventive drug therapy following acute myocardial infarction (AMI) is recommended to reduce the risk of new cardiovascular events. The aim of this nationwide cohort study was to examine the initiation and long-term use of secondary preventive drugs after AMI.

Methods: The prescription of drugs in 42,707 patients < 85 years discharged alive from hospital after AMI in 2009–2013 was retrieved by linkage of the Norwegian Patient Register, the Norwegian Prescription Database, and the Norwegian Cause of Death Registry. Patients were followed for up to 24 months.

Results: The majority of patients were discharged on single or dual antiplatelet therapy (91 %), statins (90 %), beta-blockers (82 %), and angiotensin-converting enzyme inhibitors (ACEI)/angiotensin receptor II blockers (ARB) (60 %). Patients not undergoing percutaneous coronary intervention (PCI) (42 %) were less likely to be prescribed secondary preventive drugs compared with patients undergoing PCI. This was particular the case for dual antiplatelet therapy (43 % vs. 87 %). The adherence to prescribed drugs was high: 12 months after index AMI, 84 % of patients were still on aspirin, 84 % on statins, 77 % on beta-blockers and 57 % on ACEI/ARB. Few drug and dose adjustments were made during follow-up.

Conclusion: Guideline-recommended secondary preventive drugs were prescribed to most patients discharged from hospital after AMI, but the percentage receiving such therapy was significantly lower in non-PCI patients. The long-time adherence was high, but few drug adjustments were performed during follow-up. More attention is needed to secondary preventive drug therapy in AMI patients not undergoing PCI.

Keywords: Acute myocardial infarction, Secondary prevention, Medication adherence

Background

Ischemic heart disease is a common cause of death in industrialized countries and accounts for a large proportion of hospital admissions in Norway [1]. Approximately 13,000 men and women are diagnosed annually with acute myocardial infarction (AMI) [2]. Secondary preventive drug therapy, e.g. platelet inhibitors, statins, beta-blockers and angiotensin-converting enzyme inhibitors (ACEI)/ angiotensin receptor II blockers (ARB), is recommended following AMI to reduce the risk of new cardiovascular events and death [3–7]. However, an underuse of secondary preventive drugs has previously been observed following AMI, especially in patients not undergoing percutaneous coronary intervention (PCI) [8]. Despite their elevated cardiovascular risk [9], still many AMI patients are not treated according to guidelines [10]. This may be related to under-prescription, reduced adherence, and/or under-dosing of secondary preventive drug therapy [11, 12]. A potential source for the underuse of recommended secondary preventive drugs could be the shift of treatment responsibility from the hospitals to the general practitioners in the primary care setting. The extent to which the hospital-initiated treatment is continued as initially prescribed, the doses adjusted or drugs switched to another type of drug within the same drug class, is not known. Comprehensive analyses of

* Correspondence: sigrun.h@online.no
[1]Department of Cardiology, Oslo University Hospital Ulleval and University of Oslo, Postboks 4956, Nydalen 0424, Oslo, Norway
Full list of author information is available at the end of the article

initiation and adherence in different patient populations are essential to improve long-term use of secondary preventive drugs and cardiovascular outcomes [13].

The aim of this nationwide cohort study was to examine the initiation and long-term use of secondary preventive drug in patients hospitalized with AMI in Norway during the years 2009 to 2013.

Methods

Data sources

This observational, historical cohort study was based on data from three Norwegian national registries: 1) The Norwegian Patient Register covering all hospital admissions and including diagnoses according to the International Classification of Diseases, 10th revision, Clinical Modification (ICD-10-CM) [14]; 2) the Norwegian Prescription Database registering all pharmacy dispenses [15]; and 3) the Norwegian Cause of Death Registry registering all deaths [16]. The prescription of drugs in patients discharged alive from hospital after AMI in 2009–2013 was retrieved by linkage of the Norwegian Patient Register, the Norwegian Prescription Database, and the Norwegian Cause of Death Registry. Patients were followed for up to 24 months. The Norwegian Institute of Public Health performed the data linkage. Data were anonymised before further analysis. The linked database was managed by The Norwegian University of Science and Technology, Trondheim, Norway.

Study population

All patients below 85 years of age who were admitted to hospital with a primary diagnosis of AMI (index AMI) (ICD-10: I21) between 1 January 2009 and 30 November 2013 and alive 30 days after discharge were included in this study. Patients 85 years or older were excluded for two reasons: 1) their likelihood of long-term use of secondary preventive drugs might be extensively confounded by fragility; 2) older patients have an increased risk of long-term institutional stays where the drug use cannot be captured by the available registries. Patients were classified as PCI and non-PCI patients depending on whether PCI was performed or not up to 30 days after index-AMI. The study population was further stratified into two groups; ≤75 years and 76–84 years.

Index AMI was defined as the first recorded primary diagnosis of AMI for a patient during the specified time-period (not necessarily the patient's first AMI). All residents in Norway are covered by a national health security system with a universal tax-funded access to primary and secondary health care, including secondary preventive drugs recommended after AMI.

Follow-up

Observational data on drug prescriptions were collected up to 24 months following AMI, or until 31 December 2014 or death (whichever occurred first).

Drug treatment and adherence

Drug treatment at discharge for index AMI were calculated from dispensed drugs from pharmacies one year within and until 30 days after the index AMI; either a prior dispensing covering day 0 to day 30 or a new dispensing within day 0 to day 30. Drug adherence was defined as the proportion of patients on the treatment of interest at each day from 12 months prior to the date of hospitalization for AMI until a maximum of 24 months after. The calculation of drug use (days on treatment) was based on the prescribed dose and on the number of pills collected or delivered from the pharmacies. Whether or not the pills were taken by the patients, were not assessed. If a patient had a gap in collection of drugs, the patient was defined as a non-user from last calculated day with available drug. Furthermore, if a patient after a gap, again collected the same drug from the pharmacy, the patient was defined as a user from that actual date, and if a patient was switched to another type of drug within the same drug class after the index AMI episode, the patient was defined as a user.

In the separate analysis of the adherence to the P_2Y_{12}-antagonists clopidogrel, prasugrel or ticagrelor during the first 18 months after AMI, the proportion of all patients still alive continuing on the same P_2Y_{12} antagonist as at discharge was estimated.

In order to describe changes in drug treatment over time, treatment at discharge for index AMI was compared to treatment in the post AMI period (dispensed during 12 18 months after the AMI).

Statistical analyses

Data are presented as mean with standard deviation for continuous variables and absolute and relative frequencies for categorical variables. Patients were stratified by age (≤75 years or 75–84 years) and by PCI status (PCI or no PCI). Statistical analyses were performed using SAS version 9.3 (SAS Institute Inc, Cary, NC, USA) and R version 3.2.2 [17].

Results

A total of 57,106 individuals were admitted to Norwegian hospitals for AMI during the study period, of whom 45,838 (80.3 %) were younger than 85 years. Of these, 42,707 (93.2 %) were alive 30 days after hospital discharge and could be included in the study (Fig. 1). Overall, 70 % of the patients were men and mean age was 65.8 years (standard deviation 11.8) (Table 1). A total of 58 % of the patients underwent PCI, with an increasing proportion

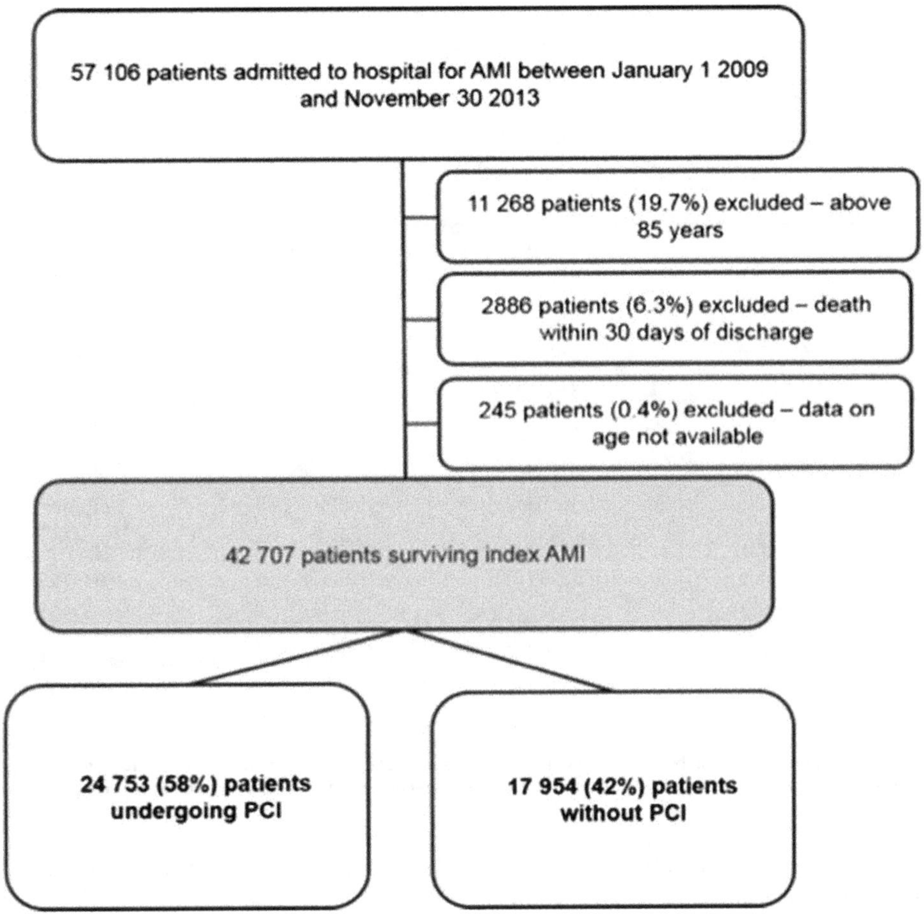

Fig. 1 Flow chart of the study population

during the study period (from 53 % to 63 %) (Additional file 1, Table 1). Patients undergoing PCI were younger and more often male compared with the medically treated patients (Table 1).

Initiation of secondary preventive drugs

The prescription of secondary preventive drugs at discharge is shown in Tables 1 and 2. The majority of patients were discharged on single or dual antiplatelet therapy (DAPT) (19 % and 72 %, respectively), statins (90 %), beta-blockers (82 %), and ACEI/ARB (60 %). The percentage receiving these drugs were slightly lower in patients 75–84 years compared to patients ≤75 years, except for ACEI/ARB which was prescribed slightly more often in the elderly (Table 1).

Patients undergoing PCI were prescribed secondary preventive drug therapy more often than patients not undergoing PCI (Table 1). This was the case both for patients <75 years and patients 75–84 years. The difference in prescriptions was largest with respect to DAPT, which was prescribed in 92 % of the PCI patients vs. 45 % of patients not undergoing PCI (Table 1, Figs. 2 and 3). In contrast, non-PCI patients were prescribed other kinds of antithrombotic therapy more often than PCI patients: Aspirin monotherapy in 28 % vs. 2 %, oral anticoagulant (OAC) monotherapy in 4 % vs. 0 %, or OAC in combination with single antiplatelet therapy in 6 % vs. 1 %, respectively. However, 14 % of the non-PCI patients were discharged with neither antiplatelet drugs nor OAC, compared to 2 % of the PCI patients. Surprisingly, the differences in prescription pattern between PCI and non-PCI patients were found also with respect to other types of secondary preventive drugs (Table 1).

The mean dose of statins at discharge was 37 mg for simvastatin (55 % of patients) and 57 mg for atorvastatin (40 % of patients). The mean doses of ACEI/ARB and beta-blocker at discharge were 35-60 % and 30-50 % of maximal recommended doses, respectively (Table 2).

Adherence to secondary preventive drugs

The overall long-time adherence was high among all patients initiated on treatment with statins, beta-blockers and ACEI/ARB (Figs. 2 and 3, Table 2). The proportions of patients using statins, ACEI/ARB and beta-blockers

Table 1 Drug treatment at discharge after index AMI. Patients stratified by age (≤75 years or 75–84 years) and by PCI status (PCI or no PCI)

	Age ≤75 years *n* = 30 843		Age 75–84 years *n* = 11 864		Total *n* = 42 707
	PCI *n* = 19 835 (64.3)	No PCI *n* = 11 008 (35.7)	PCI *n* = 4918 (29.3)	No PCI *n* = 6946 (70.7)	
Women	4065 (20.5)	3478 (31.6)	1819 (37.0)	3357 (48.3)	12 719 (29.8)
Age, mean (SD)	59.8 (9.1)	61.6 (9.6)	79.0 (2.8)	80.0 (2.8)	65.8 (11.8)
DAPT	17 505 (88.3)	5107 (46.4)	3877 (78.8)	2597 (37.4)	29 086 (68.1)
Only $P2Y_{12}$ inhibitor	668 (3.4)	354 (3.2)	202 (4.1)	295 (4.3)	1519 (3.6)
Only ASA	288 (1.5)	3105 (28.2)	151 (3.1)	1860 (26.7)	5404 (12.3)
Only OAC	21 (0.1)	312 (2.8)	15 (0.3)	339 (4.9)	687 (1.6)
OAC + DAPT	925 (4.7)	241 (2.2)	473 (9.6)	165 (2.4)	1804 (4.2)
OAC + $P2Y_{12}$ inhibitor	58 (0.3)	40 (0.4)	28 (0.6)	58 (0.8)	184 (0.4)
OAC + ASA	43 (0.2)	520 (4.7))	32 (0.7)	529 (7.6)	1124 (2.6)
No antiplatelet or OAC	327 (1.7)	1329 (12.1)	140 (2.9)	1103 (15.9)	2899 (6.8)
Statins	19 168 (96.6)	9224 (83.8)	4574 (93.0)	5262 (75.7)	38 228 (89.5)
Beta-blockers	16 763 (84.5)	8529 (77.5)	4238 (86.2)	5456 (78.6)	34 986 (81.9)
ACE inhibitors	7977 (40.3)	3478 (31.7)	2027 (41.2)	2497 (36.0)	15 988 (37.4)
ARB	4822 (24.3)	2945 (26.8)	1597 (32.5)	2072 (29.8)	11 346 (26.8)

Numbers in parentheses are percentages of total number of patients in the group. *SD* denotes standard derivation, *DAPT* dual antiplatelet therapy, *AMI* Acute myocardial infaction, *ASA* Acetylsalicylic acid, *OAC* Oral anticoagulants, *ACE* Angiotensin-converting enzyme, *ARB* Angiotensin II receptor blocker

were reduced by 6 %, 3 % and 4 %, respectively, after one year. No major differences in drug adherence was observed between PCI and non-PCI patients, or between patients ≤75 and 76–84 years. When primary health care physicians took over the prescription responsibility for these patients (approximately 3 months after the AMI), no overall change in adherence was found. Approximately 20 % of patients changed to another drug within the same drug class, or changed the dose of statin, beta-blocker and ACEI/ARB within 12–18 months after the AMI (Table 2).

The adherence to antiplatelet drugs was also high (Figs. 2 and 3). After 12 months, 84 % of patients were still on aspirin; 83 % after 18 months. The adherence to P_2Y_{12} inhibitors are shown in more detail in Fig. 4 and Additional file 1: Table S2. Patients not undergoing PCI had a shorter length of time on treatment with a P_2Y_{12} inhibitor compared with PCI patients, with a substantial proportion of these patients discontinuing treatment already after three months. The majority of the PCI patients treated with ticagrelor and prasugrel maintained the treatment through 12 months. Many PCI patients on clopidogrel discontinued P_2Y_{12} inhibitor after nine months.

Discussion

This nationwide observational cohort study, including all patients younger than 85 years surviving an AMI in Norway during the years 2009 to 2013, showed a generally high long-term adherence to the prescribed treatment with antiplatelet drugs, statins, beta-blockers and ACEI/ARB. The shift of responsibility for prescribing secondary preventive drugs from hospital to primary health care showed a sustained high use of the originally prescribed drugs. Only few patients switched to another type of statin or changed the dose of statin, beta-blocker and ACEI/ARB during the first two years after the AMI. For patients not undergoing PCI, a smaller proportion was discharged with secondary preventive drugs following their AMI compared with patients undergoing PCI, and less than half were prescribed DAPT at discharge.

Contemporary national level data describing long-term adherence to secondary preventive medications, i.e. antiplatelet drugs, statins, beta-blockers, and ACEI/ARB in AMI populations comparing younger vs. older and PCI vs. non-PCI patients are scarce. Furthermore, little is known on the impact of change in drug treatment responsibilities as AMI patients are transferred from hospital care to primary health care.

The initiation of secondary preventive drugs in our study was considerably higher than was found in a previous Danish nationwide study [12]. In patients admitted with a first AMI between 1995 and 2002 in Denmark, only 58 % received beta-blockers, 29 % ACE-inhibitors, and 34 % statins at discharge [12].

Table 2 Secondary preventive drugs at discharge from hospital for index AMI and 12-18 months later; patients <85 years

	Secondary preventive drugs at discharge for index AMI (*n* = 42 707)		Secondary preventive drugs 12–18 months after index AMI (*n* = 28 767)			
	n (%)	Mean dose (mg)	*n* (%)	Mean dose (mg)	*n* (%) switched to another drug within same drug class in post-AMI period	*n* (%) changed dose of actual drug in post-AMI period
Statins	38 228 (89.5)		24 062 (83.6)			
Simvastatin	23 528 (55.1)	37.2	12 478 (43.4)	38.4	2571 (15.7)	1415 (8.7)
Atorvastatin	17 084 (40.0)	56.9	10 913 (37.9)	52.1	592 (6)	1755 (17.8)
Rosuvastatin	225 (0.5)	17.7	367 (1.3)	19.6	10 (9.6)	13 (12.5)
Pravastatin	1158 (2.7)	33.5	651 (2.3)	33.5	120 (20.9)	39 (6.8)
ACEI/ARB[a]	25 445 (59.6)		16 274 (56.6)			
Losartan	3658 (8.6)	66.6	2049 (7.1)	66.5	153 (6.9)	238 (10.8)
Candersartan	4157 (9.7)	13.1	2778 (9.7)	13.5	145 (5.4)	467 (17.4)
Valsartan	1503 (3.5)	124.9	865 (3.0)	125.2	68 (7.2)	127 (13.4)
Irbesartan	1530 (3.6)	235.6	770 (2.7)	237.3	72 (7.8)	61 (6.6)
Enalapril	2951 (6.9)	11.8	1657 (5.8)	11.9	170 (8.9)	324 (16.9)
Ramipril	11 492 (26.9)	3.5	6999 (24.3)	4.5	733 (8.8)	2156 (25.8)
Lisinopril	1753 (4.1)	11.3	949 (3.3)	11.3	121 (10.3)	207 (17.5)
Beta-blockers	34 986 (81.9)		22 061 (76.7)			
Metoprolol	30 874 (72.3)	60.6	18 920 (65.8)	62.3	702 (3.2)	4452 (20.3)
Atenolol	1381 (3.2)	52.4	457 (1.6)	51.0	117 (21.6)	54 (10)
Propranolol	305 (0.7)	66.2	82 (0.3)	80.4	26 (26.3)	6 (6.1)
Sotalol	358 (0.8)	80.3	138 (0.5)	75.9	49 (33.3)	14 (9.5)
Bisoprolol	2477 (5.8)	4.1	1856 (6.5)	4.4	64 (4)	310 (19.3)
Carvedilol	1298 (3.0)	15.8	813 (2.8)	15.6	73 (9.1)	123 (15.3)

Numbers in parentheses are percentages of total number of patients in the group

ACEI Angiotensin-converting enzyme inhibitor, *AMI* Aciute myocardial infraction, *ARB* Angiotensin II receptor blocker

[a]some patients were prescribed both ACEI and ARB

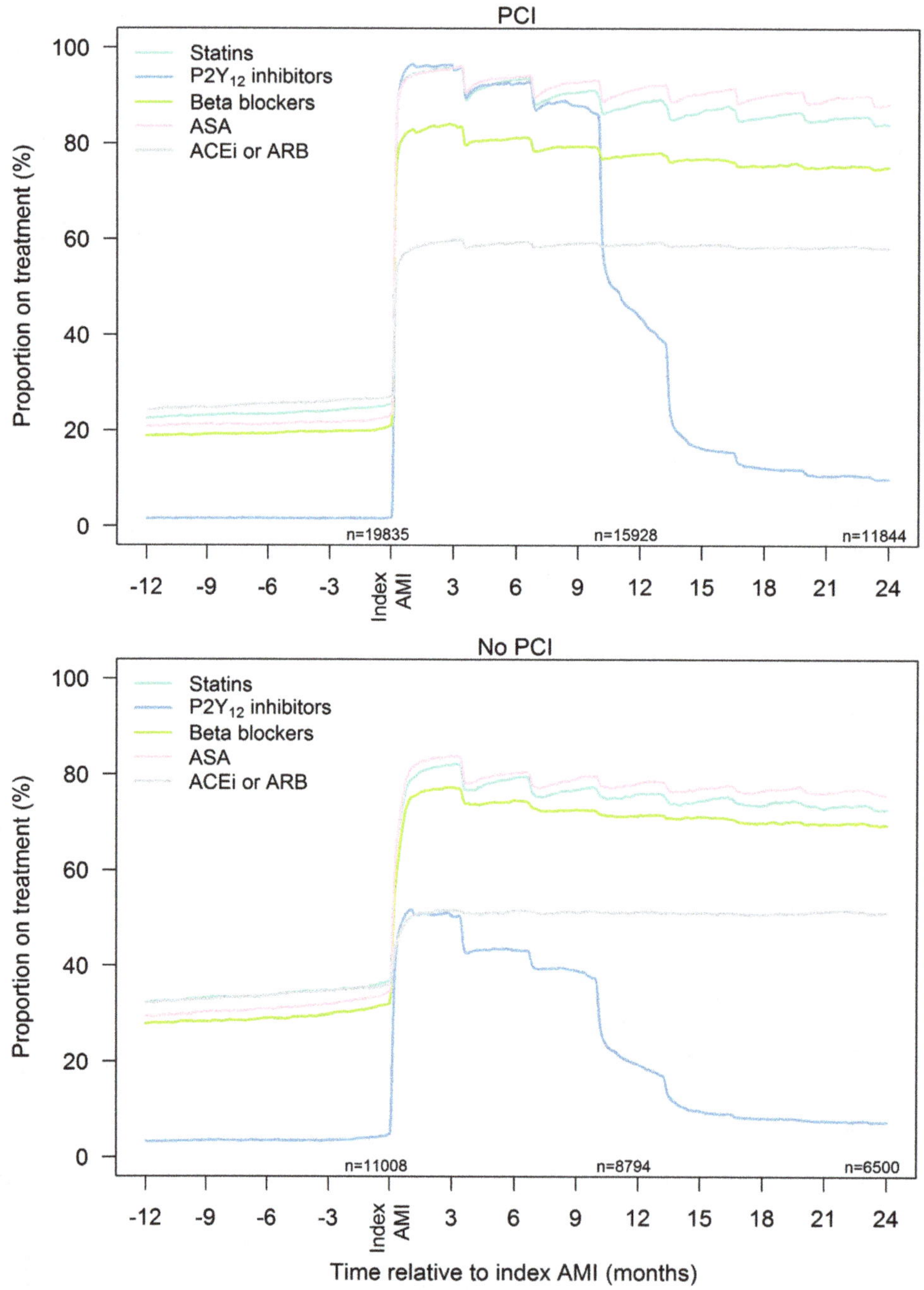

Fig. 2 Adherence to secondary preventive drugs over time in AMI patients ≤75 years with or without PCI. Norway 2009–2013. *Abbreviations:* ASA, acetylsalicylic acid; ACEI, angiotensin-converting enzyme inhibitor; AMI, acute myocardial infarction; ARB, angiotensin II receptor blocker; PCI, percutaneous coronary intervention

Although long-term compliance was reasonably good, patients who did not start treatment shortly after discharge had a low probability of starting treatment later [12]. In a more recent Swedish study, both initiation and long-term adherence to secondary preventive drug therapy was higher and similar to our findings: 82 % of AMI patients were still on aspirin 12 months post AMI, 73 % on statins and 80 % on beta-blockers [18].

A high degree of initiation of secondary preventive drug therapy was also observed in a recent study from the United States [13]. However, when patients were divided into risk groups based on the Global Registry of Acute Coronary Event (GRACE) risk score at hospital discharge, high-risk patients had a lower likelihood of receiving all appropriate therapies at discharge compared with low-risk patients.

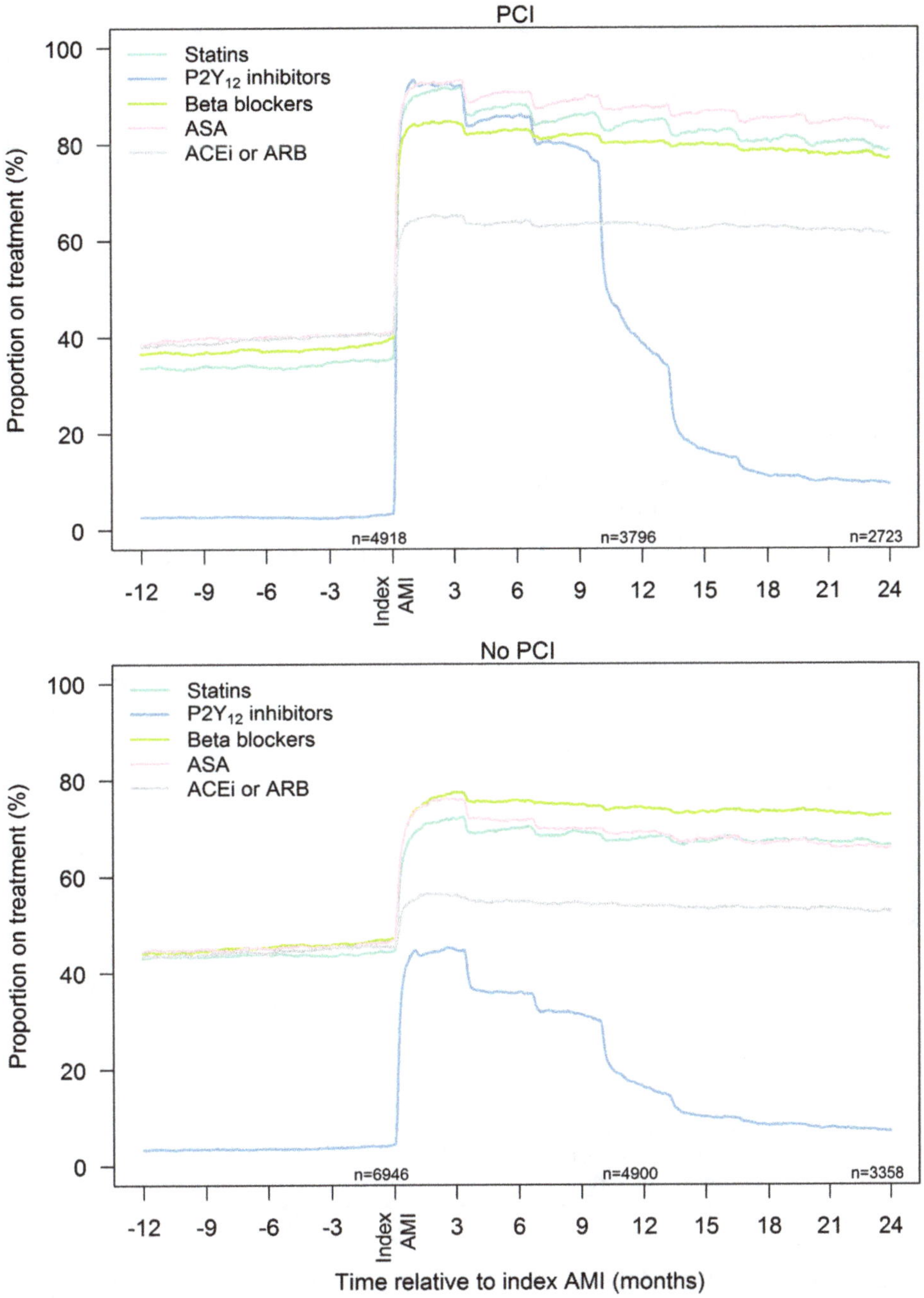

Fig. 3 Adherence to secondary preventive drugs over time in AMI patients 76–84 years with and without PCI. Norway 2009–2013. *Abbreviations*: ASA, acetylsalicylic acid; ACEI, angiotensin-converting enzyme inhibitor; AMI, acute myocardial infarction; ARB, angiotensin II receptor blocker; PCI, percutaneous coronary intervention

Our data may indicate that if secondary preventive drug therapy after AMI is not prescribed at hospital discharge, the likelihood of receiving such treatment is limited. Thus, initiation of guideline-recommended secondary preventive drug therapy after AMI seems to depend on the hospital physicians, in accordance with the previous observations from Denmark [12]. The present study further demonstrates that only minor dose adjustments for drugs prescribed at discharge were performed by the primary care physicians during follow-up. Thus, Norwegian primary care physicians seemed reluctant to changing already prescribed secondary preventive drug therapies after AMI.

This finding further underscores the importance of drug prescription prior to discharge of AMI patients from hospitals. Not only should AMI patients be prescribed guideline-recommended secondary preventive drugs, but the hospital

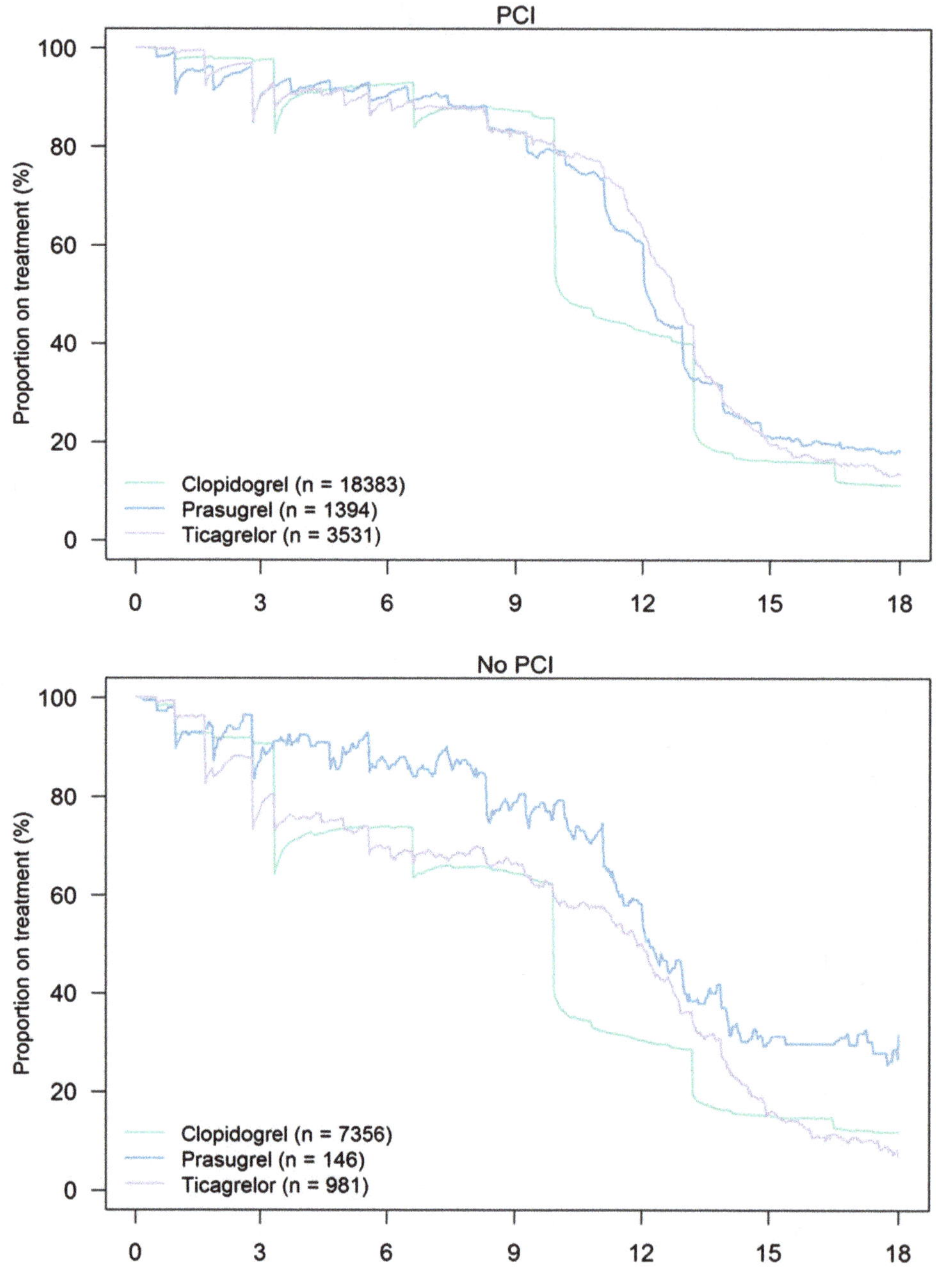

Fig. 4 Adherence to treatment with different $P2Y_{12}$ inhibitors in AMI patients <85 years with and without PCI. Norway 2009–2013. *Abbreviations*: AMI, acute myocardial infarction; PCI, percutaneous coronary intervention

physicians could also advice on further up-titration and the target doses of the prescribed drugs in the discharge summary sent to the patient's general practitioner. It is also important that the general practitioners are updated on current guidelines and take the responsibility for optimizing secondary preventive treatment after AMI. Interestingly, patients not undergoing PCI were less likely to receive guideline-recommended secondary preventive drugs compared with patients undergoing PCI. For example, a 10–20 % higher use of statins and beta-blockers was seen in PCI patients vs. patients not undergoing PCI. Furthermore, a larger portion of patients not undergoing PCI was discharged without a $P2Y_{12}$ inhibitor (48 % and 55 %, respectively, in patients ≤75 or 76–84 years) compared with PCI patients (4 % and 7 %). The reasons for this undertreatment of non-PCI patients are not known. We might speculate that a higher degree of comorbidities might be present in these patients, making the physicians more selective in their prescription of secondary preventive drugs.

The mean doses of both ACEI, ARB and beta-blockers in our study were lower than the target doses in randomized trials studying the efficacy and safety of these drugs. The reasons for the choice of these lower doses, or the lack of up-titration of doses after hospital discharge, are unknown. These drugs are used for a variety of indications, and since we have limited data on weight, blood pressure, heart rate, ejection fraction, comorbidities and on the specific indications for the various drugs (e.g. for ACEI/ARB), we find it difficult to draw any firm conclusions regarding target doses and whether the doses used in our study were too low or not. With respect to statin treatment, it should be noted that during most of our study period, no specific statin dose was recommended and statins were prescribed mainly according to LDL-cholesterol levels.

We observed a generally short duration of P_2Y_{12} inhibitor treatment for patients not undergoing PCI (Fig. 4), with a significant proportion of patients treated for only three months as also observed in a recent study from Sweden [19]. One possible reason for the longer treatment duration after PCI may be that $P2Y_{12}$ inhibition is regarded particularly important after stent implantation to avoid stent thrombosis. However, ESC guidelines recommend P_2Y_{12} inhibition for 12 months in all ACS patients [3–6].

A large proportion of patients discontinued P_2Y_{12} inhibitor after nine months; mainly patients on clopidogrel treatment. One likely explanation to this finding was the nine months' limited reimbursement of clopidogrel in Norway until September 2011 [20]. Prasugrel and ticagrelor have not had such reimbursement limitations. This finding demonstrates the influence the health authorities have on medical treatment by determining the prescription rules for reimbursements of various drugs.

Limitations

Our data set provides a unique possibility to examine adherence to antiplatelet therapy, statins, beta-blockers and ACEI/ARB. It includes nationwide data from all patients hospitalized in Norway for AMI in 2009–2013, allowing analyses of a complete and unselected cohort of patients, and also allowing differentiation between younger and older patients and between patients undergoing PCI or not. This reduces potential problems arising from selection bias due to inclusion of selected hospitals, regions, or health care insurance systems. Furthermore, by restricting the inclusion to patients below 85 years of age, this study focuses on patients who normally would be considered to be treated according to guidelines. However, this register-based analysis also has certain limitations. As our analysis relied on ICD-10 codes, the possibility of coding errors cannot be ruled out, although the primary diagnoses of AMI previously have been shown to have high sensitivity and specificity [21]. A further subclassification of patients into those presenting with and without persistent ST-segment elevation on the electrocardiogram could not be performed due to non-validated ICD-10 coding specification at this level.

Further, due the study aim describing secondary drug adherence in a nationwide patient population, patients were included based on their first AMI during the observational period, i.e. not necessarily their first time AMI. Thus, the patient population changed during the inclusion period. While patients included early in the inclusion period may have had a recent history of AMI, patients included towards the end of the study period had to be event-free for a longer time. Following from this study design, the yearly numbers of included AMIs in our study decreased during the observational period (Additional file 1, Table 1). Furthermore, how a recent prior AMI episode would affect selection for invasive treatment and secondary prevention drugs is difficult to predict, but it cannot be excluded that these patients would receive a higher attention, and thus a higher likelihood of receiving guideline-recommended treatment.

The registry data were collected for administrative purposes and we did not have any information on smoking patterns, weight, blood pressure, laboratory data or socioeconomic status. Furthermore, the Norwegian Patient Register has only had nationwide coverage since 2009 and medical history from previous hospitalizations was not available.

Conclusions

This nationwide observational study, including all patients in Norway below 85 years of age being alive 30 days after AMI during the years 2009 to 2013, showed a generally high long-term adherence to antiplatelet therapy, as well as treatment with statins, beta-blockers and ACEI/ARB. To a large extent, PCI patients received guideline-recommended treatment with secondary preventive drugs. Patients not undergoing PCI were less likely to be discharged with the recommended drugs. The shift of responsibility for prescribing drug treatment from hospital to primary health care did not to any major extent alter the already prescribed treatments. Thus, the majority of AMI patients remained on the secondary preventive treatment originally prescribed, further underlining the importance of prescribing guideline-recommended drug treatment at hospital discharge, and preferably including specialist guidance on future target doses in the discharge summary. The present study also indicates a need for more careful attention to secondary preventive drug therapy in AMI patients not undergoing PCI.

Abbreviations

ACEI, angiotensin-converting enzyme inhibitor; AMI, acute myocardial infarction; ARB, angiotensin II receptor blocker; ASA, acetylsalicylic acid; DAPT, dual antiplatelet therapy; ICD-10-CM, International Classification of Diseases, 10th revision, Clinical Modification; OAC, oral anticoagulant; PCI, percutaneous coronary intervention.

Funding

This work was supported by AstraZeneca. Project management was provided by AstraZeneca. The statistical analysis was agreed upon by the study steering committee, and data analysis was performed by the study database owner in collaboration with AstraZeneca. AstraZeneca took part as members of the study steering committee in the interpretation of the data and the drafting of the manuscript.

Authors' contributions

S. Halvorsen, J. Jortveit, P. Hasvold, M. Thuresson, and E. Øie, participated equally in the study conception, design, and statistical analysis planning. M. Thuresson was responsible for the statistical analyses and S. Halvorsen for the manuscript draft and finalization. All authors had access to study data, and had authority over manuscript preparation, approval of the final version, and the decision to submit for publication.

Competing interests

All authors have completed the Unified Competing Interest form at http://www.icmje.org/coi_disclosure.pdf (http://www.icmje.org/coi_disclosure.pdf) (available on request from the corresponding author). SH declare support from AstraZeneca for the submitted work, and personal fees from AstraZeneca, Pfizer, BMS, Eli Lilly, Sanofi, Novartis and MSD outside of the submitted work. JJ declare support from AstraZeneca for the submitted work, and personal fees from AstraZeneca, Pfizer and Sanofi outside of the submitted work. PH is employed by AstraZeneca. MT is employed by an independent statistical consultant company, Statisticon, for which AstraZeneca is a client. EØ declare support from Astra Zeneca for the submitted work, and personal fees from AstraZeneca, Pfizer, BMS, Takeda, Novartis, Sanofi and MSD outside of the submitted work.

Author details

[1]Department of Cardiology, Oslo University Hospital Ulleval and University of Oslo, Postboks 4956, Nydalen 0424, Oslo, Norway. [2]Department of Cardiology, Sørlandet Hospital, Arendal, Norway. [3]AstraZeneca NordicBaltic, Södertälje, Sweden. [4]Statisticon, Uppsala, Sweden. [5]Department of Internal Medicine, Diakonhjemmet Hospital, and Center for Heart Failure Research, University of Oslo, Oslo, Norway.

References

1. Patient statistics, 2014. Available at: https://www.ssb.no/en/helse/statistikker/pasient. Accessed 1 Oct 2015.
2. Jortveit J, Govatsmark RE, Digre TA, Risøe C, Hole T, Mannsverk J, Slørdahl SA, Halvorsen S. Myocardial infarction in Norway in 2013. Tidsskr Nor Legeforen. 2014;134:1841–6.
3. Task Force for Diagnosis and Treatment of Non-ST-Segment Elevation Acute Coronary Syndromes of European Society of Cardiology, Bassand JP, Hamm CW, Ardissino D, Boersma E, Budaj A, et al. Guidelines for the diagnosis and treatment of non-ST-segment elevation acute coronary syndromes. Eur Heart J. 2007;28:1598–660.
4. Hamm CW, Bassand JP, Agewall S, Bax J, Boersma E, Bueno H, Caso P, Dudek D, Gielen S, Huber K, Ohman M, Petrie MC, Sonntag F, Uva MS, Storey RF, Wijns W, Zahger D. ESC Committee for Practice Guidelines ESC Guidelines for the management of acute coronary syndromes in patients presenting without persistent ST-segment elevation: The task force for the management of acute coronary syndromes (ACS) in patients presenting without persistent ST-segment elevation of the European Society of Cardiology. Eur Heart J. 2011;32:2999–54.
5. Van de Werf F, Bax J, Betriu A, Blomstrom-Lundqvist C, Crea F, Falk V, Filippatos G, Fox K, Huber K, Kastrati A, Rosengren A, Steg PG, Tubaro M, Verheugt F, Weidinger F, Weis M. ESC Committee for Practice Guidelines (CPG). Management of acute myocardial infarction in patients presenting with persistent ST-segment elevation: the Task Force on the Management of ST-Segment Elevation Acute Myocardial Infarction of the European Society of Cardiology. Eur Heart J. 2008;29:2909–45.
6. Steg PG, James SK, Atar D, Badano LP, Blömstrom-Lundqvist C, Borger MA, Di Mario C, Dickstein K, Ducrocq G, Fernandez-Aviles F, Gershlick AH, Giannuzzi P, Halvorsen S, Huber K, Juni P, Kastrati A, Knuuti J, Lenzen MJ, Mahaffey KW, Valgimigli M, van't Hof A, Widimsky P, Zahger D. ESC Guidelines for the management of acute myocardial infarction in patients presenting with ST-segment elevation. Eur Heart J. 2012;33:2569–19.
7. Jneid H, Anderson JL, Wright RS, Adams CD, Bridges CR, Casey Jr DE, Ettinger SM, Fesmire FM, Ganiats TG, Lincoff AM, Peterson ED, Philippides GJ, Theroux P, Wenger NK, Zidar JP, Anderson JL. American College of Cardiology Foundation; American Heart Association Task Force on Practice Guidelines. 2012 ACCF/AHA focused update of the guideline for the management of patients with unstable angina/Non-ST-elevation myocardial infarction (updating the 2007 guideline and replacing the 2011 focused update): a report of the American College of Cardiology Foundation/American Heart Association Task Force on practice guidelines. Circulation. 2012;126:875–910.
8. Sørensen R, Gislason GH, Fosbøl EL, Rasmussen S, Køber L, Madsen JK, Torp-Pedersen C, Abildstrom SZ. Initiation and persistence with clopidogrel treatment after acute myocardial infarction: a nationwide study. Br J Clin Pharmacol. 2008;66:875–84.
9. Varenhorst C, Jensevik K, Jernberg T, Sundstrom A, Hasvold P, Held C, Lagerqvist B, James S. Duration of dual antiplatelet treatment with clopidogrel and aspirin in patients with acute coronary syndrome. Eur Heart J. 2014;35:969–78.
10. Hambraeus K, Tydén P, Lindahl B. Time trends and gender differences in prevention guideline adherence and outcome after myocardial infarction: Data from the SWEDEHEART registry. Eur J Prev Cardiol. 2015. [Epub ahead of print]
11. Kotseva K, Wood D, De Backer G, De Bacquer D, Pyörälä K, Keil U. EUROASPIRE Study Group EUROASPIRE III: a survey on the lifestyle, risk factors and use of cardioprotective drug therapies in coronary patients from 22 European countries. Eur J Cardiovasc Prev Rehabil. 2009;16:121–37.
12. Gislason GH, Rasmussen JN, Abildstrøm SZ, Gadsbøll N, Buch P, Friberg J, Rasmussen S, Køber L, Stender S, Madsen M, Torp-Pedersen C. Long-term compliance with beta-blockers, angiotensin-converting enzyme inhibitors, and statins after acute myocardial infarction. Eur Heart J. 2006;27:1153–8.
13. Shore S, Jones PG, Maddox TM, Bradley SM, Stolker JM, Arnold SV, Parashar S, Peterson P, Bhatt DL, Spertus J, Ho PM. Longitudinal persistence with secondary prevention therapies relative to patient risk after myocardial infarction. Heart. 2015;101:800–7.
14. Bakken IJ, Nyland K, Halsteinli V, Kvam U, Skjeldestad F. Norsk pasientregister: administrativ database med mange forskningsmuligheter. Nor Epidemiol. 2004; 14:65–9.
15. Furu K, Wettermark B, Andersen M, Martikainen JE, Almarsdottir AB, Sørensen HT. The Nordic countries as a cohort for pharmacoepidemiological research. Basic Clin Pharmacol Toxicol. 2010;106:86–94.
16. The Cause of Death Register. https://www.ssb.no/en/helse/statistikker/pasient10. Accessed 1 Oct 2015.
17. Core Team R. R Foundation for Statistical Computing. Vienna: Austria. URL; 2015. R: A language and environment for statistical computing, https://www.r-project.org/.
18. Jernberg T, Hasvold P, Henriksson M, Hjelm H, Thuresson M, Janzon M. Cardiovascular risk in post-myocardial infarction patients: nationwide real world data demonstrate the importance of a long-term perspective. Eur Heart J. 2015;36:1163–70.
19. Angerås O, Hasvold P, Thuresson M, Deleskog A, Braun O. Treatment pattern of contemporary dual antiplatelet therapies after acute coronary syndrome: a Swedish nationwide population-based cohort study. Scand Cardiovasc J. 2016;50:99–107.
20. Nytt om legemidler. http://tidsskriftet.no/Ekstra/Nytt-om-legemidler/Nytt-om-legemidler-2011. Accessed 1 Oct 2015.

10

Strategies to reduce hospital 30-day risk-standardized mortality rates for patients with acute myocardial infarction

Elizabeth H Bradley[1,2*], Heather Sipsma[1], Amanda L Brewster[1], Harlan M Krumholz[1,2,3,4] and Leslie Curry[1,2]

Abstract

Background: Survival rates after acute myocardial infarction (AMI) vary markedly across U.S. hospitals. Although substantial efforts have been made to improve hospital performance, we lack contemporary evidence about changes in hospital strategies and features of organizational culture that might contribute to reducing hospital AMI mortality rates. We sought to describe current use of several strategies and features of organizational culture linked to AMI mortality in a national sample of hospitals and examine changes in use between 2010 and 2013.

Methods: We conducted a cross-sectional survey of 543 hospitals (70% response rate) in 2013, and longitudinal analysis of a subsample of 107 hospitals that had responded to a survey in 2010 (67% response rate).

Results: Between 2010 and 2013, the use of many strategies increased, but the use of only two strategies increased significantly: the percentage of hospitals providing regular training to Emergency Medical Service (EMS) providers about AMI care increased from 36% to 71% (P-value < 0.001) and the percentage of hospitals using computerized assisted physician order entry more than doubled (P-value < 0.001). Most, but not all, hospitals reported having environments conducive to communication, coordination and problem solving.

Conclusions: We found few significant changes between 2010 and 2013 in hospital strategies or in key features of organizational culture that have been associated with lower AMI mortality rates. Findings highlight several opportunities to help close remaining performance gaps in AMI mortality among hospitals.

Keywords: Hospitals, Management, Quality improvement, Acute myocardial infarction

Background

Survival rates after acute myocardial infarction differ markedly across hospitals [1] despite overall reductions in AMI mortality nationally [2]. During 2006–2009, 30-day risk-standardized mortality rates (RSMR) after AMI varied from 13.2% to 18.4% at the 5th and 95th percentiles of hospitals, respectively [3]. With more than 800,000 people in the U.S. hospitalized with myocardial infarctions each year [4], closing the performance gap in hospitals could save many lives.

* Correspondence: elizabeth.bradley@yale.edu
[1]Department of Health Policy and Management, Yale School of Public Health, 60 College Street, PO Box 208034, New Haven, CT 06520-8034, USA
[2]Robert Wood Johnson Clinical Scholars Program, Department of Medicine, Yale University School of Medicine, New Haven, CT, USA
Full list of author information is available at the end of the article

Previous research has identified hospital strategies that have been associated with lower hospital RSMRs and has highlighted key features of organizational culture that are prominent among hospitals with top performance as measured by RSMR [5-8]. Although the presence of these strategies and features of organizational cultural were somewhat limited in 2010, substantial efforts have been made nationally to improve quality, particularly in the wake of public reporting on 30-day mortality rates after AMI [9]. Nevertheless, we lack contemporary evidence about changes in the use of these strategies and features of organizational culture in hospitals nationally.

Accordingly, we sought to describe current use of several strategies and features of organizational culture in a national sample of hospitals, and examine change between

2010 and 2013. We report data on a set of commonly recommended strategies and characteristics that describe organizational culture and compare the current prevalence to that reported by a subsample of the hospitals for which we had similar data from 2010. Findings can help clinicians, policy makers, and researchers seeking to improve quality of care nationally identify what has improved and where additional gaps in practice may persist and require greater attention.

Methods

Study design and sample

We conducted a cross-sectional analysis of 378 hospitals (reflecting a 70% response rate among 543 eligible hospitals surveyed between January and November 2013), and a longitudinal analysis of a subsample of 72 hospitals (reflecting a 67% response rate among the 107 hospitals that had also responded to a survey between April and December 2010). We used the data to examine the current prevalence of commonly recommended hospital strategies used to lower mortality rates among patients with AMI as well as features of organizational culture.

For the 2013 survey, we contacted a random sample of 600 hospitals that were part of the American College of Cardiology's Acute Coronary Treatment and Intervention Outcomes Network (ACTION) registry and treated at least 12 patients with ST-segment elevation acute myocardial infarction per year [9]. This sample size had been previously determined based on the conservative assumption of a 58% response rate in order to have 80% power to detect a difference in RSMR of 1.0 percentage points between 2 groups of 10% of responding hospitals. We sent a letter of invitation to participate in the study to the chief executive officer at all hospitals. We asked the chief executive officer to identify the person most involved in AMI quality improvement efforts, who we contacted to participate in a Web-based survey. Respondents were instructed to coordinate with other relevant staff to complete a single survey reflecting a hospital-level response. Of the 600 hospitals, 54 had ended their participation in the ACTION registry and 3 additional hospitals had closed, leaving 543 hospitals eligible for the follow-up survey. Of these, 378 hospitals (70%) completed a survey between January and November 2013. Additionally, 72 hospitals among the 378 respondents had been previously surveyed as part of our earlier study from April to December 2010 [5]. Among hospitals previously surveyed (N = 107), 35 were non-respondent at follow up (response rate 67%). The 72 hospitals previously surveyed did not differ statistically from the other respondent hospitals in our full sample with respect to teaching status, number of staffed beds, census region, urban/rural location, ownership type, or multihospital affiliation (all P-values > 0.05). We used the subsample of hospitals to explore changes in hospital strategies and organizational culture characteristics between 2010 and 2013.

Measures

Hospitals responded to a modified version of the survey previously described [5] (See Additional file 1 for questionnaire). Measures included a set of strategies (e.g., employing quality improvement teams focused on post-hospital mortality, physician and nurse champions, pharmacist rounding) as well as features of organizational culture (e.g., communication and coordination across departments, creative problem solving). We also obtained data on hospital characteristics from the 2010 American Hospital Association (AHA) annual survey. Variables included hospital size (total number of hospital beds), teaching status (Council of Teaching Hospitals (COTH)/has accredited residency program/non-teaching), ownership (for-profit/nonprofit/government) and multihospital affiliation (yes/no). We determined census regions from the U.S. Census Bureau and ascertained area type (urban/suburban/rural) using the 2003 Urban Influence Codes.

Statistical Analysis

We generated frequencies to describe hospital characteristics among our overall and subsample of hospitals. We compared characteristics of these two samples using chi-square tests. We then generated frequencies to describe the current use of hospital strategies and features of organizational culture among the overall sample of hospitals. Last, we generated frequencies of hospital strategies used among the subsample of hospitals for 2010 and 2013 and compared these differences using McNemar's chi-square tests. A complete case analysis was conducted because only a low proportion of data was missing. We used a significance threshold of P-value < 0.01 given the multiple comparisons. All analyses were completed with SAS 9.3 (Cary, NC). We obtained Internal Review Board exemption (protocol number 1207010622) for our study; participant consent was waived because no identifying participant information was obtained.

Results

Hospital sample

Almost 40% of respondents for which data were available on hospital characteristics (N = 358) were teaching hospitals, 73% had fewer than 399 staffed beds, and 90% were in urban locations (Table 1). The hospitals were distributed among all Census regions. The subsample of 72 hospitals that was surveyed in both 2010 and 2013 was not significantly different from the overall sample in terms of teaching status, number of beds, region, geographic location, ownership type, or multihospital affiliation.

Table 1 Hospital characteristics, weighted by hospital volume

	Overall: 2013 survey (N = 358)[1]	Subsample: 2010 and 2013 surveys (N = 72)[2]	Remaining sample: 2013 survey only (N = 286)	P-value[3]
Hospital teaching status				0.445
Council of teaching	54 (15.2%)	14 (19.7%)	40 (14.0%)	
Hospitals member				
Has accredited residency training	88 (24.7%)	18 (25.4%)	70 (24.6%)	
	214 (60.1%)	39 (54.9%)	175 (61.4%)	
Nonteaching				
Number of staffed beds				0.115
< 200 beds	115 (32.3%)	21 (29.6%)	94 (33.0%)	
200–399 beds	143 (40.2%)	24 (33.8%)	119 (41.8%)	
400–599 beds	65 (18.3%)	20 (28.2%)	45 (15.8%)	
600+ beds	33 (9.3%)	6 (8.5%)	27 (9.5%)	
Census region				0.795
New England	7 (2.0%)	2 (2.8%)	5 (1.8%)	
Middle Atlantic	30 (8.5%)	5 (7.0%)	25 (8.8%)	
East North Central	68 (19.2%)	11 (15.5%)	57 (20.1%)	
West North Central	34 (9.6%)	5 (7.0%)	29 (10.2%)	
South Atlantic	85 (23.9%)	18 (25.4%)	67 (23.6%)	
East South Central	20 (5.6%)	5 (7.0%)	15 (5.3%)	
West South Central	45 (12.7%)	10 (14.1%)	35 (12.3%)	
Mountain	23 (6.5%)	3 (4.2%)	20 (7.0%)	
Pacific	43 (12.1%)	12 (16.9%)	31 (10.9%)	
Geographic location				0.993
Urban	321 (90.4%)	64 (90.1%)	257 (90.5%)	
Suburban	15 (4.2%)	3 (4.2%)	12 (4.2%)	
Rural	19 (5.4%)	4 (5.6%)	15 (5.3%)	
Ownership type				0.182
For-profit	65 (18.3%)	18 (25.4%)	47 (16.5%)	
Nonprofit	255 (71.6%)	45 (63.4%)	210 (73.7%)	
Government	36 (10.1%)	8 (11.3%)	28 (9.8%)	
Multihospital affiliation				0.913
Yes	254 (71.0%)	50 (70.4%)	204 (71.1%)	
No	104 (29.1%)	21 (29.6%)	83 (28.9%)	

[1]20 hospitals missing all AHA data.
[2]1 hospital missing all AHA data.
[3]P-values derived from independent chi-square tests.

Current strategies

In terms of strategies pertaining to quality improvement and monitoring, the vast majority of hospitals had quality improvement teams devoted to improving inpatient mortality in patients with AMI, had a designated person or group to review deaths of patients with AMI that occurred during hospitalization, and belonged to a regional effort or consortium to improve AMI care (Table 2). In contrast, less than half of hospitals had a quality improvement team focusing on post-discharge deaths or a review process for deaths that occurred within 30 days of admission. In terms of strategies for pre-hospital and inpatient care, several of the strategies were used by less than half of the hospitals, including meeting at least monthly with Emergency Medical Services (EMS) providers to review AMI care, not cross-training nurses to cover in the catheterization laboratory, and having pharmacists rounding on patient with AMI.

Several features of organizational culture were prominent in the full sample of hospitals surveyed in 2013. For instance, 87% of hospitals reported that clinicians were

Table 2 Description of current strategies used by sample (N = 378 Hospitals)[1]

Survey item	N (%)
Quality Improvement and Monitoring	
Hospital had a QI team devoted to improving inpatient mortality in patients with AMI	289 (79.8%)
Hospital had QI team for improving post-discharge mortality in patients with AMI	163 (45.3%)
Hospital had a designated person or group to review deaths of patients with AMI that occurred during hospitalization	301 (88.8%)
Hospital had a designated person or group to review deaths of patients with AMI that occurred within 30 days of admission	121 (33.9%)
Hospital had a regular morbidity and mortality conferences (or another educational session) to discuss individual cases of patients with AMI	192 (53.9%)
Hospital was part of a regional effort or consortium of hospitals to improve AMI care	289 (80.5%)
Strategies for Pre-Hospital and In-Patient Care	
Hospital provided training to EMS providers about AMI care monthly or quarterly	195 (54.5%)
Clinicians from your hospital met with EMS providers to review the care of patients with AMI	
Yes, about monthly	125 (38.8%)
Other than monthly	197 (61.2%)
Hospital had 1 or more physician or nurse champions focused on improving either inpatient or 30-day mortality in patients with AMI	
Neither physician nor nurse champion	87 (24.3%)
Nurse champion only	17 (4.8%)
Physician champion only	40 (11.2%)
Both physician and nurse champion	214 (59.8%)
On inpatient units, hospital had computerized assisted physician order entry	274 (76.3%)
Non-interventional or interventional cardiologists or cardiology fellows were at the hospital 24-hours/day and 7-days/week	90 (24.7%)
Nurses in at least one of your critical care areas were cross-trained to cover in the catheterization laboratory	52 (14.5%)
Which of the following best describes the role of pharmacists in caring for patients with AMI during this time?	
Pharmacists round on all patients in the CCU or with AMI	162 (48.8%)
Pharmacists do not round, but review the medications of all patients with AMI	102 (30.7%)
Pharmacists do not have a specific role in care of patients with AMI	68 (20.5%)
Organizational Culture	
Clinicians are encouraged to creatively solve problems related to AMI care processes.	
Never, rarely, or sometimes	47 (13.1%)
Usually or always	311 (86.9%)
There is good coordination among the different departments involved with the care of patients with AMI.	
Never, rarely, or sometimes	36 (10.1%)
Usually or always	322 (89.9%)
Clinicians caring for patients with AMI share new evidence-based approaches with the AMI team.	
Never, rarely, or sometimes	69 (19.3%)
Usually or always	288 (80.7%)
Departments caring for patients with AMI (e.g., cardiology, emergency medicine) communicate easily with each other.	
Never, rarely, or sometimes	32 (9.0%)
Usually or always	325 (91.0%)
Mistakes have led to positive changes in AMI care processes at the hospital.	
Never, rarely, or sometimes	89 (25.1%)
Usually or always	265 (74.9%)

[1]Number of missing responses ranged generally from 14 to 22, with two items that had 46 and 56 missings, respectively.

Table 3 Description of baseline and follow-up strategies (N = 72 Hospitals)

Survey Item	Baseline[1] 2010 survey N (%)	Follow up[2] 2013 survey N (%)	McNemar's P-value
Quality Improvement and Monitoring			
Hospital had a QI team devoted to improving inpatient mortality in patients with AMI	45 (62.5%)	54 (77.1%)	0.108
Hospital had QI team to improve post-discharge mortality in patients with AMI	17 (23.6%)	30 (43.5%)	0.024
Hospital had a designated person or group to review deaths of patients with AMI that occurred during hospitalization	63 (87.5%)	58 (84.1%)	0.607
Hospital had a designated person or group to review deaths of patients with AMI that occurred within 30 days of admission	16 (22.2%)	25 (36.2%)	0.163
Hospital had a regular 'morbidity and mortality' conferences (or another educational session) for discussing individual cases involving patients with AMI	40 (55.6%)	35 (51.5%)	0.851
Hospital was part of a regional effort or consortium of hospitals to improve AMI care	53 (73.6%)	56 (81.2%)	0.442
Strategies for Pre-Hospital and In-Patient Care			
Hospital provided training to EMS providers about AMI care monthly or quarterly	26 (36.1%)	42 (60.9%)	<0.001
Clinicians from your hospital met with EMS providers to review the care of patients with AMI			0.458
Yes, about monthly	29 (40.3%)	32 (51.6%)	
Other than monthly	43 (59.7%)	30 (48.4%)	
Hospital had 1 or more physician or nurse champions focused on improving either inpatient or 30-day mortality in patients with AMI			0.518[3]
Neither physician nor nurse champion	23 (31.9%)	17 (24.6%)	
Nurse champion only	4 (5.6%)	1 (1.5%)	
Physician champion only	9 (12.5%)	11 (15.9%)	
Both physician and nurse champion	36 (50.0%)	40 (58.0%)	
On the inpatient units, hospital had computerized assisted physician order entry	24 (33.3%)	57 (82.6%)	<0.001
Non-interventional or interventional cardiologists or cardiology fellows were at the hospital 24-hours/day and 7-days/week	10 (14.5%)	16 (23.2%)	0.238
Nurses in at least one of your critical care areas were cross-trained to cover in the catheterization laboratory	12 (16.7%)	8 (11.6%)	0.607
Which of the following best describes the role of pharmacists in caring for patients with AMI during this time?			0.915[3]
Pharmacists round on all patients in the CCU or with AMI	32 (45.7%)	31 (46.3%)	
Pharmacists do not round, but review the medications of all patients with AMI	24 (34.3%)	23 (34.3%)	
Pharmacists do not have a specific role in the care of patients with AMI	14 (20.0%)	13 (19.4%)	
Organizational Culture			
Clinicians are encouraged to creatively solve problems related to AMI care processes.			1.000
Never, rarely or sometimes	12 (16.7%)	12 (17.7%)	
Usually or always	60 (83.3%)	56 (82.4%)	
There is good coordination among the different departments involved with the care of patients with AMI.			0.012
Never, rarely, or sometimes	3 (4.2%)	11 (16.2%)	
Usually or always	69 (95.8%)	57 (83.8%)	
Clinicians caring for patients with AMI share new evidence-based approaches with the AMI team.			1.000
Never, rarely, or sometimes	14 (19.4%)	12 (17.7%)	
Usually or always	58 (80.6%)	56 (82.4%)	
Departments caring for patients with AMI (e.g., cardiology, emergency medicine) communicate easily with each other.			0.035
Never, rarely or sometimes	4 (5.6%)	12 (17.9%)	
Usually or always	68 (94.4%)	55 (82.1%)	

Table 3 Description of baseline and follow-up strategies (N = 72 Hospitals) *(Continued)*

Mistakes have led to positive changes in AMI care processes at the hospital.			0.557
Never, rarely, or sometimes	19 (26.4%)	23 (33.8%)	
Usually or always	53 (73.6%)	45 (66.2%)	

[1]Number of missing responses range from 0 to 3.
[2]Number of missing items range from 3 to 5; one item missing 10.
[3]Tests of symmetry used.

encouraged to creatively solve problems related to AMI care processes, and easy communication among departments caring for patients with AMI was reported by 91% of hospitals (Table 2). In terms of collaboration and coordination with partners outside of the hospital, 39% of hospitals held monthly meetings between clinicians and EMS providers to review the care of AMI patients. Somewhat more hospitals (55%) provided training to Emergency Medical Service (EMS) providers monthly or quarterly.

Changes in strategies

Between 2010 and 2013, the use of many strategies increased but only three increased significantly; the percentage of hospitals that had a quality improvement team to improve post-discharge mortality in patients with AMI increased from 23.6% to 43.5% (P-value = 0.024), and the percent of hospitals providing training to EMS providers about AMI care at least monthly or quarterly increased from 36.1% to 60.9% (P-value < 0.001). The percentage of hospitals using computerized assisted physician order entry increased from 33.3% to 82.6% (P-value < .001) (Table 3). A couple of features of organizational culture worsened, notably coordination among different departments (4.2% to 16.2% of hospitals reported they never, rarely, or sometimes versus usually or always had good coordination, P-value = 0.012), and communication across departments caring for patients with AMI (5.6% to 17.9% of hospitals reported they never, rarely, or sometimes versus usually or always had good coordination, P-value = 0.035) (Table 3).

Discussion

We observed modest changes in hospital strategies and features of organizational culture for hospitals surveyed in 2010 and 2013. The overall direction in terms of strategies used was toward improvement, although few of the changes were statistically significant. The overall direction of features of organizational culture worsened, with 2 of 5 of the organizational culture indicators being significant.

Several hospital strategies associated with lower AMI RSMR in previous research highlight room for further improvement, with levels of adoption under 60% at baseline and at follow up. These strategies largely pertained to inpatient care including having both physician and nurse champions focused on improving AMI mortality [5,10], having cardiologists or cardiology fellows on site 24 hours a day, 7 days a week [5,11,12] (or among hospitals without such cardiologist coverage, having pharmacists round on all patients with AMI [5]), and having clinicians meet with EMS providers monthly for training and to review AMI care [5,8,13]. Notably, these strategies are complex interventions that require coordination among units or organizations, and in some cases require substantial investment by hospitals. One strategy in particular, having cardiologists on site 24/7, is resource intensive and may not be feasible for many hospitals.

We found significant increases in hospitals providing regular training to EMS providers. Previous qualitative studies have suggested multiple avenues exist for engaging EMS providers in AMI care; high-performing hospitals in AMI care have been found to actively engage EMS providers in quality improvement activities, invest in strong communication and coordination with EMS agencies and maintain a high level of respect for EMS as valued professionals and colleagues [6]. Although few studies have focused on hospital interaction with EMS providers, a survey of EMS agencies indicated that greater medical supervision of agencies is associated with stronger cardiovascular care procedures [14]. Given the key contributions that EMS providers make in AMI care [15], greater attention to this aspect of care may be warranted.

Another hospital strategy that significantly increased during our study period was computerized physician order entry (CPOE), which has generally been linked to higher quality care [16] and adherence to best practices in AMI care processes [17]. Unintended negative impacts have also been documented, however, depending on the design and implementation of specific CPOE systems [18,19]. These have included in the earlier days of CPOE implementation perceived loss of control by clinicians [18] and increases in medication error risk [19]. Nevertheless, the substantial rise in CPOE between 2010 and 2013 is not surprising given the improvement in the systems, adaptation by clinicians, and financial incentives for hospitals and providers to adopt electronic health record systems over that time period [20].

Finally, more hospitals reported having quality improvement teams working on improving 30-day mortality after AMI in the follow up compared with the baseline survey. Such re-focusing requires substantial commitment of resources and acceptance of a larger role for hospitals in the post-discharge quality of care. At the same time, some features of organizational culture conducive to high quality AMI care appeared to be less prevalent in the follow up compared with the baseline survey. In particular, coordination and communication across departments caring for patients with AMI still remained a challenge for a notable minority of hospitals and was reported less commonly at follow up than in the baseline survey.

Our findings should be interpreted in light of several limitations. First, the relatively small size of our longitudinal sample means that we were only able to detect changes of large magnitude. Our data suggest that some additional strategies may have increased over time more modestly; for example, the proportion of hospitals with a quality improvement team focused on post-discharge AMI mortality increased from 24% to 44% but the result was not statistically significant. Second, the time period covered by our study, 2010–2013, was fairly short and may not have been sufficient for hospitals to implement some strategies such as monthly meetings with EMS providers. Third, the sample was drawn from hospitals participating in the ACTION registry and therefore may be more invested in quality improvement for cardiovascular care than other hospitals, and within the sample, respondents may have been those that were focusing greater attention on AMI care processes. Such effects may potentially lead to overestimates of the changes in strategy use; thus the magnitude of changes in the use of strategies examined may be more modest among other hospitals.

Conclusions

In conclusion, we found an overall trend toward greater adoption of strategies that have been found to be associated with lower 30-day AMI mortalities rates, although most changes were modest in size and non-significant, and cross-departmental communication and coordination remain challenging for a small but notable group of hospitals. Improvements may be due in part to extensive previous efforts within the ACTION registry, from which the sample of hospitals was drawn, to improve quality of AMI care. The findings nonetheless highlight important areas for future improvement. Several evidence-based strategies showed low levels of adoption which, if adopted more widely, could help close remaining performance gaps in AMI mortality among hospitals.

Abbreviations

AMI: Acute myocardial infarction; EMS: Emergency medical service; RSMR: Risk-standardized mortality rate; ACTION: Acute coronary treatment and intervention outcomes network; AHA: American hospital association; COTH: Council of teaching hospitals; CPOE: Computerized physician order entry.

Competing interests

Dr. Bradley and Dr. Curry report that they are the recipients of a research grant from The Medicines Company. Dr. Krumholz reports that he is the recipient of a research grant from Medtronic through Yale University and chairs a cardiac scientific advisory board for United Health.

Authors' contributions

EHB, LC, and HK conceptualized and designed the study. EHB and HK acquired the data. EHB, HS, ALB, HK and LC analyzed and interpreted the data. EHB, HS and AB drafted the manuscript. LC and HK critically revised the manuscript for important intellectual content. HS conducted the statistical analysis. EHB, HK and LC obtained funding for the study and EHB supervised the study. All authors read and approved the final manuscript.

Acknowledgements

Funding for this research was provided by The Commonwealth Fund, One East 75th Street, New York, NY 10021 and The Donaghue Foundation, 18 West Main Street, West Hartford, CT 06107. Dr. Horwitz is supported by the National Institute on Aging (K08 AG038336) and by the American Federation for Aging Research through the Paul B. Beeson Career Development Award Program. Dr. Horwitz is also a Pepper Scholar with support from the Claude D. Pepper Older Americans Independence Center at Yale University School of Medicine (#P30AG021342 NIH/NIA). Dr. Krumholz is supported by grant U01 HL105270-03 (Center for Cardiovascular Outcomes Research at Yale University) from the National Heart, Lung, and Blood Institute in Bethesda, MD.

Author details

[1]Department of Health Policy and Management, Yale School of Public Health, 60 College Street, PO Box 208034, New Haven, CT 06520-8034, USA. [2]Robert Wood Johnson Clinical Scholars Program, Department of Medicine, Yale University School of Medicine, New Haven, CT, USA. [3]Center for Outcomes Research and Evaluation, Yale-New Haven Hospital, New Haven, CT, USA. [4]Section of Cardiovascular Medicine, Department of Medicine, Yale University School of Medicine, New Haven, CT, USA.

References

1. Krumholz H, Wang Y, Chen J, Drye EE, Spertus JA, Ross JS, Curtis JP, Nallamothu BK, Lichtman JH, Havranek EP, Masoudi FA, Radford MJ, Han LF, Rapp MT, Straube BM, Normand ST: **Reduction in acute myocardial infarction mortality in the united states: risk-standardized mortality rates from 1995–2006.** *JAMA* 2009, **302:**767–773.
2. Yeh RW, Sidney S, Chandra M, Sorel M, Selby JV, Go AS: **Population trends in the incidence and outcomes of acute myocardial infarction.** *N Engl J Med* 2010, **362:**2155–2165.
3. Bernheim SM, Grady JN, Lin Z, Wang Y, Wang Y, Savage SV, Bhat KR, Ross JS, Desai MM, Merrill AR, Han LF, Rapp MT, Drye EE, Normand S-LT, Krumholz HM: **National patterns of risk-standardized mortality and readmission for acute myocardial infarction and heart failure update on publicly reported outcomes measures based on the 2010 release.** *Circ Cardiovasc Qual Outcomes* 2010, **3:**459–467.
4. Go AS, Mozaffarian D, Roger VL, Benjamin EJ, Berry JD, Borden WB, Bravata DM, Dai S, Ford ES, Fox CS, Franco S, Fullerton HJ, Gillespie C, Hailpern SM, Heit JA, Howard VJ, Huffman MD, Kissela BM, Kittner SJ, Lackland DT, Lichtman JH, Lisabeth LD, Magid D, Marcus GM, Marelli A, Matchar DB, McGuire DK, Mohler ER, Moy CS, Mussolino ME, *et al*: **Heart disease and stroke statistics—2013 update a report from the american heart association.** *Circulation* 2013, **127:**e6–e245.
5. Bradley EH, Curry LA, Spatz ES, Herrin J, Cherlin EJ, Curtis JP, Thompson JW, Ting HH, Wang Y, Krumholz HM: **Hospital strategies for reducing risk-standardized mortality rates in acute myocardial infarction.** *Ann Intern Med* 2012, **156:**618–W–221.
6. Cherlin EJ, Curry LA, Thompson JW, Greysen SR, Spatz E, Krumholz HM, Bradley EH: **Features of high quality discharge planning for patients following acute myocardial infarction.** *J Gen Intern Med* 2013, **28:**436–443.
7. Curry LA, Spatz E, Cherlin E, Thompson JW, Berg D, Ting HH, Decker C, Krumholz HM, Bradley EH: **What distinguishes top-performing hospitals in acute myocardial infarction mortality rates?A qualitative study.** *Ann Intern Med* 2011, **154:**384–390.

8. Landman AB, Spatz ES, Cherlin EJ, Krumholz HM, Bradley EH, Curry LA: **Hospital collaboration with emergency medical services in the care of patients with acute myocardial infarction: perspectives from Key hospital staff.** *Ann Emerg Med* 2013, **61**:185–195.
9. **ACTION Registry-GWTG for Acute Coronary Syndrome Patients.** [https://www.ncdr.com/webncdr/action/home].
10. Ellerbeck EF, Bhimaraj A, Hall S: **Impact of organizational infrastructure on β-blocker and aspirin therapy for acute myocardial infarction.** *Am Heart J* 2006, **152**:579–584.
11. Kulkarni VT, Ross JS, Wang Y, Nallamothu BK, Spertus JA, Normand S-LT, Masoudi FA, Krumholz HM: **Regional density of cardiologists and rates of mortality for acute myocardial infarction and heart failure.** *Circ Cardiovasc Qual Outcomes* 2013, **6**:352–359.
12. Abubakar I, Kanka D, Arch B, Porter J, Weissberg P: **Outcome after acute myocardial infarction: a comparison of patients seen by cardiologists and general physicians.** *BMC Cardiovasc Disord* 2004, **4**:14.
13. Travers AH, Rea TD, Bobrow BJ, Edelson DP, Berg RA, Sayre MR, Berg MD, Chameides L, O'Connor RE, Swor RA: **Part 4: CPR overview 2010 American Heart Association guidelines for cardiopulmonary resuscitation and emergency cardiovascular care.** *Circulation* 2010, **122**(18 suppl 3):S676–S684.
14. Greer S, Williams I, Valderrama AL, Bolton P, Patterson DG, Zhang Z: **EMS medical direction and prehospital practices for acute cardiovascular events.** *Prehospital Emergency Care* 2013, **17**:38–45.
15. Johnston S, Brightwell R, Ziman M: **Paramedics and pre-hospital management of acute myocardial infarction: diagnosis and reperfusion.** *Emerg Med J* 2006, **23**:331–334.
16. Kaushal R, Shojania K, Bates D: **Effects of computerized physician order entry and clinical decision support systems on medication safety: a systematic review.** *Arch Intern Med* 2003, **163**:1409–1416.
17. Swanson Kazley A, Diana M: **Hospital computerized provider order entry adoption and quality: an examination of the United States.** *Health Care Manage Rev* 2011, **36**:86–94.
18. Campbell EM, Sittig DF, Ash JS, Guappone KP, Dykstra RH: **Types of unintended consequences related to computerized provider order entry.** *J Am Med Inform Assoc* 2006, **13**:547–556.
19. Koppel R, Metlay J, Cohen A, Abaluck B, Localio AR, Kimmel SE, Strom BL: **Role of computerized physician order entry systems in facilitating medication errors.** *JAMA* 2005, **293**:1197–1203.
20. Blumenthal D, Tavenner M: **The "Meaningful Use" regulation for electronic health records.** *N Engl J Med* 2010, **363**:501–504.

11

Microvascular obstruction assessed by 3-tesla magnetic resonance imaging in acute myocardial infarction is correlated with plasma troponin I levels

Karine Pernet, Fiona Ecarnot, Romain Chopard, Marie-France Seronde, Philoktimon Plastaras, Francois Schiele and Nicolas Meneveau*

Abstract

Background: Microvascular obstruction (MVO) at the acute phase of myocardial infarction (MI) is associated with poor prognosis. We aimed to evaluate the correlation between plasma cardiac troponin I (cTnI) at the acute phase of MI and extent of no-reflow, as assessed by 3-T cardiac magnetic resonance imaging (MRI). Secondly, we defined a cut-off value for cTnI predictive of no-reflow.

Methods: 51 consecutive patients with no previous history of cardiovascular disease, presenting ST elevation MI within <12 h. Infarct size and extent of no-reflow were evaluated by 3-T MRI at day 5. Extent of no-reflow at 15 minutes (MVO) was correlated with cTnI at admission, 6, 12, 24, 48 and 72 hours. At 6 months, MRI was performed to evaluate the impact of MVO on LV remodeling.

Results: MVO was diagnosed in 29 patients (57%). Extent of MVO was significantly correlated to peak troponin, cTnI (except admission values) and area under the curve. Using Receiver-operating characteristic (ROC) curve analysis, a cut-off cTnI value >89 ng/mL at 12 h seemed to best predict presence of early MVO (sensitivity 63%, specificity 88%). At 6 months, MVO was associated with left ventricular (LV) remodeling, resulting in higher LV volumes.

Conclusion: There is a relationship between cTnI at the acute phase of AMI and extent of MVO as assessed by 3-T cardiac MRI. A cut-off cTnI value of 89 ng/mL at 12 h seems to best predict presence of MVO, which contributes to LV remodeling.

Keywords: Myocardial infarction, MRI, Troponin, Microvascular obstruction

Background

In acute ST-segment-elevation myocardial infarction (STEMI), primary percutaneous coronary intervention is the treatment of choice to restore myocardial revascularization and minimize ischemic damage to the myocardium [1]. Several studies have demonstrated that microvascular dysfunction after infarct-related artery revascularization is associated with myocardial reperfusion injury, resulting in greater infarct size [2-10], left ventricular impairment [3-5,7,11-17], recurrent MI [2-4,14], heart failure [2-4,12,14] and higher mortality [2-5,12,14,18,19]. In addition, microvascular dysfunction has a negative prognostic value, irrespective of infarct size [3]. Magnetic Resonance Imaging (MRI) is not systematically performed in routine practice, and it would thus be useful if there was a more accessible prognostic marker that could identify patients with microvascular obstruction (MVO). Cardiac troponin levels correlate well with infarct size [20] and are of prognostic value in the short and long term [21].

The aim of our study was to evaluate the relationship between plasma levels of cardiac troponin I (cTnI) and microvascular obstruction (MVO) as assessed by magnetic resonance imaging (MRI) at day 5, and to define a cut-off value for cTnI that predicts MVO.

* Correspondence: nicolas.meneveau@univ-fcomte.fr
Department of Cardiology, EA3920, University Hospital Jean Minjoz, Boulevard Fleming, Besançon 25000, France

Methods

Study population

This study was a prospective single-center study. Patients < 75 years old referred to our department for a first ST elevation MI (STEMI) and admitted within 12 hours of symptom onset were considered for inclusion. MI was defined by the guidelines of the joint Task Force of the European Society of Cardiology (ESC), the American College of Cardiology (ACC), the American Heart Association (AHA), and the World Heart Federation (WHF) [1,22]. MI was confirmed by detection of elevated cardiac biomarkers (at least one value above the 99th percentile of the upper reference limit (URL)), together with evidence of myocardial ischemia (i.e., new ST-T changes or new left bundle branch block, or development of pathological Q waves in the ECG).

Exclusion criteria were: previous cardiovascular or pulmonary diseases, cardiogenic shock and contraindication for MRI.

The study protocol was approved by the local ethics committee (Comité de Protection des Personnes Est II, University Hospital Besancon, France) and informed consent was obtained from all enrolled patients.

Angiographic evaluation

All patients were referred to the catheterization laboratory within the first 24 hours after admission for coronary angiogram, and received medication according to current guidelines [1].

The initial and post-procedural blood flow in the infarct-related artery was graded according to the Thrombolysis in Myocardial Infarction (TIMI) grading system [23]. A successful procedure was defined by a TIMI flow grade = 3 and residual stenosis < 20%.

Magnetic resonance imaging

All CE-MRI studies were conducted at 3.0 field strength (Signa HD, General Electric Healthcare, Milwaukee, WI, USA) and performed in the acute phase and repeated at 6 months. Left ventricular function was assessed by ECG-gated cine steady-state free precession (SSFP) breath-hold sequences in the two-chamber and four-chamber views as well as in the short cardiac axis from base to apex (30 phases per cardiac cycle; repetition time 3.5 ms, echo time 1.2 ms, flip angle 45°, typical voxel size 1.92 × 1.25 × 8.0 mm).

Contrast-enhancement imaging was performed at 3 and 15 min with a breath-hold ECG-gated T1-weighted sequence after the injection of a bolus of gadolinium (Dota-Gd; Guerbet, Roissy, France) at a single dose of 0.1 mmol/kg (TE = MinFull/field of view 440 mm/TI = optimised to obtain an optimal myocardial nulling/matrix 256 × 224, interpolated 256 × 256/slice thickness = 8 mm/gap = 1 mm). The number and position of slices were the same as used for functional imaging.

Image analysis was performed in a blind fashion by two operators using an off-line dedicated workstation (General Electric Healthcare, Milwaukee, WI, USA). Left ventricular (LV) ejection fraction (LVEF), end-diastolic (LVEDVI) and end–systolic volume index (LVESVI) and mass were calculated from SSFP short-axis views. MVO was assessed on the initial CE-MRI performed during in-hospital stay. Infarct size was assessed from the same initial CE-MRI and at 6 months follow-up. Infarct size and MVO (if present) were manually traced from the contrast-enhancement short-axis images [24]. Myocardial regions was considered infarcted if the infarct size signal intensity was >2 SDs above the remote myocardium. MVO was defined as a dark zone within the infarcted segments, usually located in the subendocardium. MVO and infarct size are expressed as a percentage of LV mass assuming 1.05 g/ml as the specific gravity of myocardium.

Enzyme measurement

Serum levels of troponin I (TnI), creatine kinase (CK) and creatine kinase isoenzyme myocardial and brain (CK-MB) were determined on admission, and 6, 12, 24, and 48 hours after onset of MI. cTnI was measured quantitatively using sandwich immunoassay (Dimension RXL max, SIEMENS, Germany). The lower limit of detection for this assay was 0.04 ng/ml. A value of cTnl > 0.15 ng/ml was considered indicative of myocardial necrosis for the purposes of clinical care. The peak level was determined as the highest value.

Statistical analysis

Quantitative continuous variables are expressed as mean ± standard deviation, and qualitative variables as number and percent. The Student t test and Chi square or Fisher's exact tests were used for comparisons, as appropriate. We calculated the relative change at 6 months from baseline in LV end-diastolic volume index, LV end-systolic volume index, and LV ejection fraction. The model used to take initial infarct size into account was the calculation of relative change, normalized for baseline infarct size. The correlations between serum enzyme levels and MVO at day 5 were assessed using the Spearman rank test. A receiver-operating characteristic (ROC) curve was used to define the threshold value of troponin levels predictive of MVO at day 5. A p-value <0.05 was considered statistically significant. All analyses were performed using SAS version 9.2 (SAS Institute, Cary, NC, USA).

Results

Patient characteristics

Between 2006 and 2008, 51 patients were enrolled in the study. Mean age was 54 years; there were 9 women and

42 men. Baseline and angiographic characteristics of the study population are shown in Table 1. Eighteen patients (35%) had anterior MI location. All patients underwent coronary angiogram and angioplasty within the first 24 hours. Reperfusion therapy was initiated 5.3 ± 3.2 hours after the onset of symptoms, by primary PCI in 37 patients (73%) and thrombolysis in 14 patients (27%). In patients who underwent thrombolysis, rescue PCI was performed in 6 patients (12%) and the remaining 8 underwent systematic PCI within the first 24 hours after reperfusion.

Twenty-nine patients (57%) had MVO (MVO^{pos} patients) diagnosed by MRI and 22 (43%) had no MVO (MVO^{neg} patients). MVO^{pos} and MVO^{neg} patients were comparable as regards baseline characteristics.The percentage of patients with TIMI flow grade ≤2 before PCI was significantly higher in the MVO ^{pos} group. After PCI, the rate of TIMI flow grade 3 was comparable in both groups (Figure 1).

During follow-up, there were 0 deaths, and 4 revascularisations (1 for recurrent MI due to stent thrombosis at 12 days and 3 on arteries other than the infarct-related artery).

Magnetic resonance imaging

MRI was performed at 5.7 ± 2.7 days after symptom onset and at 6 ± 1 months follow-up. MRI was not performed in 6 patients at 6 months due to patient refusal, or intervention (PCI or CABG) during the follow-up period.

At day 5, the extent of MVO was 7.3 ± 3.7%. Infarct size was 23.5 ± 8.4% in MVO^{pos} patients versus 12.7 ± 9.4% in MVO^{neg} patients (p = 0.0001). There was a significant correlation between the extent of MVO at day 5 and the infarct size at day 5 (r = 0.61, p < 0.0001). Similarly, we observed a significant correlation between extent of MVO and time to reperfusion (r = 0.43, p = 0.004).

At 6 months follow-up, a significant positive correlation was observed among MVO^{pos} patients between MVO at day 5 and infarct size at 6 months (Figure 2). In MVO^{pos} patients, the relative change in LV end-diastolic volume index (LVEDVI) and in LV end-systolic volume

Table 1 Baseline and angiographic characteristics

	All patients N = 51	Pts MVO^{neg} N = 22 (43%)	Pts MVO^{pos} N = 29 (57%)	P
Age - years	53.6 ± 9.9	56 ± 10	52.6 ± 9.4	0.27
Female (%)	9 (18)	4 (19)	5 (17.5)	0.93
Arterial hypertension (%)	18 (35)	7 (32)	11(38)	0.65
Diabetes mellitus (%)	11 (22)	5 (23)	6 (21)	0.86
Family history of CAD (%)	15 (29)	7 (32)	8 (27)	0.74
Current smoking	42 (82)	18 (82)	24 (83)	0.93
Hyperlipidemia (%)	21 (41)	9 (41)	12 (41)	0.97
Body mass index ≥30Kg/m²(%)	9 (18)	3 (14)	6 (20.6)	0.51
One vessel disease (%)	28 (55)	13 (59)	15 (52)	0.60
Multivessel disease (%)	16 (31)	7 (32)	9 (31)	0.95
Stenosis < 50% (%)	7 (14)	2 (9)	5 (17)	0.40
Anterior location (%)	18 (35)	9 (41)	9 (31)	0.46
Time from symptom onset to 1st reperfusion therapy – hours	5.3 ± 3.2	4.7 ± 2.9	5.9 ± 3.7	0.21
Fibrinolysis (%)	14 (27)	5 (23)	9 (31)	0.73
Primary PCI (%)	37 (73)	17 (77)	20 (69)	
Rescue PCI (%)	6 (12)	2 (9)	4 (14)	0.94
Aspirin	51 (100)	22 (100)	29 (100)	1
Clopidogrel loading dose (300/600 mg)	34/17	14/8	20/9	0.69
GP IIb-IIIa inhibitors (%)	22 (43)	8 (36)	14(48)	0.39
TnI peak (ng/mL) (range)	81 ± 71	53.6 (13–225)	118.5 (22–585)	0.0006
CK peak, U/L (range)	1985 ± 1522	1825 (63–9580)	2663 (160–9930)	0.006
CK-MB peak, U/L (range)	124 ± 132	145.6 (9–940)	189.1 (9–760)	0.09

Pts MVO^{neg} = patients without microvascular obstruction; Pts MVO^{pos} = patients with microvascular obstruction; CAD = coronary artery disease; PCI = percutaneous coronary intervention; TnI = troponin I; CK = creatine kinase; CK-MB = creatine kinase isoenzyme myocardial and brain.

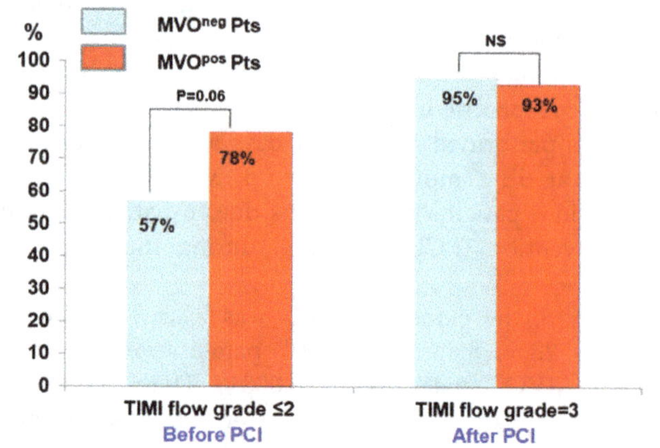

Figure 1 TIMI flow grade before and after percutaneous coronary intervention. TIMI = thrombolysis in myocardial infarction; PCI = percutaneous coronary intervention; MVO^{neg} = patients without microvascular obstruction; MVO^{pos} = patients with microvascular obstruction.

index (LVESVI) was significantly greater than in MVO^{neg} patients ($p = 0.002$ for LVEDVI, $p = 0.004$ for LVESVI) (Figure 3). There was no significant difference in relative change in LV ejection fraction (LVEF).

Enzyme measurement

Peak troponin and peak CK were significantly higher in MVO^{pos} patients (respectively $p = 0.0006$ and $p = 0.006$) (Table 1).

There was no significant difference in terms of peak troponin values between patients with TIMI flow grade 3 and those with TIMI flow ≤2 after revascularisation (peak troponin 75 ± 58 vs 83 ± 65, TIMI 3 vs ≤2 respectively, $p = 0.65$).

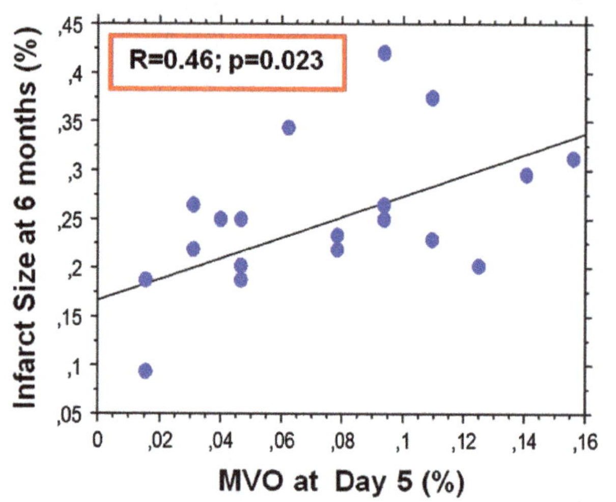

Figure 2 Relationship between MVO at Day 5 and infarct size at 6 months. MVO = microvascular obstruction; MVO^{pos} = patients with microvascular obstruction.

Correlation between the extent of MVO and troponin I levels

The extent of MVO at day 5 was significantly correlated with peak troponin (Figure 4) and troponin I levels at 6, 12, 24, 48 and 72 hours (Table 2). Infarct size was significantly correlated with peak troponin ($p < 0.0001$) and the different cTnI levels ($p < 0.001$), except cTnI at admission.

Relationship between the presence of MVO and troponin I levels

Peak troponin and all cTnI levels except cTnI at admission were significant predictors of MVO (Table 3). The Area under the curve (ROC) varied from 0.68 for troponin at 72 h to 0.766 for troponin at 12 h. Sensitivity varied from 56% for troponin at 48 h to 74% for troponin at 6 h. Specificity ranged from 65% for troponin at 6 h and 72 h to 88% for troponin at 12 h, 48 h and the AUC troponin. Using ROC curve analysis, a cTnI level > 89 ng/ml at 12 hours was found to be the best cut-off value to predict MVO with a sensitivity of 63% and a specificity of 88% ($p < 0.0002$) (Figure 5).

Discussion

We aimed to find an accessible prognostic marker that could identify patients with microvascular dysfunction after reperfusion at the acute phase of myocardial infarction. Our data demonstrated that troponin levels (except troponin at admission), and particularly peak troponin, were correlated with the extent of MVO on MRI at day 5. A troponin I level > 89 ng/ml at 12 hours was found to be the best cut-off value to predict MVO, with a sensitivity of 63% and a specificity of 88%.

The phenomenon of no-reflow [25,26] or microvascular obstruction is due to microembolization of atherosclerotic debris or thrombotic material, intimal oedema, tissue haemorrhage and/or leukocyte sticking [8,27], and is diagnosed well by MRI [3,6,13,28]. In addition, besides microvascular obstruction, intra-myocardial hemorrhage and microvascular destruction have also been shown to play an important role in this setting [29]. At the acute phase of MI, the successful restoration of epicardial coronary artery patency does not always lead to adequate reperfusion at the microvascular level. In our study, although 93 to 95% of the patients had a TIMI flow grade =3 after PCI at 24 h, MVO was diagnosed by MRI in 57% of cases at day 5. There was no significant difference in peak troponin between patients with TIMI flow grade 3 and those with TIMI flow ≤2 after revascularisation. Several studies have shown that microvascular dysfunction after infarct-related artery revascularization is associated with myocardial reperfusion injury, resulting in greater infarct size [2-10], left ventricular impairment [3-5,7,11-17], recurrent MI [2-4,14], heart failure [2-4,12,14] and higher mortality [2-5,12,14,18,19]. In

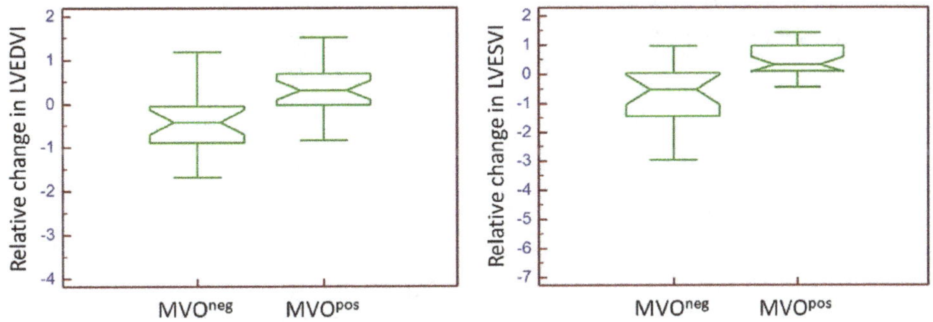

Figure 3 Relative change at 6 months from baseline in left ventricular end-diastolic volume index (LVEDVI) and left ventricular end-systolic volume index (LVESVI) normalized for baseline infarct size. MVO^{neg} = patients without microvascular obstruction; MVO^{pos} = patients with microvascular obstruction.

patients with MVO, mortality has been reported to increase by 75% at 1 month [18], 67% at 1 year [5] and 50% at 5 years [19]. In our study, MVO at day 5 was associated with LV remodelling at 6 months, as reflected by significantly increased left ventricular volumes assessed on MRI. These results are comparable to those of Orn et al. [7] at 1 year, and those of Nijveldt et al. [13] at 4 months, using the MRI technique.

This is strong evidence that both serial and single-point measurements of troponin correlate well with infarct size [8,9,20]. In routine practice, plasma levels of troponin I are used by the clinician to estimate the extent of necrosis. In our study, infarct size was significantly correlated with peak troponin and with the serial troponin I levels, except for troponin values at admission. To date, only 3 studies have investigated the relationship between MVO as assessed by MRI and serial troponin measurements, and the optimal timing for a single measurement. Our results confirm those of the literature. In the study of Neizel et al. [8], 61 patients with STEMI <24 h reperfused by fibrinolysis or PCI, underwent MRI within 4 ± 1 days and serial troponin T measurements at admission and after 24, 48, 72 and 96 hours. They found that a troponin T level > 2.52 μg/l at 24 h was a predictor for MVO with a sensitivity of 100% and a specificity of 80%. In this study, Neizel et al. used troponin T levels, and no troponin measurements were performed between admission and 24 h. Furthermore, MVO was evaluated on earlier delayed-enhancement imaging after contrast injection. Younger and al [9] enrolled 93 patients who underwent MRI on average 3.7 ± 1.4 days after medical treatment for acute ST elevation or non-ST elevation myocardial infarction. Serum troponin I concentrations were sampled at 12 h and 72 h only after admission. They found a close relationship between a single measurement of troponin I at 72 h and the extent of MVO. The early and complete reperfusion of the infarct-related artery accelerates the appearance of cardiac enzymes in the first hours after reperfusion therapy. This wash-out phenomenon is characterized by a steeper rise and an earlier peak after successful restoration of anterograde coronary blood flow. These changes are more pronounced after mechanical reperfusion, which was used in our study, than after thrombolytic therapy [8]. Therefore, the almost exclusive reliance on thrombolytic therapy

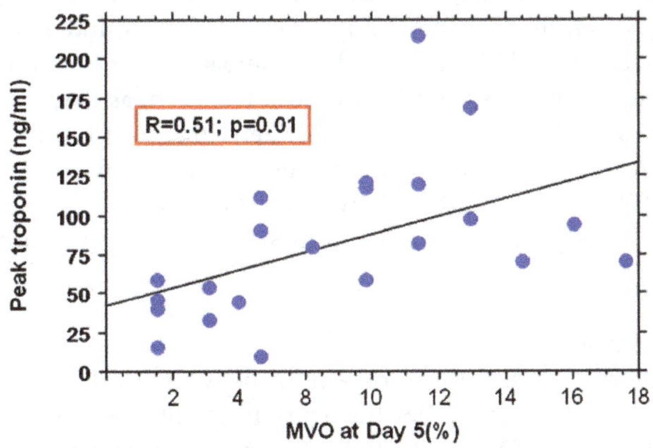

Figure 4 Relationship between MVO and Peak troponin. MVO = microvascular obstruction.

Table 2 Correlation between the extent of MVO and troponin I levels

	MVO (N = 29)	
	r	p
Troponin peak	0.51	0.01
AUC troponin	0.58	0.01
Troponin on admission	0.11	0.59
Troponin at 6H	0.57	0.01
Troponin at 12H	0.67	<0.0001
Troponin at 24H	0.46	0.02
Troponin at 48H	0.57	0.01
Troponin at 72H	0.42	0.04

MVO = microvascular obstruction; AUC = area under the curve; H = hours.

Table 3 Cut-off value of cTnI predictive of MVO

	Cut-off value (ng/ml)	Se (%)	Sp (%)	AUC ROC	p
Troponin at H6	44.6	74	65	0.729	0.0025
Troponin at H12	89	63	88	0.766	0.0002
Troponin at H24	27.4	65	81	0.703	0.0116
Troponin at H48	16.35	56	88	0.724	0.0041
Troponin at H72	7.9	71	65	0.68	0.0308
Peak troponin	79.9	63	82	0.761	0.0003
AUC Troponin	275.3	59	88	0.726	0.0057

Se = sensitivity; Sp = specificity; AUC = area under the curve; ROC = receiver operating characteristic; H = hours.

in the study of Younger and al [9] may explain the more delayed troponin release observed. In study by Mayr and al [10], MRI was performed in 118 patients within 8 days after successful interventional reperfusion of STEMI. Cardiac troponin T concentrations were measured at least 3 times during the first 24 h after admission, and subsequently on days 1, 2, 3 and 4. These authors demonstrated that a peak troponin > 4.7 µg/l was predictive of MVO with a sensitivity of 78% and a specificity of 83%.

One of the advantages of the present study is the large number of repeat troponin measures, at relatively short time intervals, which allowed more accurate determination of a threshold value that could predict MVO at the acute phase of infarction.

It has previously been shown that a longer duration of ischemia is associated with more pronounced impairment of myocardial perfusion and consequently, infarct size [30]. In our study, we observed a correlation between the extent of MVO and the time to reperfusion.

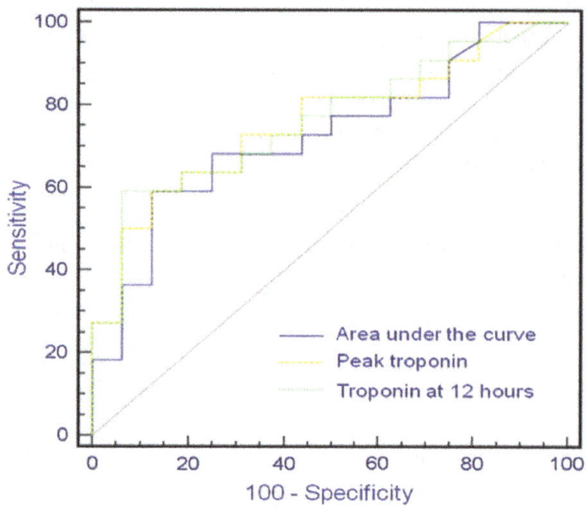

Figure 5 Cut-off value of cTnI predictive of MVO. ROC curves established for: AUC troponin (AUC $_{ROC}$ 0.726, 95% CI 0.56-0.86). Peak troponin (AUC$_{ROC}$ 0.757, 95% CI 0.59-0.88). Troponin at 12 hours (AUC$_{ROC}$ 0.763, 95% CI 0.6-0.88) cTnI = cardiac troponin I; MVO = microvascular obstruction; ROC = receiver operating characteristic; AUC = area under the curve.

Thus, the relation between troponin and the presence of MVO should be interpreted taking into account the time to reperfusion, since restoration of TIMI flow grade 3 by angioplasty does not necessarily guarantee the normalization of myocardial perfusion [31].

Newton et al. previously studied MVO on MRI in the context of non-ST elevation MI, and observed that MVO was correlated with infarct size and troponin levels. Thus, it would appear that the results observed in the context of STEMI are also applicable in NSTEMI [32].

Study limitations

This is a single-center study, with a relatively small population of highly selected patients. Nonetheless, the selection of the population made it possible to independently analyse MVO as evaluated by MRI in the absence of other cardiovascular comorbidities. Secondly, we did not evaluate blush grade, which corresponds to the angiographic evaluation of microcirculation after revascularisation. Our study focused on MVO at 5 days, which is a different phenomenon, and shown to be an independent prognostic factor in acute MI. These results merit further confirmation in a larger, prospective study. Thirdly, reperfusion strategy (primary PCI or thrombolysis) may possibly influence the occurrence of MVO. In particular, it has been shown that rescue PCI is associated with an increased thrombotic risk in this setting. However, in our study, only 6 (12%) patients underwent rescue PCI. This likely did not impact on the relation observed between MVO and peak troponin, as there was no significant difference between groups (Table 1). Fourthly, MRI could not be performed in 6 patients (11.7%) at 6 months. However, this does not impact the interpretation of the primary endpoint evaluated at 5 days.

Conclusion

Our results suggest a correlation between plasma levels of cardiac troponin I at the acute phase of AMI, and the extent of MVO as assessed by 3-T cardiac magnetic resonance imaging. The extent of MVO at 5 days post-STEMI is correlated with infarct size, and negatively impacts on

LV remodeling at 6 months. A cut-off value of 89 ng/mL for cTnI at 12 hours seems to best predict the presence of early MVO with high sensitivity and specificity. Troponin measurement is an easily accessible prognostic marker that could help identify patients with MVO and unfavorable prognosis.

Competing interests

The authors declare that they have no competing interests.

Authors' contributions

Study conception and design: KP, MFS, NM. Acquisition of data: KP, RC, MFS, PP, FS, NM. Analysis and interpretation of data: FE, RC, PP, FS, NM. Drafting of the manuscript and critical revision: All. All authors read and approved the final version of the manuscript to be published. All authors agree to be accountable for all aspects of the work in ensuring that questions related to the accuracy or integrity of any part of the work are appropriately investigated and resolved.

References

1. Van de Werf F, Bax J, Betriu A, Blomstrom-Lundqvist C, Crea F, Falk V, Filippatos G, Fox K, Huber K, Kastrati A, Rosengren A, Steg PG, Tubaro M, Verheugt F, Weidinger F, Weis M, ESC Committee for Practice Guidelines (CPG): **Management of acute myocardial infarction in patients presenting with persistent ST-segment elevation: the task force on the management of ST-segment elevation acute myocardial infarction of the European society of cardiology.** *Eur Heart J* 2008, **29:**2909–2945.
2. Cochet AA, Lorgis L, Lalande A, Zeller M, Beer JC, Walker PM, Touzery C, Wolf JE, Brunotte F, Cottin Y: **Major prognostic impact of persistent microvascular obstruction as assessed by contrast-enhanced cardiac magnetic resonance in reperfused acute myocardial infarction.** *Eur Radiol* 2009, **19:**2117–2126.
3. Hombach V, Grebe O, Merkle N, Waldenmaier S, Hoher M, Kochs M, Wohrle J, Kestler HA: **Sequelae of acute myocardial infarction regarding cardiac structure and function and their prognostic significance as assessed by magnetic resonance imaging.** *Eur Heart J* 2005, **26:**549–557.
4. Wu KC, Zerhouni EA, Judd RM, Lugo-Olivieri CH, Barouch LA, Schulman SP, Blumenthal RS, Lima JA: **Prognostic significance of microvascular obstruction by magnetic resonance imaging in patients with acute myocardial infarction.** *Circulation* 1998, **97:**765–772.
5. Ndrepepa G, Tiroch K, Keta D, Fusaro M, Seyfarth M, Pache J, Mehilli J, Schomig A, Kastrati A: **Predictive factors and impact of no reflow after primary percutaneous coronary intervention in patients with acute myocardial infarction.** *Circ Cardiovasc Interv* 2010, **3:**27–33.
6. Bogaert J, Kalantzi M, Rademakers FE, Dymarkowski S, Janssens S: **Determinants and impact of microvascular obstruction in successfully reperfused ST-segment elevation myocardial infarction: assessment by magnetic resonance imaging.** *Eur Radiol* 2007, **17:**2572–2580.
7. Orn S, Manhenke C, Greve OJ, Larsen AI, Bonarjee VV, Edvardsen T, Dickstein K: **Microvascular obstruction is a major determinant of infarct healing and subsequent left ventricular remodelling following primary percutaneous coronary intervention.** *Eur Heart J* 2009, **30:**1978–1985.
8. Neizel M, Futterer S, Steen H, Giannitsis E, Reinhardt L, Lossnitzer D, Lehrke S, Jaffe AS, Katus HA: **Predicting microvascular obstruction with cardiac troponin T after acute myocardial infarction: a correlative study with contrast-enhanced magnetic resonance imaging.** *Clin Res Cardiol* 2009, **98:**555–562.
9. Younger JF, Plein S, Barth J, Ridgway JP, Ball SG, Greenwood JP: **Troponin-I concentration 72 h after myocardial infarction correlates with infarct size and presence of microvascular obstruction.** *Heart* 2007, **93:**1547–1551.
10. Mayr A, Klug G, Schocke M, Trieb T, Mair J, Pedarnig K, Pachinger O, Jaschke W, Metzler B: **Late microvascular obstruction after acute myocardial infarction: relation with cardiac and inflammatory markers.** *Int J Cardiol* 2012, **157:**391–396.
11. Bekkers SC, Smulders MW, Passos VL, Leiner T, Waltenberger J, Gorgels AP, Schalla S: **Clinical implications of microvascular obstruction and intramyocardial haemorrhage in acute myocardial infarction using cardiovascular magnetic resonance imaging.** *Eur Radiol* 2010, **20:**2572–2578.
12. Morishima I, Sone T, Okumura K, Tsuboi H, Kondo J, Mukawa H, Matsui H, Toki Y, Ito T, Hayakawa T: **Angiographic no-reflow phenomenon as a predictor of adverse long-term outcome in patients treated with percutaneous transluminal coronary angioplasty for first acute myocardial infarction.** *J Am Coll Cardiol* 2000, **36:**1202–1209.
13. Nijveldt R, Hofman MB, Hirsch A, Beek AM, Umans VA, Algra PR, Piek JJ, van Rossum AC: **Assessment of microvascular obstruction and prediction of short-term remodeling after acute myocardial infarction: cardiac MR imaging study.** *Radiology* 2009, **250:**363–370.
14. Bolognese L, Carrabba N, Parodi G, Santoro GM, Buonamici P, Cerisano G, Antoniucci D: **Impact of microvascular dysfunction on left ventricular remodeling and long-term clinical outcome after primary coronary angioplasty for acute myocardial infarction.** *Circulation* 2004, **109:**1121–1126.
15. Larose E, Rodes-Cabau J, Pibarot P, Rinfret S, Proulx G, Nguyen CM, Dery JP, Gleeton O, Roy L, Noel B, Barbeau G, Rouleau J, Boudreault JR, Amyot M, De Larochellière R, Bertrand OF: **Predicting late myocardial recovery and outcomes in the early hours of ST-segment elevation myocardial infarction traditional measures compared with microvascular obstruction, salvaged myocardium, and necrosis characteristics by cardiovascular magnetic resonance.** *J Am Coll Cardiol* 2010, **55:**2459–2469.
16. Tarantini G, Razzolini R, Cacciavillani L, Bilato C, Sarais C, Corbetti F, Marra MP, Napodano M, Ramondo A, Iliceto S: **Influence of transmurality, infarct size, and severe microvascular obstruction on left ventricular remodeling and function after primary coronary angioplasty.** *Am J Cardiol* 2006, **98:**1033–1040.
17. Gerber BL, Rochitte CE, Melin JA, McVeigh ER, Bluemke DA, Wu KC, Becker LC, Lima JA: **Microvascular obstruction and left ventricular remodeling early after acute myocardial infarction.** *Circulation* 2000, **101:**2734–2741.
18. Brosh D, Assali AR, Mager A, Porter A, Hasdai D, Teplitsky I, Rechavia E, Fuchs S, Battler A, Kornowski R: **Effect of no-reflow during primary percutaneous coronary intervention for acute myocardial infarction on six-month mortality.** *Am J Cardiol* 2007, **99:**442–445.
19. Ndrepepa G, Tiroch K, Fusaro M, Keta D, Seyfarth M, Byrne RA, Pache J, Alger P, Mehilli J, Schomig A, Kastrati A: **5-year prognostic value of no-reflow phenomenon after percutaneous coronary intervention in patients with acute myocardial infarction.** *J Am Coll Cardiol* 2010, **55:**2383–2389.
20. Giannitsis E, Steen H, Kurz K, Ivandic B, Simon AC, Futterer S, Schild C, Isfort P, Jaffe AS, Katus HA: **Cardiac magnetic resonance imaging study for quantification of infarct size comparing directly serial versus single time-point measurements of cardiac troponin T.** *J Am Coll Cardiol* 2008, **51:**307–314.
21. Bassand JP, Hamm CW, Ardissino D, Boersma E, Budaj A, Fernandez-Aviles F, Fox KA, Hasdai D, Ohman EM, Wallentin L, Wijns W: **Guidelines for the diagnosis and treatment of non-ST-segment elevation acute coronary syndromes.** *Eur Heart J* 2007, **28:**1598–1660.
22. Thygesen K, Alpert JS, White HD, Jaffe AS, Apple FS, Galvani M, Katus HA, Newby LK, Ravkilde J, Chaitman B, Clemmensen PM, Dellborg M, Hod H, Porela P, Underwood R, Bax JJ, Beller GA, Bonow R, Van der Wall EE, Bassand JP, Wijns W, Ferguson TB, Steg PG, Uretsky BF, Williams DO, Armstrong PW, Antman EM, Fox KA, Hamm CW, Ohman EM, *et al*: **Universal definition of myocardial infarction.** *Circulation* 2007, **116:**2634–2653.
23. **The thrombolysis in myocardial infarction (TIMI) trial: phase I findings: TIMI study group.** *N Engl J Med* 1985, **312:**932–936.
24. Kim HW, Farzaneh-Far A, Kim RJ: **Cardiovascular magnetic resonance in patients with myocardial infarction: current and emerging applications.** *J Am Coll Cardiol* 2009, **55:**1–16.
25. Kloner RA, Ganote CE, Jennings RB: **The "no-reflow" phenomenon after temporary coronary occlusion in the dog.** *J Clin Invest* 1974, **54:**1496–1508.
26. Eeckhout E, Kern MJ: **The coronary no-reflow phenomenon: a review of mechanisms and therapies.** *Eur Heart J* 2001, **22:**729–739.
27. Bekkers SC, Yazdani SK, Virmani R, Waltenberger J: **Microvascular obstruction: underlying pathophysiology and clinical diagnosis.** *J Am Coll Cardiol* 2010, **55:**1649–1660.
28. Lima JA, Judd RM, Bazille A, Schulman SP, Atalar E, Zerhouni EA: **Regional heterogeneity of human myocardial infarcts demonstrated by contrast-enhanced MRI: potential mechanisms.** *Circulation* 1995, **92:**1117–1125.

29. Robbers LF, Eerenberg ES, Teunissen PF, Jansen MF, Hollander MR, Horrevoets AJ, Knaapen P, Nijveldt R, Heymans MW, Levi MM, van Rossum AC, Niessen HW, Marcu CB, Beek AM, van Royen N: **Magnetic resonance imaging-defined areas of microvascular obstruction after acute myocardial infarction represent microvascular destruction and haemorrhage.** *Eur Heart J* 2013, **34:**2346–2353.
30. Tarantini G, Cacciavillani L, Corbetti F, Ramondo A, Marra MP, Bacchiega E, Napodano M, Bilato C, Razzolini R, Iliceto S: **Duration of ischemia is a major determinant of transmurality and severe microvascular obstruction after primary angioplasty: a study performed with contrast-enhanced magnetic resonance.** *J Am Coll Cardiol* 2005, **46:**1229–1235.
31. De Luca G, Hof AW v 't, de Boer MJ, Ottervanger JP, Hoorntje JC, Gosselink AT, Dambrink JH, Zijlstra F, Suryapranata H: **Time-to-treatment significantly affects the extent of ST-segment resolution and myocardial blush in patients with acute myocardial infarction treated by primary angioplasty.** *Eur Heart J* 2004, **25:**1009–1013.
32. Mewton N, Bonnefoy E, Revel D, Ovize M, Kirkorian G, Croisille P: **Presence and extent of cardiac magnetic resonance microvascular obstruction in reperfused non-ST-elevated myocardial infarction and correlation with infarct size and myocardial enzyme release.** *Cardiology* 2009, **113:**50–58.

12

Incidence and impact on prognosis of peri-procedural myocardial infarction in 2760 elective patients with stable angina pectoris in a historical prospective follow-up study

Martin Kirk Christensen[1*], Hui Huang[2], Christian Torp-Pedersen[3], Torleif Trydal[4] and Jan Ravkilde[1]

Abstract

Background: The clinical significance of myocardial infarction related to treatment with percutaneous coronary intervention (PCI) has been subject of great discussion. This subject has been studied for many years using different definitions of peri-procedural myocardial infarction and different biomarkers, the results have varied greatly depending on methods and time of the study. This study was to determine the incidence and prognostic significance of elevated cardiac biomarkers after elective PCI in patients with stable angina pectoris using the current cut-off set by the Third Universal Definition of Myocardial Infarction and current biomarkers.

Methods: We performed a historical prospective follow-up study of all patients with stable angina pectoris who underwent elective PCI at Aalborg University Hospital, Denmark from January 1st 2000 to December 31st 2012. We stratified patients according to peak post-PCI troponin T (cTnT) and Creatine Kinase MB mass (CK-MBmass).

Results: Follow-up for time to all-cause mortality was mean 5.8 years and total 15,891 years and mean 3.7 years and total 10,160 years for the combined endpoint of all-cause mortality and new onset heart failure. During the follow up period 399 of 2760 patients died (14.5 %) and 1095 (39.7 %) suffered the combined endpoint. Post-PCI concentration of cTnT and CK-MBmass was elevated above the defined cut-off in 419 patients (15.2 %) and 113 patients (4.1 %) respectively. There was no statistically significant difference between the groups in stratified analysis of the hazard rates by time regarding all-cause mortality for cTnT nor CK-MBmass. Regarding the combined endpoint the results were ambiguous. The results were unchanged in multivariable analyses that included age and gender.

Conclusion: The incidence of elevated biomarkers after elective PCI in patients with stable angina pectoris using the defined cut-off (>5 x URL) was 15.2 % using cTnT and 4.1 % using CK-MBmass. The independent prognostic value for both cardiac biomarkers of any cut-off showed no statistical significance for all-cause mortality, whereas the combined endpoint (all-cause mortality or new-onset heart failure) were ambiguous in both short- and long-term follow-up.

Keywords: Troponin, Elective, Prognosis, Myocardial infarction, Peri-procedural, Percutaneous coronary intervention

* Correspondence: mkc@martinkc.dk
[1]Department of Cardiology, Aalborg University Hospital, Aalborg, Denmark
Full list of author information is available at the end of the article

Background

Percutaneous coronary intervention (PCI) is an established procedure for the treatment of both stable angina pectoris and acute coronary syndrome, but the procedure is not without risk. An important complication to PCI is myocardial infarction (MI). This form of MI has been defined as MI type 4a by the Third Universal Definition of Myocardial Infarction Task Force Group [1]. Despite the clear definition, it remains unclear whether the chosen cut-off for biomarker concentration post-PCI is clinically and prognostically meaningful and should lead to changes in the treatment strategy [2].

The biomarker historically used for this purpose has been creatine kinase isoenzyme MB (CK-MB) initially as a measure of activity followed by analysis of mass concentration. Previous studies have shown a proportional relationship between rise in CK-MB and 6-month all-cause mortality [3, 4]. CK-MB has been largely replaced by high sensitive cardiac troponins T or I (cTn) as the biomarkers of choice in all types of myocardial infarction due to both higher sensitivity and specificity for myocardial necrosis [1, 2].

The aims of this study were to determine the incidence of elevated biomarkers post-PCI using the cut-off set by the Third Universal Definition of Myocardial Infarction in a cohort of patients with stable angina pectoris undergoing elective PCI and to determine the prognostic significance of this arbitrarily set limit of cardiac biomarker elevation defining peri-procedural MI by evaluating primarily all-cause mortality and secondarily a combined endpoint of all-cause mortality and heart failure.

Methods

Study design and inclusion

We performed a historical prospective follow up study of a cohort of patients with stable angina pectoris who underwent elective PCI at Aalborg University Hospital, Denmark from January 1st 2000 to December 31st 2012. Patients were eligible if the procedure was elective and there was no elevation of troponin prior to the procedure. Selection of the included 2760 patients can be followed in Fig. 1. As per department routine, patients had cTnT and CK-MBmass measured immediately before or during the procedure and 3–24 h later. In patients with more than one sample post-PCI, the highest value for cTnT was included. Patients who underwent several separate procedures were only included in analysis for the first intervention. All patients with a previous diagnosis of heart failure were excluded from analysis of the secondary endpoint of new-onset heart failure. As older studies have used CK-MB and not cTn, we also analyzed peak post-PCI CK-MBmass from the same cohort included in analysis for cTnT sampled from 3–24 h after the procedure.

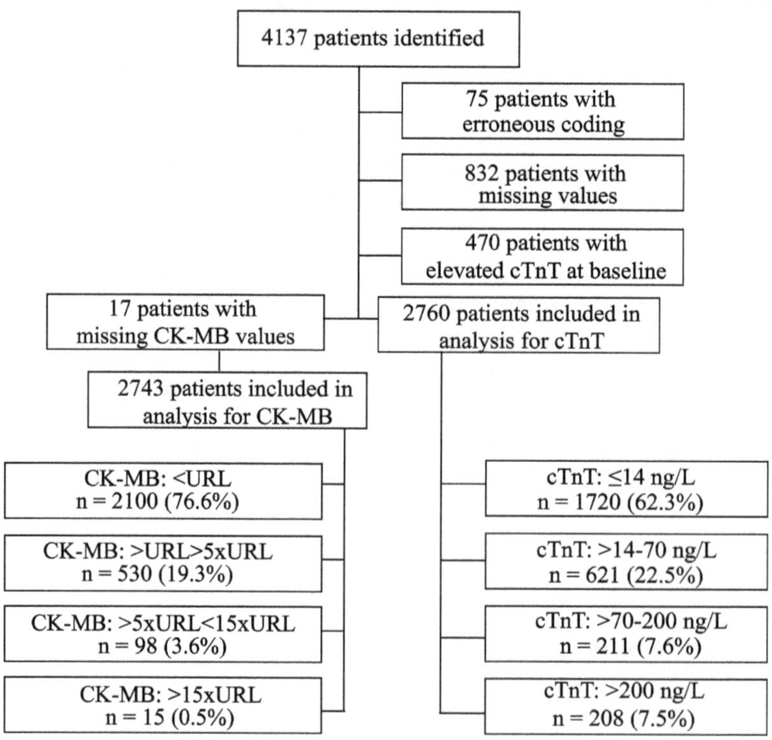

Fig. 1 Study flow chart. cTnT = peak post procedural concentration of troponin T. CK-MB = peak post procedural concentration of CK-MBmass. URL = Upper reference limit

Biochemical analysis

cTnT and CK-MBmass were measured using a chemiluminiscence assay on either Elecsys 2010, Cobas 6000 or Cobas 8000 (Roche, Mannheim, Germany). The cTnT analysis changed to the new high sensitive version (hsTnT) in June 2010. Alignment of the concentrations between the cTnT and the hsTnT measurements was done according to a comparison study and information from the provider [5]. The 99th percentile upper reference limit (URL) of hsTnT has been determined to be 14 ng/L, and the 99th percentile of 4th generation TnT analysis has been determined to less than 10 ng/L [5, 6].

Values up to 14 ng/l in hsTnT methods, or less than 10 ng/L in non-hsTnT methods, were defined as normal values. We considered that different versions of the TnT-assays had the same standardization from cTnT-values 70 ng/L and above. The cTnT value of 70 ng/L is also 5 x URL set by the Third Universal Definition Myocardial Infarction [1].

The CK-MB was measured as massconcentration and the assays underwent no change of standardization in the period in question. URL for CK-MBmass is gender specific and the current URL of 4 μg/L and 7 μg/L for woman and men (information from the provider, [6]), respectively, were used.

The analyses were performed as instructed by the provider. Internal quality controls at low and high concentrations, and external quality assessment (Labquality, Helsinki, Finland) were performed regularly throughout the period. The results were obtained from the clinical laboratory information system LABKA1 and LABKA2 databases [7].

Follow-up

In this study data from one center, Aalborg University Hospital, was included. All patients were continuously registered in the Western Denmark Heart Registry immediately after the procedure [8]. In this registry patient data are available including risk factors, previous cardiac disease, clinical data e.g., body weight, blood pressure, latest P-Creatinine, indication, priority and procedural details such as number of treated vessels and details regarding type and number of stents used. Using the Western Denmark Heart Registry we were able to restrict our cohort to PCI performed on the indication stable angina pectoris that were performed electively.

To link databases and follow the patients we extracted information from the Danish National Civil Registration System, which identifies all Danish citizens with a unique personal identification number. Death is registered in this system within 2 weeks of death. The data, including date of birth, sex and date of death is updated continuously and is considered highly valid [9]. New onset heart failure required that the patient did not have a clinical diagnosis of heart failure prior to the procedure and further did use furosemide for a period of 60 days prior to the procedure. New onset heart failure was then considered to take place if the patient collected a prescription for furosemide or was admitted to hospital with a diagnosis of heart failure. Prescriptions were identified in the Danish Register of Medicinal Product Statistics, maintained by the Danish Medicines Agency. It contains information on all dispensed prescriptions from Danish pharmacies since 1994, including dosage, dispensing date and quantity of the drug dispensed. All drugs are categorized according to the Anatomical Therapeutic Chemical classification system [10].

Endpoints were chosen to all-cause mortality and the combined endpoint of all-cause mortality and new onset heart failure.

This study complies with the Declaration of Helsinki and STROBE guidelines. According to Danish law no specific approval from a local ethics committee or informed consent from the patients was required for this registry study. Permission was obtained to use data from Western Denmark Heart Registry. The study was approved by the Danish Data Protection Agency.

Statistical analysis

Statistical analysis was performed in three and four groups after peak post-PCI concentrations of cTnT, the three groups were: ≤14 ng/L (URL), >14–70 ng/L and >70 ng/L (5x URL) and as four groups ≤14 ng/L (URL), >14–70 ng/L, >70–200 ng/L and >200 ng/L and four groups for CK-MBmass: < 4 μg/L (women) or 7 μg/L (men)), 4–20 μg/L or 7–35 μg/L; 20–60 μg/L or 35–105 μg/L and >60 μg/L or >105 μg/L for women and men, respectively. The values for CK-MBmass correspond to URL, 5 x URL and 15 x URL.

Comparison of baseline demographics was performed using rank-sum tests for continuous variables and chi-square for discrete variables. Survival curves were constructed from Kaplan Meier survival estimates and differences were analyzed using Cox Proportional Hazard Models. Analyses were performed with SAS (Statistical Analysis System, version 9.4, The SAS Institute) and R version 3.02 (R core development team) [11].

Results

From January 1st 2000 to December 31st 2012; 4137 elective PCIs were performed on the diagnosis of stable angina pectoris, from this we identified 2760 patients eligible for further analysis (Fig. 1). Seventeen additional patients were excluded from analysis for CK-MBmass due to missing values. Follow-up for time to death was mean 5.8 years and total 15,891 years and mean 3.7 years and total 10,160 years for the combined endpoint of all-cause mortality and new onset heart failure. During the follow up period 399 patients died (14.5 %) and 1095 (39.7 %)

suffered the combined endpoint. The incidence of elevated biomarkers post-PCI with cTnT exceeding URL was 1040/2760 (37.7 %) and 419/2760 (15.2 %) exceeding 5 x URL. Correspondingly for CK-MBmass 643/2743 (23.4 %) above URL and only 113/2743 (4.1 %) exceeded 5 x URL.

Table 1 shows the key elements of previous medical history, clinical and angiographic data in the four groups according to peak post-PCI cTnT. Of the 2760 included patients there was a high prevalence of risk factors for ischemic heart disease with male sex (71 %), age (mean 65 years), current smoking (25.9 %), diabetes (15.3 %), medically treated hypertension (64.3 %), medically treated hypercholesterolemia (70.8 %) and family history of coronary artery disease (49.2 %). The risk factors were evenly distributed among the groups with few statistically significant differences. The group with lowest cTnT were statistically significantly younger (64 years versus 67 years) than the other groups. Kidney function evaluated by P-Creatinine was also slightly but statistically significantly lower in the group with lowest cTnT (83 μmol/L versus 86 μmol/L). For severity of symptoms, all patients were evaluated by Canadian Cardiovascular Society classification of angina pectoris (CCS) with an even distribution and 87.7 % with angina pectoris CCS 1-2. As expected, the patients often had previous MI (26.6 %) and previous revascularization with PCI (23.4 %). There were statistically significantly more previous MIs in the group with cTnT >14–70 ng/L. With the lowest mean age in the group with cTnT ≤14 ng/L and the highest number of stents being used in the two groups with cTnT above 70 ng/L. Post-PCI peak values for cTnT were mainly distributed below the defined cut-off, but of the 2760 patients 419 (15.2 %) had elevated cTnT above 5 x URL post-PCI.

The Kaplan-Meier curve of all-cause mortality by peak concentration of troponin T showed no sign of separation between the curves until after approximately 6 years (2000 days). After this time point, there was a slight tendency towards lower all-cause mortality in the group with cTnT ≤14 ng/L, but this was not statistically

Table 1 Patient characteristics

Post-PCI peak TnT (ng/L)	≤14 (*n* = 1720)	>14-70 (*n* = 621)	>70-200 (*n* = 211)	>200 (*n* = 208)	*P* Value
Clinical data					
Age - years (IQR)	64 (57, 71)	67 (60, 74)	67 (59, 74)	67 (59, 73)	<0.0001
Male sex - no. (%)	1220 (70.9)	435 (70.0)	161 (76.3)	154 (74.0)	0.27
Angina severity CCS 1	247 (18.8)	94 (18.9)	28 (17.9)	26 (16.4)	
Angina severity CCS 2	913 (69.4)	365 (73.4)	111 (71.2)	121 (76.1)	
Angina severity CCS 3	151 (11.5)	36 (7.2)	17 (10.9)	11 (6.9)	
Angina severity CCS 4	4 (0.3)	2 (0.4)	0 (0.0)	1 (0.6)	0.34
Body Mass Index - kg/m^2 (IQR)	26.3 (23.4, 29.3)	26.6 (23.5, 30.0)	25.8 (23.1, 29.2)	27.2 (24.4, 30.5)	0.23
P-Creatinine - μmol/L median (IQR)	83 (73, 96)	84 (74, 99)	85 (74, 100)	86 (75, 101)	0.01
Risk factors					
Smoking - Current - no. (%)	454 (27.2)	132 (21.8)	44 (21.2)	55 (26.8)	0.22
Non-insulin dependent diabetes- no. (%)	177 (10.5)	54 (9.1)	21 (10.3)	20 (10.0)	
Insulin dependent diabetes - no. (%)	80 (4.8)	34 (5.7)	9 (4.4)	10 (4.9)	0.62
Medically treated hypertension - no. (%)	1038 (62.8)	399 (67.2)	133 (64.3)	134 (66.3)	0.19
Medically treated hypercholesterolemia - no. (%)	1166 (70.5)	428 (71.6)	145 (70.0)	138 (68.3)	0.92
Family history of coronary artery disease - no. (%)	822 (49.6)	289 (48.5)	91 (44.2)	94 (46.5)	0.13
Medical history					
Previous myocardial infarction - no. (%)	439 (25.5)	184 (29.6)	59 (28.0)	51 (24.5)	0.034
Previous percutaneus coronary intervention - no. (%)	397 (23.9)	146 (24.4)	54 (26.1)	48 (23.8)	0.93
Medically treated heart failure	135 (7.8)	66 (10.6)	21 (10.0)	26 (12.5)	0.11
Procedure					
Stents used: 0 - no. (%)	60 (5.2)	32 (6.2)	5 (3.1)	9 (5.4)	
Stents used: 1 - no. (%)	751 (64.7)	269 (52.1)	57 (35.8)	51 (30.7)	
Stents used: 2-3 - no. (%)	316 (27)	179 (34.7)	75 (47)	74 (45)	
Stents used: >3 - no. (%)	34 (2.9)	36 (7.0)	22 (14)	32 (19)	<0.0001

IQR Interquartile range, *CCS* Canadian Cardiovascular Society classification of angina pectoris. *P* values reflects chi-square statistics comparing the five groups

significant and there were relatively few patients available for follow up in each of the other three groups at this time (Fig. 2). The results were unchanged in multivariable analyses that included age and gender (Fig. 3). The corresponding curves for the combined endpoint of all-cause mortality and new onset heart failure showed early separation of the curves but with an unclear pattern. The group with post-PCI cTnT >70–200 ng/L was without significant separation from the group with cTnT ≤14 ng/L. However, the groups with cTnT >14–70 ng/L and above 200 ng/L did show separation of the curves throughout the follow-up period (Fig. 4).

In stratified analysis the hazard rates for time until death after post-PCI, peak cTnT was compared to the strata with cTnT < URL. There were no statistically significant differences regarding the primary endpoint of all-cause mortality with hazard ratios (HR) respectively in order of rising cTnT 1.62 (95 % confidence interval (CI) 0.97–1.63 $p = 0.07$), 0.99 (95 % CI 0.76–1.30 $p = 0.96$) and 1.21 (95 % CI 0.92–1.60 $p = 0.17$).

There were a few statistically significant differences when analyzing the combined endpoint of all-cause mortality or new onset heart failure the HRs in stratified analysis. The HR were respectively in order of rising cTnT 1.28 (95 % CI 1.04–1.58 $p = 0.02$), 1.18 (95 % CI 0.94–1.48 $p = 0.16$) and 1.31 (95 % CI 1.03–1.67 $p = 0.03$). There was trend towards higher cTnT being

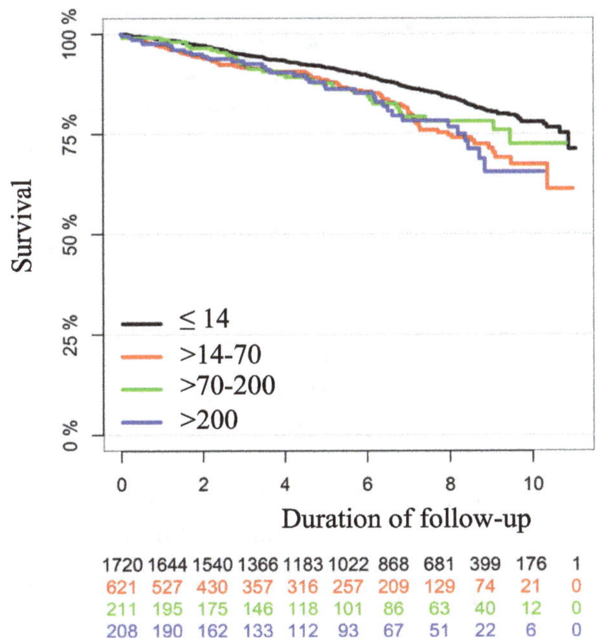

Fig. 2 Kaplan-Meier curve of all-cause mortality by peak concentration of troponin T in ng/L. Each colored line representing one group according to peak concentration of troponin T. Duration of follow up in years from index procedure. Below the Kaplan-Meier curve is the number of patients still available for follow-up in each group

associated with higher risk. However, the group with cTnT 70–200 ng/L was not statistically significant. To further examine this, we additionally re-grouped values into three groups by peak post cTnT and compared the group with cTnT ≤14 ng/L to a group with cTnT >14–70 ng/L (HR 1.1 (95 % CI 0.97–1.34 $p = 0.11$) and a group with cTnT above 70 ng/L (HR 0.92 (95 % CI 0.78–1.09 $p = 0.35$). When grouped in three groups there was no statistically significant differences.

There was no significant difference regarding all-cause mortality when analyzed in four groups after peak post-PCI CK-MBmass: <URL, between URL and 5 x URL (HR 1.96 (95 % CI 0.76–5.05 $p = 0.16$), between 5 and 15 x URL (HR 1.16 (95 % CI 0.55–2.44 $p = 0.69$) and above 15 x URL (HR 0.87 (95 % CI 0.55–1.37 $p = 0.55$) (Fig. 5). The results were unchanged in multivariable analyses that included age and gender. There was no clear pattern regarding the combined endpoint of all-cause mortality and new onset heart failure when analyzed in four groups after peak post-PCI CK-MBmass.: <URL, between URL and 5 x URL (HR 1.97 (95 % CI 1.19–3.27 $p = 0.0088$), between 5 and 15 x URL (HR 1.15 (95 % CI 0.77–1.72 $p = 0.50$) and above 15 x URL (HR 0.88 (95 % CI 0.68–1.15 $p = 0.36$). The results were unchanged in multivariable analyses that included age and gender.

Discussion

The aim of this study was to examine the incidence of cardiac biomarker elevation according to the definition of peri-procedural MI given by the European Society of Cardiology-guidelines "Third Universal definition of MI" type 4a myocardial infarction, and to determine whether this carries independent prognostic value. The elevation of cTnT could be linked directly to the procedure, since only patients with normal baseline cTnT were included. Our population had an even distribution of patient characteristics with few differences and the differences in kidney function and previous MI do not seem clinically relevant since they do not have a clear pattern, and the differences are small. The only statistically significant and clinically meaningful differences between the groups were age and number of stents used. The incidence in our population using the cTnT cut off >5 x URL (cTnT >70 ng/L) was 15.2 %,

For the primary endpoint of all-cause mortality, we did not find that any interval of troponin was associated with an increased all-cause mortality. However, we did find a possible association between elevation of cTnT and the combined endpoint of new onset heart failure and all-cause mortality with the groups with cTnT >14–70 ng/L and >200 ng/L since these groups had borderline statistically significantly higher risk compared to the group with cTnT ≤14 ng/L. Regarding the combined endpoint of new onset heart failure and all-cause mortality and CKMB there was also a seemingly isolated risk

Variable	Hazard ratio (95% confidence interval)	p-value
cTnT≤14ng/L	1	
cTnT>14-70ng/L	1.26 (0-98-1.63)	0.07
cTnT>70-200ng/L	0.99 (0.76-1.30)	0.96
cTnT>200ng/L	1.21 (0.92-1.60)	0.17
Age	1.08 (1.07-1.09)	
Sex	1.00 (0.81-1.23)	1.00

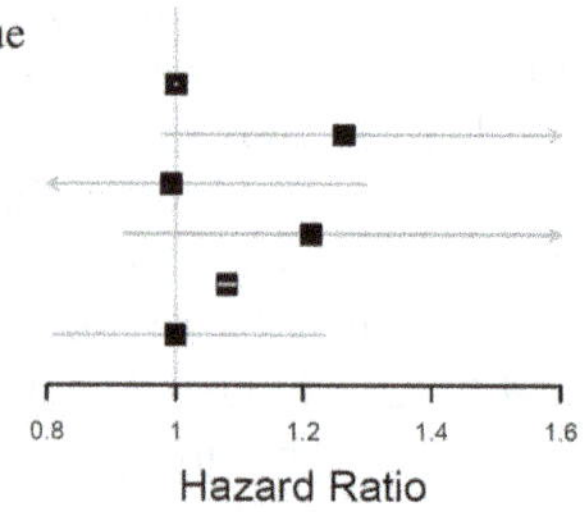

Fig. 3 Forest Plot displaying Multivariate Cox Regression analysis for all-cause mortality. cTnT = peak post procedural concentration of troponin T in ng/L. Age signifies risk pr. year and sex risk associated with being male

associated with values between URL and 5x URL, but not with higher levels of CK-MB.

When using CK-MBmass the fraction of patients with elevated cardiac biomarkers was much lower than for cTnT (15.2 % versus 4.1 % respectively). The reason for this is probably, that cTnT is a more sensitive biomarker than CKMB mass. In contrast to some previous studies, we found that CK-MBmass was not an independent marker for prognosis [3, 4]. However, in our study we used CKMBmass, which is a more sensitive biomarker than CKMBcatalytic activity, and the >5 URL of CKMBmass corresponds to approximately an increase in CKMBcatalytic activity of 1–2 times URL; which in these studies did not show any prognostic information.

The fraction of elevated cardiac biomarkers found in our study is slightly higher than previously reported in meta-analysis by Testa et al. [12] They showed a detectable elevation of cTn after scheduled PCI in 28.7 % of 7578 patients (compared to 37.7 % in our study), and in 14.5 % of the patients cTn exceeded 3 x 99th percentile URL (the previously used cut-off value) [13]. The data used by Testa et al. was of a more heterogeneous population with 7 studies including unstable angina and different assays including both cTnT and cTnI. Furthermore, different cut-off values for cTnT were allowed including 100 ng/L which even with 3 x URL (=300 ng/L) is far above the presently supported 70 ng/L. It seems

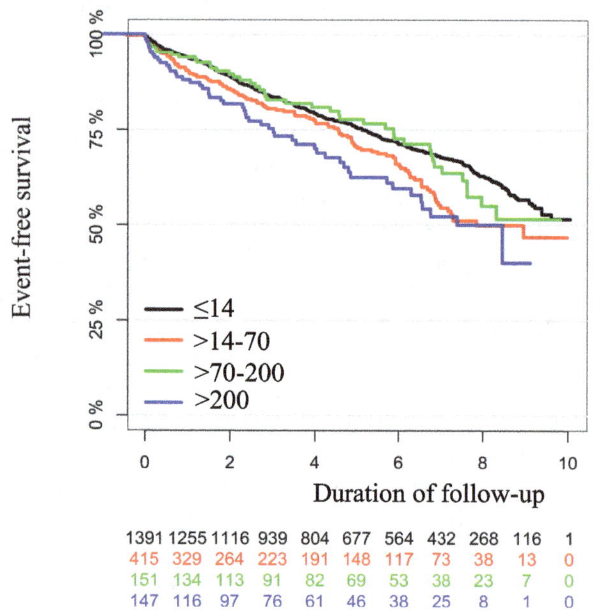

Fig. 4 Kaplan-Meier curve of the combined endpoint of all-cause mortality or new onset heart failure by peak concentration of troponin T in ng/L. Each colored line representing one group according to peak concentration of troponin T. Duration of follow-up in years from index procedure. Below the Kaplan-Meier curve is shown the number of patients still available for follow-up in each group

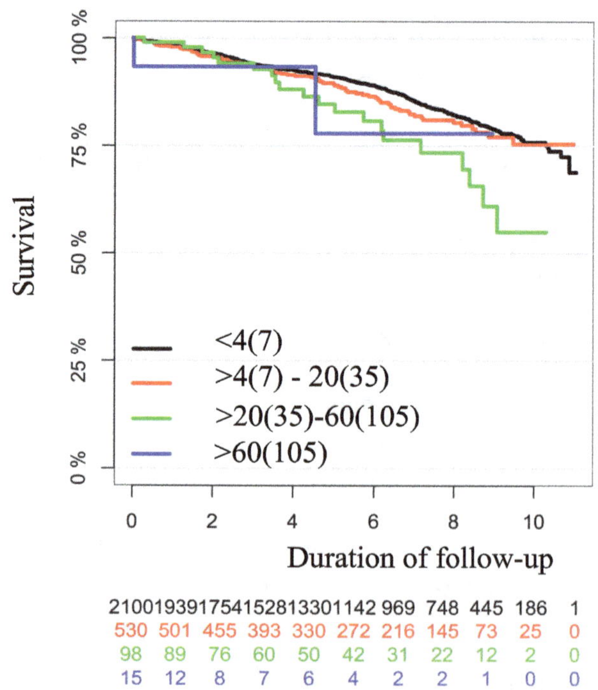

Fig. 5 Kaplan-Meier curve of all-cause mortality by peak post procedural concentration of CK-MBmass. The values for women in μg/L are shown in the figure with values for men in parentheses. Duration of follow-up in years from index procedure. Below the Kaplan-Meier curve is shown the number of patients still available for follow-up in each group

likely, that these differences explain the lower occurrence of cTn above URL. In their meta-analysis there was a significant risk associated with elevation of cTn above 3 x URL, but this conclusion seems uncertain in our study of a more homogenous patient group. We found no association between biomarker elevation and all-cause mortality but a possible association between the combined endpoint of all-cause mortality and new onset heart failure. There is little doubt when examining the combined data that the presently used hsTnT is indeed highly sensitive and the present cut-off makes cTn elevation corresponding to peri-procedural MI a very common occurrence following elective PCI.

Peri-procedural MI can be difficult to rule out - as the symptoms, electrocardiographic changes, angiography and other imaging modalities can be uncertain due to older ischemic injuries and discomfort associated with the procedure itself. A study showed that on angiography only approximately 60 % of peri-procedural MI could be explained [14]. Clinicians must therefore rely considerably on cardiac biomarkers. However, this is not without difficulties, as a definite cut-off value for prognostic significance has not been established for the present sensitive cardiac biomarkers, and the nature of the association between elevated biomarkers after PCI and prognosis is still under discussion [2, 3, 15–21]. The question is whether increased all-cause mortality is caused by acute PCI-related myocardial necrosis or whether the elevations of biomarkers is due to diffuse cTn release functioning as a general indicator of increased risk. In a meta-analysis the relationship between elevated cTnI or cTnT above URL after elective PCI and all-cause mortality was shown to be statistically significant with increased long-term (3–67 months) all-cause mortality of 5.8 % compared to 4.4 % in the group without elevated cTn [22]. These studies were performed before the Third Universal definition of peri-procedural MI – type 4a – was defined. Furthermore, cut-offs of TnI or TnT were not given in the meta-analysis.

The issue is further opaqued by the diversity of PCI related causes of increased cTn such as re-perfusion of an already injured area, distal embolization, coronary dissection, coronary spasm, occlusion of a sidebranch or even major coronary artery, microvascular plugging, disruption of collateral flow, slow flow or no-reflow [23]. Some of these specific causes might be prognostically significant, but this might be overlooked, when all causes are examined as one general group with elevated biomarkers. In non-elective PCI the post-PCI elevation might be caused by a pre-PCI injury and an already rising baseline value as seen in acute coronary syndrome [15, 20, 21, 24]. It has been hypothesized that there are multiple risk factors. Marked elevations of biomarkers after elective PCI could be associated with large infarction area, which is known to be associated to increased risk of death by heart failure and malignant arrhythmias with worsening prognosis [25, 26]. On the contrary, smaller elevations might not represent an actually MI, but be an indicator of extensive coronary atherosclerosis and high procedural complexity, this is however, also known to be related to poorer long term outcome [18, 22, 27]. In previous studies, prognostic significance was demonstrated for post-PCI elevation of CK-MB [23, 28, 29]. However, cTn is now accepted as a more sensitive marker of myocyte necrosis than CK-MB [1, 18, 24] and therefore, it can be assumed that peri-procedural MI diagnosed on the basis of CK-MB had relatively larger probability of representing a severe MI than if based on cTn. However, in our study, there is no indication that CK-MBmass is a significant prognostic indicator, probably due to absolute low concentrations at >15 times URL in comparison to older studies, or superior to TnT.

To the best of our knowledge, the numerous studies previously describing elevated biomarkers after PCI all have considerably shorter follow up. Assuming that the prognostic significance of peri-procedural MI is due to myocardial scarring followed by development of heart failure and/or malignant arrhythmias, it seems reasonable that the difference in prognosis should progress over time. The shorter follow up of previous studies might lead to underestimation of risk, but based on our data this is a not the case.

Limitations

Our study is a historic follow-up and is not able to report on any causality between peri-procedural MI and adverse events. Furthermore no data regarding symptoms, electrocardiographic changes or imaging is available to the study group so we cannot conclude whether the patients found with elevated cTnT ≥ 5 x URL also fulfilled the other defined criteria in the Third Universal Definition of Myocardial Infarction which includes patient reported symptoms, electrocardiographic or imaging suggestive of myocardial ischemia [1]. Due to the design of the study, it was necessary to use a surrogate marker for new-onset heart failure. Using hospitalization for heart failure as endpoint, was considered too insensitive, as a diagnosis of heart failure is known to be an unreliable marker with a sensitivity of about 25 % [30]. We expect most cases of overt heart failure to receive furosemide in Denmark, but acknowledge that some patients with obstructive lung disease and kidney disease may also receive this treatment, but it was deemed the best marker available when combined with hospital admittance due to heart failure.

It should be noted, that our data is from a strictly stable population and not "non-emergent" as used in many previous studies. Emergent is typically defined as procedures that have to be performed within hours of symptom onset.

This group can include both recent non-ST-elevation myocardial infarction (NSTEMI) and unstable angina. NSTEMI can cloud the issue due to a rising baseline of cTn and also represents a higher risk of procedural complications. Therefore, the conclusions from this study should only be applied with great care to other than truly stable patients.

Conclusion

The incidence of elevated biomarkers after elective PCI in patients with stable angina pectoris using the cut-off set by the Third Universal Definition of Myocardial Infarction (>5 x URL) was 15.2 % using cTnT and 4.1 % using CK-MBmass. The independent prognostic value of any cutoff for both cardiac biomarkers does not seem certain in neither short-term nor in long-term follow-up.

Our data suggest that routine measurement of cardiac biomarkers after elective PCI is not relevant unless procedural complications occur. We acknowledge that clinically driven measurement and observation after PCI in patients with stable angina pectoris is still relevant.

Abbreviations

CCS, Canadian Cardiovascular Society classification of angina pectoris; CI, confidence interval; CK-MBmass, creatine kinase isoenzyme MB mass concentration; cTn, cardiac troponins; cTnT, troponin T; HR, hazard ratio; hsTnT, high sensitive troponin T; MI, myocardial infarction; NSTEMI, non-ST-segment elevation myocardial infarction; PCI, percutaneous coronary intervention; URL, upper reference limit.

Acknowledgements

Simon Lykkeboe, Department of Clinical Biochemistry, Aalborg University Hospital, Denmark for help with data retrieval and verification.

Funding

No funding was obtained for this study.

Authors' contributions

MKC participated in design of the study, data acquisition, statistical analysis and drafted the manuscript. HH participated in drafting of the manuscript and revised for key intellectual content. TT participated in study design, data acquisition and drafting of the manuscript. CTP participated in data acquisition, revision for key intellectual content and performed statistical analysis. JR participated in drafting of the manuscript, key revision and designed the study. All authors read and approved the final manuscript.

Competing interests

Dr. Huang, Dr. Trydal and Dr. Ravkilde have no competing interests. Dr. Kirk Christensen reports minor personal fees from AstraZenaca A/S, Boehringer-Ingelheim A/S and Bayer A/S outside the submitted work. Dr. Torp-Pedersen reports grants and personal fees from Cardiome, grants and personal fees from Merck, grants and personal fees from Sanofi, grants and personal fees from Daiichi, grants from BMS, outside the submitted work.

Author details

[1]Department of Cardiology, Aalborg University Hospital, Aalborg, Denmark. [2]General Hospital of Ningxia Medical University, Yinchuan, China and Visiting Doctor at Department of Cardiology, Aalborg University Hospital, Aalborg, Denmark. [3]Department of Health Science and Technology, Aalborg University, Aalborg, Denmark. [4]Department of Clinical Biochemistry, Aalborg University Hospital, Aalborg, Denmark.

References

1. Thygesen K, Alpert JS, Jaffe AS, Simoons ML, Chaitman BR, White HD. ESC/ACCF/AHA/WHF Expert Consensus Document Third Universal Definition of Myocardial Infarction. 2012.
2. Moussa ID, Klein LW, Shah B, Mehran R, Mack MJ, Brilakis ES, Reilly JP, Zoghbi G, Holper E, Stone GW. Consideration of a new definition of clinically relevant myocardial infarction after coronary revascularization: an expert consensus document from the Society for Cardiovascular Angiography and Interventions (SCAI). J Am Coll Cardiol. 2013;62:1563–70.
3. Akkerhuis KM, Alexander JH, Tardiff BE, Boersma E, Harrington RA, Lincoff AM, Simoons ML. Minor myocardial damage and prognosis: are spontaneous and percutaneous coronary intervention-related events different? Circulation. 2002;105:554–6.
4. Abdelmeguid AE, Whitlow PL, Sapp SK, Ellis SG, Topol EJ. Long-term outcome of transient, uncomplicated in-laboratory coronary artery closure. Circulation. 1995;91:2733–41.
5. Giannitsis E, Kurz K, Hallermayer K, Jarausch J, Jaffe AS, Katus HA. Analytical validation of a high-sensitivity cardiac troponin T assay. Clin Chem. 2010;56:254–61.
6. Apple FS, Quist HE, Doyle PJ, Otto AP, Murakami MM. Plasma 99th percentile reference limits for cardiac troponin and creatine kinase MB mass for use with European Society of Cardiology/American College of Cardiology consensus recommendations. Clin Chem. 2003;49:1331–6.
7. Grann AF, Erichsen R, Nielsen AG, Frøslev T, Thomsen RW. Existing data sources for clinical epidemiology: The clinical laboratory information system (LABKA) research database at Aarhus University, Denmark. Clin Epidemiol. 2011;3:133–8.
8. Schmidt M, Maeng M, Jakobsen C-J, Madsen M, Thuesen L, Nielsen PH, Bøtker HE, Sørensen HT. Existing data sources for clinical epidemiology: The Western Denmark Heart Registry. Clin Epidemiol. 2010;2:137–44.
9. Pedersen CB. The Danish Civil Registration System. Scand J Public Health. 2011;39(7 Suppl):22–5.
10. Kildemoes HW, Sørensen HT, Hallas J. The Danish National Prescription Registry. Scand J Public Health. 2011;39(7 Suppl):38–41.
11. R Development Core Team. R: A Language and Environment for Statistical Computing. Vienna, Austria: the R Foundation for Statistical Computing; 2011.
12. Testa L, Van Gaal WJ, Biondi Zoccai GGL, Agostoni P, Latini RA, Bedogni F, Porto I, Banning AP. Myocardial infarction after percutaneous coronary intervention: a meta-analysis of troponin elevation applying the new universal definition. QJM. 2009;102:369–78.
13. Thygesen K, Alpert JS, White HD. Universal definition of myocardial infarction. Eur Heart J. 2007;28:2525–38.
14. Muschart X, Slimani A, Jamart J, Chenu P, Dangoisse V, Gabriel L, Guédès A, Marchandise B, Schröder E. The different mechanisms of periprocedural myocardial infarction and their impact on in-hospital outcome. J Invasive Cardiol. 2012;24:655–60.
15. White HD. The prequel: defining prognostically important criteria in the periprocedural PCI troponin saga. Circ Cardiovasc Interv. 2012;5:142–5.
16. Prasad A, Rihal CS, Lennon RJ, Singh M, Jaffe AS, Holmes DR. Significance of periprocedural myonecrosis on outcomes after percutaneous coronary intervention: an analysis of preintervention and postintervention troponin T levels in 5487 patients. Circ Cardiovasc Interv. 2008;1:10–9.
17. Cavallini C, Verdecchia P, Savonitto S, Arraiz G, Violini R, Olivari Z, Rubartelli P, De Servi S, Plebani M, Steffenino G, Sbarzaglia P, Ardissino D. Prognostic value of isolated troponin I elevation after percutaneous coronary intervention. Circ Cardiovasc Interv. 2010;3:431–5.
18. Prasad A. Slow but steady progress towards understanding peri-procedural myocardial infarction. Eur Heart J. 2013;34:1615–7.
19. Selvanayagam JB, Porto I, Channon K, Petersen SE, Francis JM, Neubauer S, Banning AP. Troponin elevation after percutaneous coronary intervention directly represents the extent of irreversible myocardial injury: insights from cardiovascular magnetic resonance imaging. Circulation. 2005;111:1027–32.

20. Califf RM, Abdelmeguid AE, Kuntz RE, Popma JJ, Davidson CJ, Cohen EA, Kleiman NS, Mahaffey KW, Topol EJ, Pepine CJ, Lipicky RJ, Granger CB, Harrington RA, Tardiff BE, Crenshaw BS, Bauman RP, Zuckerman BD, Chaitman BR, Bittl JA, Ohman EM. Myonecrosis after revascularization procedures. J Am Coll Cardiol. 1998;31:241–51.
21. Lee C-H, Tse H-F. Microvascular obstruction after percutaneous coronary intervention. Catheter Cardiovasc Interv. 2010;75:369–77.
22. Feldman DN, Kim L, Rene AG, Minutello RM, Bergman G, Wong SC. Prognostic value of cardiac troponin-I or troponin-T elevation following nonemergent percutaneous coronary intervention: a meta-analysis. Catheter Cardiovasc Interv. 2011;77:1020–30.
23. Park D-W, Kim Y-H, Yun S-C, Ahn J-M, Lee J-Y, Kim W-J, Kang S-J, Lee S-W, Lee CW, Park S-W, Park S-J. Frequency, causes, predictors, and clinical significance of peri-procedural myocardial infarction following percutaneous coronary intervention. Eur Heart J. 2013;34:1662–9.
24. Jaffe AS, Apple FS, Lindahl B, Mueller C, Katus HA. Why all the struggle about CK-MB and PCI? Eur Heart J. 2012;33:1046–8.
25. Hallén J. Troponin for the estimation of infarct size: what have we learned? Cardiology. 2012;121:204–12.
26. Savonitto S, Granger CB, Ardissino D, Gardner L, Cavallini C, Galvani M, Ottani F, White HD, Armstrong PW, Ohman EM, Pieper KS, Califf RM, Topol EJ. The prognostic value of creatine kinase elevations extends across the whole spectrum of acute coronary syndromes. J Am Coll Cardiol. 2002;39:22–9.
27. Kanaparti PK, Brown DL. Atherosclerotic Plaque Burden and Percutaneous Coronary Intervention. Am J Cardiol. 2000;86:619–22.
28. Jeremias A, Baim DS, Ho KKL, Chauhan M, Carrozza JP, Cohen DJ, Popma JJ, Kuntz RE, Cutlip DE. Differential mortality risk of postprocedural creatine kinase-MB elevation following successful versus unsuccessful stent procedures. J Am Coll Cardiol. 2004;44:1210–4.
29. Lindsey JB, Kennedy KF, Stolker JM, Gilchrist IC, Mukherjee D, Marso SP, Pencina MJ, Kleiman NS, Cohen DJ. Prognostic implications of creatine kinase-MB elevation after percutaneous coronary intervention: results from the Evaluation of Drug-Eluting Stents and Ischemic Events (EVENT) registry. Circ Cardiovasc Interv. 2011;4:474–80.
30. Kümler T, Hilmar G, Kirk V, Bay M, Nielsen OW, Køber L, Torp-pedersen C. Accuracy of a heart failure diagnosis in administrative registers. Eur J Heart Fail. 2008;10(7):658–660.

13

Stable phase post-MI patients have elevated VEGF levels correlated with inflammation markers, but not with atherosclerotic burden

Barbara Eržen[1*], Mira Šilar[2] and Mišo Šabovič[1]

Abstract

Background: The role of vascular endothelial growth factor (VEGF) in patients in the stable phase after myocardial infarction (MI) has not yet been explored. Therefore, we compared the values of VEGF in post-MI patients with those obtained in healthy controls. Furthermore, we investigated whether the values of VEGF correlate to either inflammation markers or the atherosclerotic burden.

Methods: 41 male patients (on average 44 years old) in the stable phase after MI (on average 20.5 months after MI) were recruited, while 25 healthy age-matched males served as controls. Plasma levels of VEGF and several markers of inflammation were measured by standard procedures. The atherosclerotic burden was determined by the angiographic severity of coronary atherosclerosis, endothelial dysfunction (measured by ultrasound measurement of the flow mediated dilation of the brachial artery), the intima-media thickness of the common carotid artery and the ankle-brachial pressure index.

Results: VEGF values were significantly elevated in post-MI patients compared to the controls (53.8 ± 42.7 pg/ml vs. 36.3 ± 8.9 pg/ml, $p = 0.014$). The elevated VEGF values significantly correlated to the (increased) values of the inflammatory molecules interleukin 6 and 8 ($r = 0.37$, $p = 0.017$; and $r = 0.45$, $p = 0.003$; respectively). In contrast, no correlation was found between VEGF and the parameters of the atherosclerotic burden, although FMD and IMT were significantly impaired in patients.

Conclusions: We found that plasma levels of VEGF are increased in the stable phase after MI and correlate with inflammation cytokines, but not with the atherosclerotic burden. Thus, this suggests that increased levels of VEGF are a part of ongoing inflammatory activity. Since VEGF in these patients stimulates neovascularization of inflamed plaques and induces their destabilization, the VEGF level can have an important negative prognostic value. Clearly, further studies are needed to clarify the role of VEGF as a prognostic marker.

Keywords: Vascular endothelial growth factor, Inflammation markers, Interleukin 6, Interleukin 8, Endothelial dysfunction, Myocardial infarction, Young adult patients

Background

VEGF induces angiogenesis in several physiological conditions (for example embryogenesis), as well as in pathological states (for example tumour growth). VEGF induces angiogenesis through the formation of new vessels as a compensatory process in myocardial ischemia, but on the other hand, it can also be a mechanism producing destabilization of atherosclerotic plaques in coronary arteries [1-5]. Understanding of these evidently different roles of VEGF is still insufficient. Besides VEGF, several other angiogenic markers are known such as angiogenin, hepatocyte growth factor and basic fibroblast growth factor, though undoubtedly VEGF is the key angiogenic molecule. However, as mentioned above, its ability to assume either a pro-atherosclerotic or an anti-atherosclerotic role is somewhat confusing and still insufficiently explained.

There is only scare and conflicting data about the role of VEGF in coronary artery disease. Studies have shown

* Correspondence: erzen_b@yahoo.com
[1]Department of Vascular Disease, University Clinical Centre, Ljubljana 1000, Slovenia
Full list of author information is available at the end of the article

that VEGF levels are increased in the acute phase of MI, as a response to myocardial ischemia. In acute MI patients who successfully underwent primary percutaneous intervention (PCI), VEGF levels reach their peak at day 7 [6-9], and return to normal after about 6 months [10]. There are conflicting data about the prognostic meaning of VEGF levels in the acute phase after MI. In a recently published Japanese prospective multicentre study it was shown that low levels of VEGF in the acute phase of MI are associated with a worse 6 months prognosis. In this study the incidence of recurrent acute coronary syndrome and stroke were significantly higher in the low VEGF group [6]. On the other hand, and in complete contrast, a European study showed that high VEGF levels in the acute phase of MI are related to an adverse outcome during a 6 months follow-up [11]. Discussing these conflicting results one could only conclude that VEGF may have an important prognostic value, but one which surprisingly may be positive or negative. From the clinical point of view it is even more important to investigate the role of VEGF in the stable phase of the disease.

Therefore the aim of the present study was to investigate whether VEGF is increased in the stable phase of coronary artery disease and to explore its role in this period. For this purpose we compared serum levels of VEGF in young post-MI patients and healthy age-matched controls. Furthermore, we were interested whether VEGF is related to the severity of inflammation (indicated by increased levels of serum inflammatory molecules) or to the degree of atherosclerotic burden. If associated with inflammation it could be deduced that VEGF probably has a negative angiogenic role in the inflammatory process inducing destabilization of plaques, whereas if associated with the atherosclerotic burden this suggests that it has a positive angiogenic role inducing angiogenesis in ischemic areas.

Methods

Study population

The study group consisted of 41 patients with coronary heart disease. In all patients MI was defined by a positive troponin level, ECG changes and obstructive coronary lesions confirmed by angiography. Inclusion criteria were male gender, age at the time of myocardial infarction less than 50 years, more than 6 months and less than 3 years from the time of MI to the time of the trial performance (an average of 20.5 months), and coronary artery disease in the stable period (absence of unstable AP). Exclusion criteria were malignancy, heart failure, an acute inflammation state 14 days before the study, a history of diabetes mellitus, anticoagulant therapy, and the use of any other drugs except ACE inhibitors, beta blockers, antiplatelet drugs and statins. We divided the patients into three groups (one, two or three vessel disease) according to the number of diseased vessels seen on the coronarography at the time of MI. Significant stenosis was determined as stenosis above 50%.

The control group consisted of 25 healthy male volunteers, who did not differ from the patients regarding age and had no manifested atherosclerotic disease.

All subjects were informed about the study protocol and gave their informed consent. The study protocol conformed to the ethical guidelines of the 1975 Declaration of Helsinki, and was approved by the State Ethics Committee of Slovenia.

Clinical examination and laboratory procedures

One visit by the subjects was necessary at which their medical history was recorded, and a clinical examination, biochemical tests and ultrasound measurements were performed. All ultrasound measurements were performed in the morning. Patients were on their regular therapy and had taken their usual dose of morning medicine. Any smokers abstained from smoking on that day.

A detailed family and personal history was recorded, and a clinical examination performed according to a questionnaire. Systolic and diastolic blood pressures were measured with a mercury sphygmomanometer after a minimum of 10-min rest in the sitting position. The average of three measurements was taken. Anthropometric parameters were determined, and BMI was calculated as weight in kilograms divided by the square of the height in meters, and WHR was calculated as waist size divided by hip size.

Blood for laboratory analysis was collected in the morning after a 12-hour overnight fast. Samples were drawn from the antecubital vein. Blood for the analysis of glucose and lipids was collected without additives, centrifuged and samples of serum were analysed. Concentrations of glucose, total cholesterol, high density lipoprotein (HDL) cholesterol and triglycerides were determined by standard colorimetric assays from the fresh samples of serum (Ektachem 250 Analyzer, Eastman Kodak Company, Rochester, USA). Low density lipoprotein (LDL) cholesterol was calculated using Friedewald's formula. High sensitivity CRP (hsCRP) was measured with a fully automated, latex-enhanced nephelometric immunoassay (N High Sensitivity CRP, Dade Behring Marburg, Germany).

Concentrations of VEGF, angiogenin and interleukin-8 (IL-8were measured by Cytometric Bead Array (BD Biosciences Pharmingen, San Diego, CA, USA) containing microparticles dyed to different fluorescence intensities. The anaphylatoxin-captured beads were incubated with standards (purified from human plasma) or test samples followed by a wash and incubation with phycoerythrin-conjugated detection antibodies to form sandwich complexes. Flow cytometric analysis was performed using a FACSCalibur flow cytometer (Becton Dickinson Immunocytometry Systems, BDIS,

BD Biosciences, San Jose, CA, USA). Data were acquired and analysed using the Beckton Dickinson Cytometric bead array (CBA) software.

Serum tumour necrosis factor- α (TNF-α) (Quantikine® HS Human TNF- α Immunoassay, R&D Systems, USA), interleukin-6 (IL-6) (Quantikine® Human IL-6 Immunoassay, R&D Systems, USA) and the serum cell adhesion molecules ICAM-1, VCAM-1, selectin-P, selectin-E (Parameter® ICAM-1, Parameter® VCAM-1, Parameter® selectin-P, Parameter® selectin-E, R&D Systems UK) were determined by enzyme-linked immunosorbent assays.

Vascular studies

a.) Measurement of endothelial dysfunction (ED); Flow mediated (FMD) (endothelium-dependent) and glyceryl trinitrate (GTN)-induced dilation (endothelium-independent) of the right brachial artery were studied using a high-resolution B mode Diasonics VST ultrasound system with a 10 MHz linear array transducer. The subjects rested in the supine position for ten minutes before hemodynamic measurements were performed. The right brachial artery was scanned in the longitudinal section 2 to 15 cm above the elbow to find the clearest images of the anterior and posterior wall layers. The mean arterial diameter was measured at the end of the diastole, which was determined by simultaneous monitoring of the electrocardiogram (concurrent with onset of the QRS complex). At least three cardiac cycles were analysed for each scan and the measurements averaged. The flow velocity was measured at a fixed incident angle of 68° to the vessel with the range gate of 1.3 mm located in the centre of the artery. The baseline blood flow was estimated by multiplying the velocity time integral of the Doppler flow signal (corrected for incident angle) by the vessel cross-sectional area. Hyperemic flow increase was induced by inflation of a blood pressure tourniquet placed around the forearm to a pressure of 300 mmHg for 4.5 minutes. Hyperemic flow was recorded for the first 15 seconds and diameter measurements were taken 45–60 seconds after cuff deflation. The endothelium-dependent dilation was expressed as the percentage change of the diameter after reactive hyperaemia, relative to the baseline scan. Ten minutes were allowed for vessel recovery, after which a further resting scan was taken. A sublingual tablet of 0.5 mg of GTN was then administered, and 4.5 minutes later, the final scan was performed. The endothelium-independent dilation was expressed as the percentage change in diameter after GTN administration, relative to the baseline scan. The same investigator, who was blind to the subjects' characteristics, carried out all measurements. To assess the reproducibility of the measurements, 40 subjects were selected randomly for repeated vascular studies. The correlation coefficient between the absolute differences and mean values of paired measurements was 0.92, $p < 0.05$.

b.) Measurement of intima-media thickness; IMT of the common carotid artery (CCA) was assessed by the B-mode ultrasound technique. Measurements of IMT were obtained from the far wall of the distal part of the CCA (immediately proximal to the carotid bulb) on both sides. All studies were performed on a single ultrasound machine (Diasonics VST ultrasound system) using a linear-array 10-MHz scan head with standardized image settings, including resolution mode, depth of field, gain, and transmit focus. All sonograms were obtained with the patient in the supine position and their head turned slightly to the contra lateral side. Each ultrasound examination was performed as an independent study, without any knowledge of the history of MI and risk factors. The IMT was measured as the distance from the leading edge of the near-field (intimal-luminal surface) and far-field (medial-adventitial) arterial wall. An average of three measurements on both sides was derived. The mean IMT was calculated as the average of the left and right CCA.

c.) Measurement of ankle-brachial pressure index (ABPI); the systolic blood pressure in both arms was taken with a blood pressure cuff and Doppler probe, after a minimum of 10-min rest in the sitting position, averaged, and divided into the systolic blood pressure in the posterior tibial or dorsalis pedis artery in the leg. The higher reading was used to determine the ABPI. ABPI was calculated separately for each leg. The mean ABPI was calculated as the average of the left and right leg.

Statistical analysis

Variables showing a normal distribution, as determined by the Kolmogorov-Smirnov test, were expressed as means and standard deviations. Differences between the two groups were tested for significance by Student's t-test for normally-distributed variables with equal variances, or by the Welch t-test for variables with unequal variances. Correlation between normally distributed variables was tested with the Pearson correlation coefficient. The criterion for statistical significance was a p value of less than 0.05. We constructed a multiple linear regression model to predict VEGF in patients on the basis of classical coronary risk factors, inflammatory parameters and functional and structural characteristics of the arterial wall. All calculations were performed by the IBM SPSS statistics 19 computer program.

A power analysis was performed to calculate the appropriate sample size to detect significant differences between the two groups at adequate power. All calculations, except the power analysis which was performed with the PASS 11 statistical program, were performed by the IBM SPSS statistics 19 computer program.

Results

Characteristics of the patients and controls at the time of trial performance

There were no differences in the age of patients and controls. BMI, but not WHR, was increased in post-MI patients in comparison to healthy controls. All patients were taking anti-platelet therapy, 19 (90%) statins (simvastatin or atorvastatin), 19 (90%) beta-blockers, and 19 (90%) patients ACE-inhibitors. Subjects in the control group were not taking any medication. Because of their medication, patients had significantly lower values of LDL cholesterol and lower systolic blood pressure in comparison to the controls. The characteristics of the patients and of the controls at the time of the trial performance are shown in Table 1.

VEGF, angiogenin and inflammatory molecules in the patients and controls at the time of trial performance

The patients had significantly higher levels of VEGF in comparison to the controls (53.8 ± 42.7 pg/ml vs. 36.3 ± 8.9 pg/ml, p = 0.014). The mean values of VEGF ± one standard deviation in patients and controls are shown in Figure 1. There were no statistically significant differences in angiogenin levels between the patients and controls (1.37 ± 0.46 pg/ml vs. 1.42 ± 0.38 pg/ml, p = 0.318).

The patients had significantly increased IL-6 and hsCRP in comparison to the controls. The values are shown in Table 2.

Table 1 Characteristics of the subjects and laboratory parameters at the time of the trial performance

Parameter	Controls (N = 25)	Patients (N = 41)	p
Age (years)	42.2 (4.9)	44.8 (5.4)	ns
BMI (kg/m^2)	25.4 (3.4)	27.3 (2.7)	0.02
Waist-hip ratio (rel.)	0.93 (0.04)	0.94 (0.05)	ns
Systolic blood pressure (mmHg)	133 (13)	125 (14)	0.02
Diastolic blood pressure (mmHg)	87 (11)	82 (10)	ns
Total cholesterol (mmol/l)	4.99 (0.78)	4.55 (1.0)	ns
LDL-cholesterol (mmol/l)	3.11 (0.73)	2.6 (0.87)	0.02
HDL-cholesterol (mmol/l)	1.18 (0.26)	1.02 (0.28)	0.02
TG (mmol/l)	1.50 (0.57)	2.18 (1.57)	0.04
Blood glucose (mmol/l)	5.4 (1.3)	5.9 (1.7)	ns
Smokers (N)	4 (16%)	11 (27%)	ns
Ex-smokers (N)	4 (16%)	23 (56%)	<0.01
Family history (N)	2 (8%)	14 (34%)	0.01

Values are shown as means and standard deviations; p-for the difference between the two groups, ns-not significant, N-number, BMI-body mass index, rel.-relative, LDL-low density cholesterol, HDL-high density cholesterol, TG-triglycerides.

Vascular studies

In the patients both FMD and IMT were significantly increased in comparison to the controls. There were no significant differences in ABPI between the two groups. The data are shown in Table 3.

Correlation analysis, multiple linear regression model and power analysis

In the group of patients, a significant positive correlation was observed between VEGF and IL-6 (r = 0.37, p = 0.017) and between VEGF and IL-8 r = 0.45, p = 0.003. The correlations are plotted in Figures 2 and 3. No correlations between VEGF and parameters of atherosclerotic burden were obtained.

A multiple linear regression model was constructed to predict VEGF in the patients on the basis of classical coronary risk factors, inflammatory parameters and functional and structural characteristics of the arterial wall. Only factors that were significant in the univariant analysis were included in the model (IL-6 and IL-8). The adjusted R^2 of this model was 0.226, with a high significance (p = 0.008). After adjustment only IL-6 (β = 0.338, p = 0.025) proved to be an independent determinant of VEGF.

We performed post-hoc power and sample size analysis for comparison between the controls and the patients regarding the level of VEGF, which was the main discovery and was found to be significant in our study. The group sample sizes of 25 and 41 achieve a 74% power to detect a difference of 17.6 between the null hypothesis that the both group means are 53.9 and the alternative hypothesis that the mean of group two is 36.3, with known group standard deviations of 42.7 and 8.9 and with a significance level (alpha) $a = 0.05$ using a two-sided two-sample t-test.

Discussion

The aim of the present study was to explore the role of VEGF in the stable phase of coronary artery disease. We found that VEGF was increased in post-MI patients and furthermore that VEGF values correlated with inflammatory cytokines (IL-6 and IL-8), but not with parameters associated with the extent of the atherosclerotic burden. These results suggest that VEGF in the stable phase after MI is a part of the inflammatory response and very likely contributes to worsening of atherosclerosis by inducing plaque instability. If VEGF were to be involved in neovascularization as a compensatory mechanism to ischemia, it would certainly correlate with parameters of the atherosclerotic burden, but that was not the case.

It has been shown in clinical trials and animal models that VEGF promotes the development of collateral blood vessels in response to hypoxia [3,12-14]. All our patients were in the acute phase of MI, successfully vascularized (percutaneous trans-luminal angioplasty), and at the time

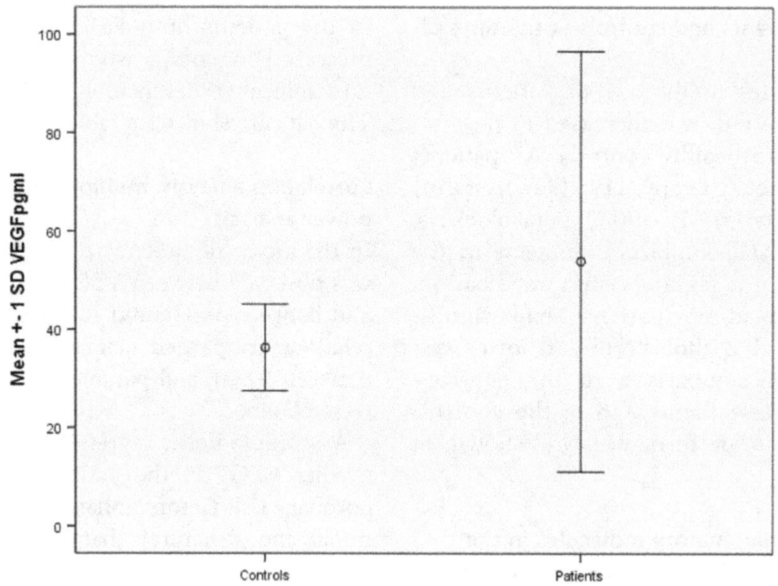

Figure 1 VEGF in patients and controls. *Legend: VEGF- vascular endothelial growth factor, SD-standard deviation.*

of the trial were asymptomatic, stable and without symptoms of angina pectoris. It is therefore interesting that they had increased VEGF levels. Although only a few studies have explored VEGF in patients with coronary artery disease, almost all were performed to determine the role of VEGF in the acute phase of MI where increased levels of VEGF were found. In one study the peak level for VEGF was reached during acute MI. After successful recanalization, the serum levels of VEGF rapidly (within 20–30 minutes) returned almost completely to the normal control range [15]. Other studies showed that VEGF returns to normal values after about three weeks or after 6 months [9,10]. The differences in VEGF normalization time are most probably the result of different methods of treating AMI (PCI, or conservative treatment with heparin, which can reduce serum VEGF), as well as different study populations. There is no data for a period longer than 6 months.

Table 2 Angiogenic and inflammation markers of subjects at the time of the trial

Parameter	Controls (N = 25)	Patients (N = 41)	p
VEGF (pg/ml)	36.3. ±8.9	53.8 ± 42.7	0.014
Angiogenin (pg/ml)	1.42 ± 0.38	1.37 ± 0.46	0.318
hs CRP (mg/l)	1.5 +/- 1.4	3.5 +/- 8.1	0.038
IL-6 (ng/ml)	2.5 ± 3.4	4.9 ± 4.1	0.016
IL-8	5.4 +/- 1.3	6.3+/- 3.0	0.102
IL-8 (pg/ml)	5.4 ± 1.3	6.3 ± 3.0	0.102
hs CRP (mg/ml)	1.5 ± 1.4	3.5 ± 8.1	0.038
VCAM-1 (ng/ml)	286.5 ± 60.1	283.3 ± 52.1	0.336
ICAM-1 (ng/ml)	182.3 ± 50.3	190.9 ± 44.9	0.775
Selectin-P (ng/ml)	52.9 ± 10.9	55.1 ± 13.4	0.373
Selectin-E (ng/ml)	44.7 ± 12.5	47.4 ± 14.8	0.112
TNF-α (ng/ml)	1.19 ± 1.12	0.93 ± 1.0	0.780

Values are shown as means and standard deviations; VEGF-vascular endothelial growth factor, IL-6 – interleukin 6, IL-8 – interleukin 8, hsCRP – high sensitive C-reactive protein, VCAM-1 – vascular cell adhesion molecule-1, ICAM-1 – intra-cellular adhesion molecule-1, TNF-α – tumour necrosis factor α.

Thus we explored the values of VEGF in patients on average 20.5 months after MI and found them to be increased, which is a new result. However, its explanation is quite complex. Hence, to clarify this we investigated the associations of VEGF with both inflammatory molecules and the atherosclerotic burden, and studied the levels of angiogenin, another angiogenic factor. The values of angiogenin were similar in the patients and controls and did not follow the increase of VEGF, thereby confirming the pivotal role of VEGF as an angiogenic factor. Furthermore, to obtain an appropriate answer to the basic question of the role of VEGF we analysed a very broad range of both inflammatory molecules and parameters of the atherosclerotic burden.

Atherosclerosis is a chronic inflammatory disease. In this context, we were interested whether VEGF is related to a possible on-going inflammation process. Namely,

Table 3 Vascular studies

Parameter	Controls (N = 25)	Patients (N = 41)	p
FMD (%)	8.8 ± 6.5	5.5 ± 4.3	0.017
IMT (mm)	0.68 ± 0.13	0.87 ± 0.17	<0.001
ABPI (rel)	1.17 ± 0.11	1.11 ± 0.13	0.052

FMD-flow mediated dilation, IMT- intima-media thickness, ABPI- ankle brachial pressure index, p- for the difference between groups.

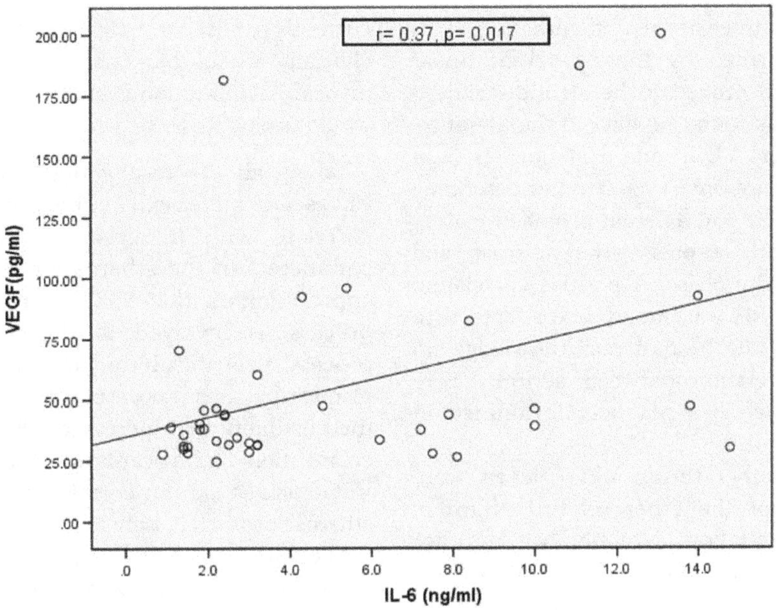

Figure 2 Correlation between VEGF and IL-6 in patients. *Legend: IL-6 - interleukin 6, VEGF- vascular endothelial growth factor, r - correlation coefficient, p - statistical significance.*

VEGF is believed to be a key molecule that connects angiogenesis with inflammatory response. In the context of this study the connection between angiogenesis and the intravascular arterial wall is of great interest. Therefore, the intensity of arterial wall inflammation was measured by the serum levels of different pro-inflammatory markers (IL-8, IL-6, hsCRP, VCAM1, ICAM1, p-selectin, e-selectin and TNFα). Importantly, in comparison to the controls, patients had significantly increased levels of IL-6 and hsCRP, whereas the values of the other inflammatory molecules were not elevated. Thus, one can conclude that IL-6 and hsCRP are the best markers of on-going arterial wall inflammation in the stable phase after MI. On evaluating the existence of possible associations, we found significant positive correlations between VEGF and IL-6, and between VEGF and IL-8. Thus, these

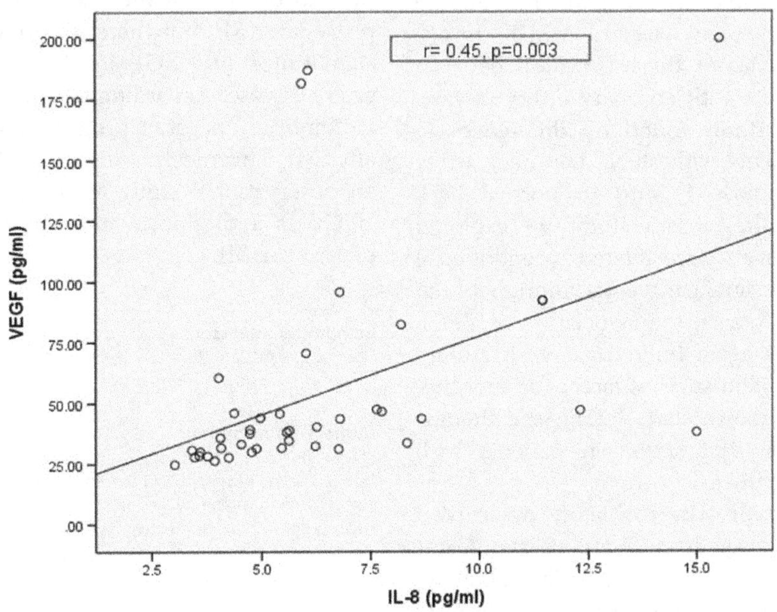

Figure 3 Correlation between VEGF and IL-8 in patients. *Legend: IL-8 - interleukin 8, VEGF- vascular endothelial growth factor, r - correlation coefficient, p - statistical significance.*

results form a strong basis for stating that serum VEGF levels are related to the intensity of inflammation. This statement is also confirmed by the model of linear regression in which IL-6 proved to be an independent determinant of VEGF. We found no data in the literature on a correlation between VEGF and IL-6 and IL-8 in coronary patients. There are only a few studies describing a correlation between VEGF and different proinflammatory molecules in patients with coronary artery disease, and even then only in the acute phase. A positive correlation between VEGF and hsCRP was found in patients with acute MI [9,16]. But to the best of our knowledge no studies describe a correlation between serum VEGF and IL-6 and IL-8, which has not been examined in the stable period after MI.

We also explored whether serum VEGF levels were related to parameters of the atherosclerotic burden, but did not find any relation. Notably, we did not find a correlation between VEGF and the severity of coronary artery disease, classified as one-, two- or three-vessel coronary artery disease found on the coronarograph. There are only some small and conflicting studies dealing with VEGF and the extent of coronary artery disease. Some studies found no correlation between serum VEGF levels and the severity (extent) of coronary atherosclerosis in patients measured on the 7th day after MI, in patients with stable AP and in patients with chest pain undergoing coronary angiography [17-19]. On the other hand, in a small Polish study, serum VEGF levels were higher in AMI patients with multi-vessel disease than in patients with single-vessel disease [16]. Larger studies are needed to clarify this relationship. Similarly, we found no correlation between IMT, measured on the common carotid artery, and serum VEGF levels. There are very few data about the association between IMT and VEGF in patients with coronary artery disease. In a small study, the authors found no differences in VEGF levels among patients with stable coronary artery disease and increased (above 1 mm) or normal IMT (below 1 mm) [20]. In the present study, we explored whether plasma VEGF levels were related to endothelial function, but found no significant correlation between FMD and VEGF levels. Data on the association of VEGF with vascular function is again limited. In vitro studies showed that VEGF is a potent survival factor for endothelial cells [21,22]. It was shown that VEGF gene therapy may improve endothelial dysfunction in patients with end-stage coronary artery disease [9].

It is well-known that biomarkers of acute myocardial ischemia (acute coronary syndrome) are of significant clinical value and already in clinical use. The following markers for acute coronary syndrome are FDA-approved: creatin kinase, myoglobin and cardiac troponin. All three have become the gold standard for confirmation of acute coronary syndrome. Several other possible biomarkers are currently under investigation. However, in contrast, no clinically useful biomarker for prediction of recurrent myocardial infarction is currently available. Such a marker would undoubtedly be very valuable.

Taking all the results together we found that VEGF values are increased in the stable phase after MI and correlate with inflammatory markers but not with parameters of the atherosclerotic burden. Therefore, it appears logical that VEGF, driven by the inflammatory process, is involved in the on-going atherosclerosis process, probably inducing destabilization of coronary plaques by their neovascularization. On the other hand, the possibility that increased VEGF levels induce neovascularization in myocardium is much less probable since VEGF values did not correlate with the parameters of the atherosclerotic (i.e. ischemic) burden.

The limitations of the present study are that it was cross-sectional and not prospective and had a relatively small sample size. However the power of the study was quite large (74%) and the mentioned limitation did not affect the main finding of the study, which is increased VEGF levels in young male patients in the stable phase after MI.

Conclusions

Several biomarkers that predict the clinical prognosis of patients with acute AMI have been identified. The relevance of our study is in using VEGF as an additional cardiovascular biomarker in the chronic stable phase of coronary artery disease. Conflicting data exists about the prognostic significance of VEGF levels in the acute phase after MI, but there is no data about the prognostic significance of VEGF in the stable phase of coronary artery disease. According to our findings, VEGF can have an important negative prognostic value in the stable phase after MI. This mechanistic study should be followed up by an observational study to definitively clarify the role of VEGF as a prognostic marker in patients in the stable phase after MI.

Competing interests

The authors declare that they have no competing interests.

Authors' contributions

BE participated in the study design, carried out the measurements and drafted the manuscript. Mira S performed the VEGF analysis. Miso S participated in the study design, drafted the manuscript and revised it critically for important intellectual content. All authors read and approved the final manuscript.

Acknowledgments

The Slovenian Ministry of Science and Technology supported the study through grant no. 3311-01-831/463.

Author details
[1]Department of Vascular Disease, University Clinical Centre, Ljubljana 1000, Slovenia. [2]Laboratory for Clinical Immunology & Molecular Genetics, University Clinic of Respiratory and Allergic Diseases, Golnik, Slovenia.

References

1. Taniguchi T, Sawada T: **Significance of measuring plasma vascular endothelial growth factor in patients with acute myocardial infarction.** *Circ J* 2012, **76**(6):1331–1332.
2. Ferrara N, Gerber HP, LeCouter J: **The biology of VEGF and its receptors.** *Nat Med* 2003, **9**:669–676.
3. Shinohara K, Shinohara T, Mochizuki N, Mochizuki Y, Sawa H, Kohya T, Fujita M, Fujioka Y, Kitabatake A, Nagashima K: **Expression of vascular endothelial growth factor in human myocardial infarction.** *Heart Vessels* 1996, **11**(3):113–122.
4. Celletti FL, Waugh JM, Amabile PG, Brendolan A, Hilfiker PR, Dake MD: **Vascular endothelial growth factor enhances atherosclerotic plaque progression.** *Nat Med* 2001, **7**:425–429.
5. Soeki T, Tamura Y, Shinohara H, Tanaka H, Bando K, Fukuda N: **Role of circulating vascular endothelial growth factor and hepatocyte growth factor in patients with coronary artery disease.** *Heart Vessels* 2000, **15**(3):105–111.
6. Matsudaira K, Maeda K, Okumura N, Yoshikawa D, Morita Y, Mitsuhashi H, Ishii H, Kondo T, Murohara T: **Impact of low levels of vascular endothelial growth factor after myocardial infarction on 6-month clinical outcome: results from the Nagoya Acute Myocardial Infarction Study.** *Circ J* 2012, **76**(6):1509–1516.
7. Ye L, Zhang W, Su LP, Haider HK, Poh KK, Galupo MJ, Songco G, Ge RW, Tan HC, Sim EK: **Nanoparticle based delivery of hypoxia-regulated VEGF transgene system combined with myoblast engraftment for myocardial repair.** *Biomaterials* 2011, **32**(9):2424–2431.
8. Shintani S, Murohara T, Ikeda H, Ueno T, Honma T, Katoh A, Sasaki K, Shimada T, Oike Y, Imaizumi T: **Mobilization of endothelial progenitor cells in patients with acute myocardial infarction.** *Circulation* 2001, **103**(23):2776–2779.
9. Soeki T, Tamura Y, Shinohara H, Tanaka H, Bando K, Fukuda N: **Serial changes in serum VEGF and HGF in patients with acute myocardial infarction.** *Cardiology* 2000, **93**(3):168–174.
10. Kranz A, Rau C, Kochs M, Waltenberger J: **Elevation of vascular endothelial growth factor-A serum levels following acute myocardial infarction. Evidence for its origin and functional significance.** *J Mol Cell Cardiol* 2000, **32**(1):65–72.
11. Heeschen C, Dimmeler S, Hamm CW, Boersma E, Zeiher AM, Simoons ML: **Prognostic significance of angiogenic growth factor serum levels in patients with acute coronary syndromes.** *Circulation* 2003, **107**(4):524–530.
12. Hoeben A, Landuyt B, Highley MS, Wildiers H, Van Oosterom AT, De Bruijn EA: **Vascular endothelial growth factor and angiogenesis.** *Pharmacol Rev* 2004, **56**(4):549–580.
13. Gruchala M, Roy H, Bhardwaj S, Yla-Herttuala S: **Gene therapy for cardiovascular diseases.** *Curr Pharm Des* 2004, **10**:407–423.
14. Shweiki D, Itin A, Soffer D, Keshet E: **Vascular endothelial growth factor induced by hypoxia may mediate hypoxia-initiated angiogenesis.** *Nature* 1992, **359**(6398):843–845.
15. Seko Y, Imai Y, Suzuki S, Kamijukkoku S, Hayasaki K, Sakomura Y, Tobe K, Kadowaki T, Maekawa H, Takahashi N, Yazaki Y: **Serum levels of vascular endothelial growth factor in patients with acute myocardial infarction undergoing reperfusion therapy.** *Clin Sci* 1997, **92**(5):453–454.
16. Wojakowski W, Maslankiewicz K, Ochala A, Wyderka R, Zuk-Popiolek I, Flak Z, Mroz I, Tendera M: **The pro- and anti-inflammatory markers in patients with acute myocardial infarction and chronic stable angina.** *Int J Mol Med* 2004, **14**(2):317–322.
17. Kawamoto A, Kawata H, Akai Y, Katsuyama Y, Takase E, Sasaki Y, Tsujimura S, Sakaguchi Y, Iwano M, Fujimoto S, Hashimoto T, Dohi K: **Serum levels of VEGF and basic FGF in the subacute phase of myocardial infarction.** *Int J Cardiol* 1998, **67**(1):47–54.
18. Chung NA, Lydakis C, Belgore F, Li-Saw-Hee FL, Blann AD, Lip GYH: **Angiogenesis, thrombogenesis, endothelial dysfunction and angiographic severity of coronary artery disease.** *Heart* 2003, **89**(12):1411–1415.
19. Alber HF, Frick M, Dulak J, Do¨rler J, Zwick R-H, Dichtl W, Pachinger O, Weidinger F: **Vascular endothelial growth factor (VEGF) plasma concentrations in coronary artery disease.** *Heart* 2005, **91**:365–366.
20. Alioglu E, Turk U, Cam S, Abbasaliyev A, Tengiz I, Ercan E: **Polymorphisms of the methylenetetrahydrofolate reductase, vascular endothelial growth factor, endothelial nitric oxide synthase, monocyte chemoattractant protein-1 and apolipoprotein E genes are not associated with carotid intima-media thickness.** *Can J Cardiol* 2009, **25**(1):e1–e5.
21. Gerber HP, McMurtrey A, Kowalski J, Yan M, Keyt BA, Dixit V, Ferrara N: **Vascular endothelial growth factor regulates endothelial cell survival through the phosphatidylinositol 3'-kinase/Akt signal transduction pathway: requirement for Flk-1/KDR activation.** *J Biol Chem* 1998, **273**:30336–30343.
22. Deuse T, Peter C, Fedak PW, Doyle T, Reichenspurner H, Zimmermann WH, Eschenhagen T, Stein W, Wu JC, Robbins RC, Schrepfer S: **Hepatocyte growth factor or vascular endothelial growth factor gene transfer maximizes mesenchymal stem cell-based myocardial salvage after acute myocardial infarction.** *Circulation* 2009, **120**(11 Suppl):S247–S254.

14

High-sensitive Troponin T assay for the diagnosis of acute myocardial infarction: an economic evaluation

Anil Vaidya[1,2*], Johan L Severens[3,4], Brenda WC Bongaerts[5], Kitty BJM Cleutjens[5], Patty J Nelemans[8], Leonard Hofstra[6], Marja van Dieijen-Visser[7] and Erik AL Biessen[5]

Abstract

Background: Delayed diagnosis and treatment of Acute Myocardial Infarction (AMI) has a major adverse impact on prognosis in terms of both morbidity and mortality. Since conventional cardiac Troponin assays have a low sensitivity for diagnosing AMI in the first hours after myocardial necrosis, high-sensitive assays have been developed. The aim of this study was to assess the cost effectiveness of a high-sensitive Troponin T assay (hsTnT), alone or combined with the heart-type fatty acid-binding protein (H-FABP) assay in comparison with the conventional cardiac Troponin (cTnT) assay for the diagnosis of AMI in patients presenting to the hospital with chest pain.

Methods: We performed a cost-utility analysis (quality adjusted life years-QALYs) and a cost effectiveness analysis (life years gained-LYGs) based on a decision analytic model, using a health care perspective in the Dutch context and a life time time-horizon. The robustness of model predictions was explored using one-way and probabilistic sensitivity analyses.

Results: For a life time incremental cost of 30.70 Euros, use of hsTnT over conventional cTnT results in gain of 0.006 Life Years and 0.004 QALY. It should be noted here that hsTnT is a diagnostic intervention which costs only 4.39 Euros/test more than the cTnT test. The ICER generated with the use of hsTnT based diagnostic strategy comparing with the use of a cTnT-based strategy, is 4945 Euros per LYG and 7370 Euros per QALY. The hsTnT strategy has the highest probability of being cost effective at thresholds between 8000 and 20000 Euros per QALY. The combination of hsTnT and h-FABP strategy's probability of being cost effective remains lower than hsTnT at all willingness to pay thresholds.

Conclusion: Our analysis suggests that hsTnT assay is a very cost effective diagnostic tool relative to conventional TnT assay. Combination of hsTnT and H-FABP does not offer any additional economic and health benefit over hsTnT test alone.

Keywords: Cost-effectiveness, Decision model, Acute myocardial infarction, High-sensitive troponin T

Background

Acute coronary syndrome (ACS) is a major cause of morbidity and mortality around the world. The most common manifestation of ACS is acute myocardial infarction (AMI). It is widely accepted that early detection and treatment of AMI has a major impact on AMI morbidity and mortality and therefore on associated costs [1-3]. According to the current guidelines, AMI is diagnosed on the basis of presenting symptoms (chest pain, shortness of breath epigastric discomfort etc.), electrocardiographic (ECG) findings and dedicated blood biomarkers of cardiac necrosis [4]. However, less than 25% symptomatic patients are finally diagnosed with AMI [5], while ECG alone may remain non diagnostic in up to 50% of cases [6]. This makes cardiac biomarker testing an important additional measure for the diagnosis of AMI.

In current clinical practice cardiac troponin T (cTnT) is the preferred biochemical marker for myocardial cell necrosis [4]. Since elevated cTnT levels are detected only 8–12 hours after onset of ischemic symptoms, the low sensitivity of cTnT assay at time of presentation is a major drawback in its use [7]. The life threatening nature of AMI and the

* Correspondence: a.vaidya@maastrichtuniversity.nl
[1]Department of Clinical Epidemiology and Medical Technology Assessment (KEMTA), Maastricht University Medical Centre, PO Box 5800, Maastricht 6202 AZ, The Netherlands
[2]School for Public Health and Primary Care (CAPHRI), Maastricht University, Maastricht, The Netherlands
Full list of author information is available at the end of the article

known inconsistency in cTnT test results at its early phase lead to over-triage of patients and substantial costs to the health system [2,8].

A recently published study has concluded that high-sensitive Troponin T (hsTnT) is a useful prognostic biomarker in patients with symptoms of chest discomfort suspected for ACS [9]. Two multi centre studies have suggested that high-sensitivity Troponin assays offer superior diagnostic accuracy for the early diagnosis of AMI compared to the conventional cTnT assay [7,10]. Another AMI biomarker, heart-type fatty acid-binding protein (H-FABP), was reported to appear in the blood within one hour of myocardial necrosis and peaks after 3–4 hours [11]. Although H-FABP is not recommended as stand-alone test for diagnosis of AMI[12], combined sensitivity of cardiac troponin and H-FABP is reported to be higher than cardiac Troponin alone [13].

In this study we assessed the cost effectiveness of the hsTnT assay and combination of hsTnT (fifth generation TnT assay) and H-FABP assays for the early diagnosis of AMI in comparison with the currently in clinical practice conventional fourth generation TnT assay. To the best of our knowledge, no economic evaluation study has yet been published in Eurozone on the conventional TnT assay based diagnostic approach versus new alternatives involving hsTnT and H-FABP assays.

Methods

Decision analytic model tree

This study was done in the Dutch context using a health care perspective. A decision tree was constructed to compare the costs and outcomes associated with three diagnostic strategies under evaluation in a hypothetical cohort (Figure 1).

Diagnostic strategies

1. cTnT assay at <6 hours of symptom onset, which will be repeated after <12 hours of symptom onset, in the case of negative test result and continuing symptoms.
2. hsTnT assay at <6 hours of symptom onset, which will be repeated after <12 hours of symptom onset, in the case of negative test result and continuing symptoms.
3. hsTnT and H-FABP assays at <6 hours of symptom onset, which will be repeated after <12 hours of symptom onset, in the case of negative test result and continuing symptoms.

Correct or incorrect diagnosis of AMI and subsequent events in the model are followed for patients with chest pain presenting to the hospital. This diagnostic work up

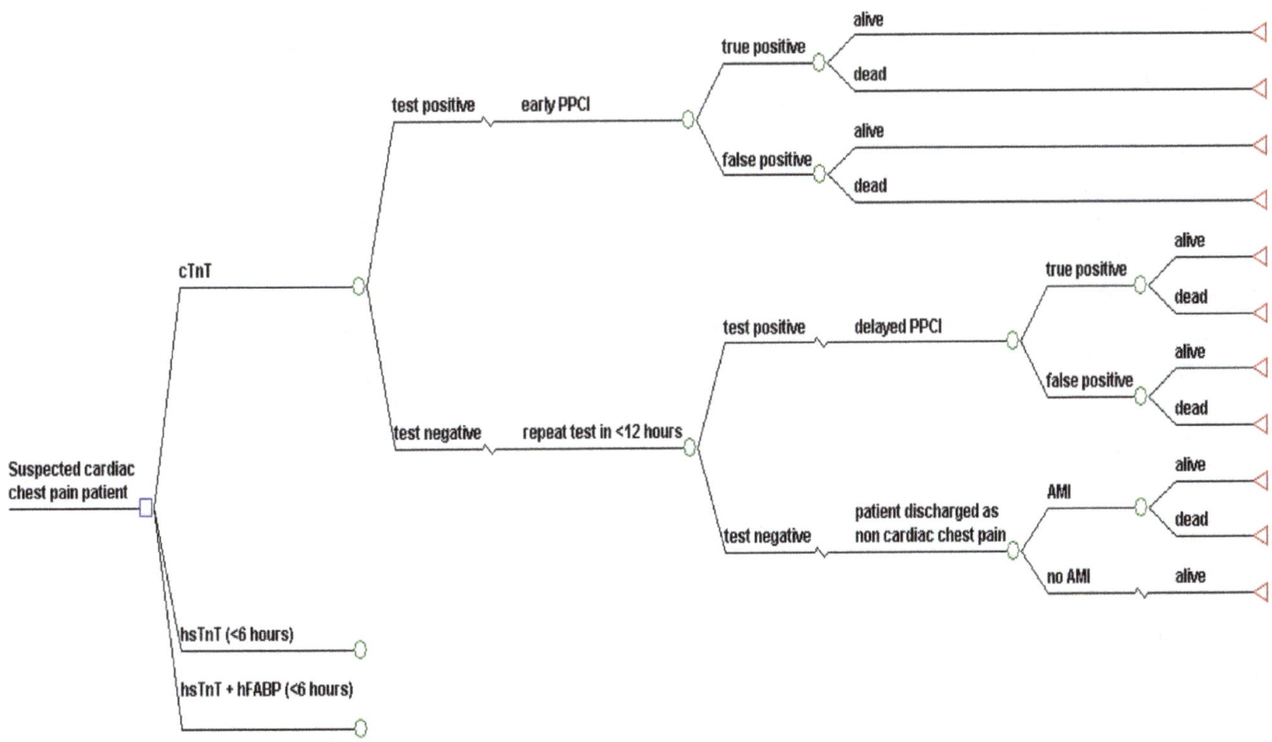

Figure 1 Decision Tree Structure for Diagnosis of AMI. Square node is decision node where patient is assigned to one of the competing strategy. Circles represent chance nodes or probabilities. Triangular terminal nodes represent the end of the paths from left to right through decision tree. Patient is discharged alive from the hospital or dies during hospitalization. Patient survives AMI lives life expectancy of AMI survivor.

of a chest pain patient by one of the above strategies will guide the treating physician to employ the therapeutic intervention i.e. primary percutaneous coronary intervention (PPCI). PPCI is the preferred therapeutic modality to treat AMI and in The Netherlands majority of patients are treated with PPCI [14,15].

The whole process will culminate into either death or survival of the patient during hospital admission. Patient endpoint can be either alive at the end of hospitalization or dead, after presenting to hospital for suspected cardiac chest pain. For the theoretical AMI survivor an average life expectancy was assigned from the literature [16], indicating the time horizon for this modelling study to be life time. Although the exact moment in time is unknown, patients who died during the period of hospitalization were assigned a life expectancy of zero. We assumed that the diagnosis of AMI is excluded in those patients who remained negative after 2 consecutive testing.

Model input parameters

Beside life expectancy and utility values, other parameters used in this model are probabilities of events and costs. Parameters fed into the model are computed from raw parameters obtained from the existing literature and from financial affairs department of Maastricht university medical centre (MUMC) (Table 1). The data for test accuracy of cTnT, hsTnT and hsTnT-H-FABP was determined from the diagnostic testing on the preserved blood samples

Table 1 Model input parameters

Parameter	Deterministic values (min – max range)	Distribution	Source
Costs & event occurrence			
Cost of conventional cTnT test	€17.11(12.8-21.4)	Beta PERT	Commercial price at MUMC
Cost of new hsTnT test	€31.5 (23.6-39.4)	Beta PERT	Time & motion study*
Cost of AMI in 1st year	€ 12446 (9334–15557)	GAMMA	[21]
Cost of AMI in subsequent year	€ 2092 (1569–2615)	GAMMA	[21]
Utility score for AMI	0.725 (0.544-0.906)	BETA	[19]
Discount rate: cost	0.4	Fixed	[23]
Discount rate: Effect	0.15	Fixed	[23]
Prevalence of AMI among patients presenting with chest pain	0.30 (0.23 -0.38)	Beta PERT	[5]
Risk adjusted mortality ratio among inappropriately discharged AMI patients	1.9 (1.43 -2.38)	Beta PERT	[20]
Life expectancy of AMI survivor (years)	8.3 (6.23-10.38)	Beta PERT	[16]
Diagnostic accuracy			
cTnT sensitivity at ≤6 hours	0.44 (0.32-0.56)	BETA	
cTnT sensitivity at ≤12 hours	0.93 (0.85-0.97)	BETA	
cTnT specificity at ≤6 hours	0.92 (0.88-0.95)	BETA	
cTnT specificity at ≤12 hours	0.85 (0.76-0.91)	BETA	
hsTnT sensitivity at ≤6 hours	0.94 (0.87-0.98)	BETA	
hsTnT sensitivity at ≤12 hours	0.95 (0.91-0.98)	BETA	
hsTnT specificity at ≤6 hours	0.52 (0.39-0.65)	BETA	[17]
hsTnT specificity at ≤12 hours	0.51 (0.40-0.62)	BETA	
hsTnT + hFABP sensitivity at ≤6 hours	0.97 (0.90-0.99)	BETA	
hsTnT + hFABP sensitivity at ≤12 hours	0.97 (0.93-0.99)	BETA	
hsTnT + hFABP specificity at ≤ 6 hours	0.39 (0.27-0.51)	BETA	
hsTnT + hFABP specificity at ≤ 12 hours	0.38 (0.27-0.49)	BETA	
Event occurrence			
Average of AMI mortality among patients given PPCI within 4 hours of presentation	0.062 (0.0468-0.0780)	Beta PERT	Calculated from [3]
AMI mortality among patients given PPCI after 4 hours of presentation	0.103 (0.077-0.1288)	Beta PERT	[3]
PPCI procedure related mortality	0.0072 (0.0054-0.009)	Beta PERT	[18]

*Time & Motion study done at Pathology Laboratory, MUMC.

from Bad Nauheim Acute Coronary Syndrome II Registry, Germany as presented by Bongaerts et al. [17].

Event probability calculation

Application of Bayes' Theorem allows us to interpret the test results. Pre-test probability or prior probability of presence/absence of a disease is calculated using Bayesian revision. Prevalence of AMI among symptomatic patients presenting at hospital and diagnostic test sensitivity and specificity are used to calculate various event probabilities. Prevalence of AMI among symptomatic patients presenting to hospital as reported in a large multi-centre study [5] is used in our model.

Post PPCI mortality among AMI patients is abstracted from the literature. Mortality increases with delay in PPCI and is reported from 15 minutes until 240 minutes delay in PPCI after presentation [3]. Average mortality, calculated from mortality reported at different points of time between 15 minutes to 240 minutes, is used in our model after initial biomarker testing at presentation. Average mortality for patients given PPCI within 4 hours of presentation is 6.24%. Mortality among patients in whom PPCI is delayed by ≥4 hours is assumed to be 10.3% based on the mortality figure reported in the literature for PPCI at 240 minutes.

Procedural mortality related to PPCI [18], post AMI life expectancy [16] utility score for AMI survivors [19] and mortality among inappropriately discharged AMI patients in comparison to hospitalized patients [20] are taken from the published literature.

Cost calculation

The cost of diagnostic cTnT test was 17.11 Euros (data obtained from the financial affairs department of Maastricht university medical centre (MUMC) database. MUMC publishes standard prices of health care products available at the MUMC every year in a freely available database [21]. Cost estimates for the new diagnostic tests hsTnT/hFABP (i.e. 21.50 euro), were based on the database, consultation with experts and an in-house time and motion study performed by a senior laboratory technician at the Pathology department of the MUMC who recorded the various stages of test procedure in a time sheet. The unit costs of resources identified for performing the assay was used to calculate the total cost per diagnostic test. Costs incurred in the first year of AMI survival are higher as the primary cost driver is PPCI as a therapeutic intervention. The Dutch costs for the AMI survivors for first year and subsequent years were taken from the published literature [22]. All costs used in the model were converted to Year 2012 costs using harmonized index of consumer prices data from the Dutch bureau of statistics [23].

Longer term costs and outcomes are discounted as per the Dutch pharmacoeconomic guidelines [24].

Outcome measures

The effectiveness of diagnostic test strategies is measured in terms of survival probabilities in AMI patients during hospitalization and incremental life years gained (LYGs) by AMI survivors. Quality adjusted life years (QALYs) are derived by multiplying LYGs with the Post AMI utility score reported in the literature [19].

Analyses

The expected costs and outcomes of all the three strategies were calculated and incremental cost effectiveness ratios were determined. Cost effectiveness analysis(CEA) and cost-utility analysis (CUA) are approaches to compare the costs and health outcomes of a new intervention with the existing practice [25]. An incremental cost effectiveness Ratio (ICER) is calculated by dividing differential costs with differential effects between existing practice and the new health technology. When more than one, 'new technologies' are under evaluation then the more costly technology is compared with the less costly technology [26].

The probabilistic sensitivity analysis (PSA) considers uncertainties in all the model parameters simultaneously. Probabilistic sensitivity analysis quantifies the uncertainty in the ICER, by placing a probability distribution over parameter values. Test accuracy parameter values were varied in the full range of their reported 95% confidence interval (CI). Other parameter values were varied between 75% and 125% of their point estimates. The model parameters were assigned BETA distribution and BETA Pert distribution was used if confidence intervals or standard errors were not reported in the source literature. BETA Pert distribution is a version of the Beta distribution. The costs of AMI treatment were assigned GAMMA distribution. Probabilistic sensitivity analysis of the model parameters with 1,000 iterations using Monte Carlo simulation technique yields a range of health outcome results. Net monetary benefit (NMB) framework was applied to Monte Carlo simulation data to construct the cost effectiveness acceptability curves (CEACs). This framework offers an advantage of unambiguously sorting out the acceptability of an individual simulation trial on cost effectiveness plane, for a range of 'willingness to pay' values [25,27].

We performed one way sensitivity analyses to assess the degree of change in results with variation of one model input parameter value at a time. All parameters were were varied in the full range of their reported 95% confidence interval (CI) or between 75% and 125% of their point estimates.

Results

Base case

The expected values for the three strategies namely conventional cTnT, hsTnT and combination of hsTnT and

Table 2 Base-case results costs and effects

	Diagnostic strategies			Increments		
	cTnT	hsTnT	hsTnT + H-FABP	hsTnT vs cTnT	hsTnT + H-FABP vs cTnT	hsTnT + H-FABP vs hsTnT
Discounted cost	€ 15115.62	€ 15137.2	€ 15187.74	€ 30.70	€ 86.61	€ 55.91
Discounted LYGs	2.286	2.292	2.296	0.006	0.010	0.0037
Discounted QALYs	1.657	1.662	1.664	0.004	0.007	0.0025
ICER						
	Incremental cost per LYG			**Incremental cost per QALY**		
cTnT	Reference strategy			Reference strategy		
hsTnT vs cTnT	€ 4945			€ 7370		
hsTnT + H-FABP vs cTnT	€ 8780			€ 13084		
hsTnT + H-FABP vs hsTnT	€ 15286			€ 22781		

H-FABP, regarding costs and outcomes are shown in Table 2. The constructed model predicts that when a diagnosis is made using hsTnT instead of conventional TnT, a hypothetical AMI survivor will live 0.006 years (Life Year Gain-LYG) longer and will have additional 0.004 QALYs for an incremental cost of 30.70 Euros. It should be noted here that hsTnT is a diagnostic intervention which costs only 4.39 Euros/test more than the cTnT test. The ICER generated with the use of hsTnT based diagnostic strategy comparing with the use of a cTnT-based strategy, is 4945 Euros per LYG and 7370 Euros per QALY. Combination strategy of the hsTnT assay with the H-FABP assay is the next more costly new technology and as per the decision modelling guidelines it is compared with less costly hsTnT [26]. Comparison of combination arm with hsTnT alone arm shows 0.0037 and 0.0025 additional LYGs and QALYs respectively, at an incremental cost of 55.91 Euros leading to an ICER of 15286 per LYG and 22781 Euros per QALY. Details of costs, outcomes and increments for all strategies are presented in the Table 2.

Probabilistic sensitivity analysis

The probabilistic results of the decision model are similar to the deterministic results hsTnT as cost effective diagnostic strategy. Figure 2 shows the probability in the PSA that each strategy is cost effective at various thresholds of willingness to pay ranging from zero to 20000 Euros. hsTnT strategy has the highest probability of being cost effective at thresholds between 8000 and 20000 Euros per QALY. The combination of hsTnT and h-FABP strategy's probability of being cost effective remains lower than hsTnT at all willingness to pay thresholds and was not analysed further by one way sensitivity analysis.

One way sensitivity analysis

The constructed model was robust to all one way sensitivity analyses and ICER remains less than 12000 Euros per QALY which is far below the acceptable willingness to pay per QALY limit of 20000 Euros in The Netherlands. The results of one way sensitivity analyses are graphically displayed as a tornado diagram in the Figure 3. This figure

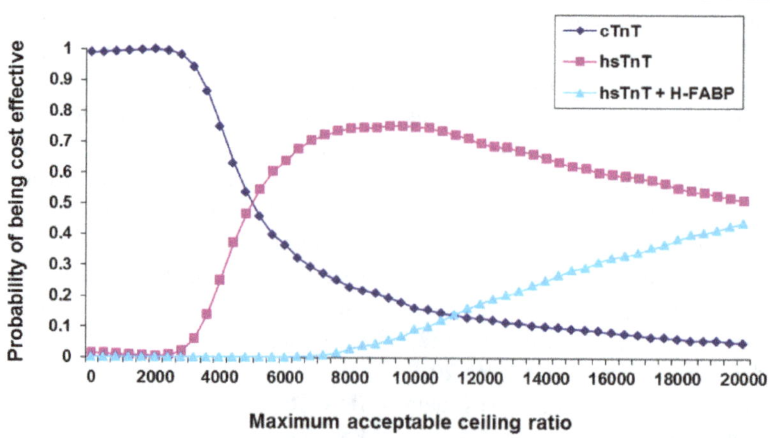

Figure 2 Cost effectiveness acceptability curve(s) shows likelihood that a strategy would be cost effective for a range of maximum acceptable ceiling ratios society is willing to pay for the gain of one QALY, assessed with 1000 Monte Carlo simulations.

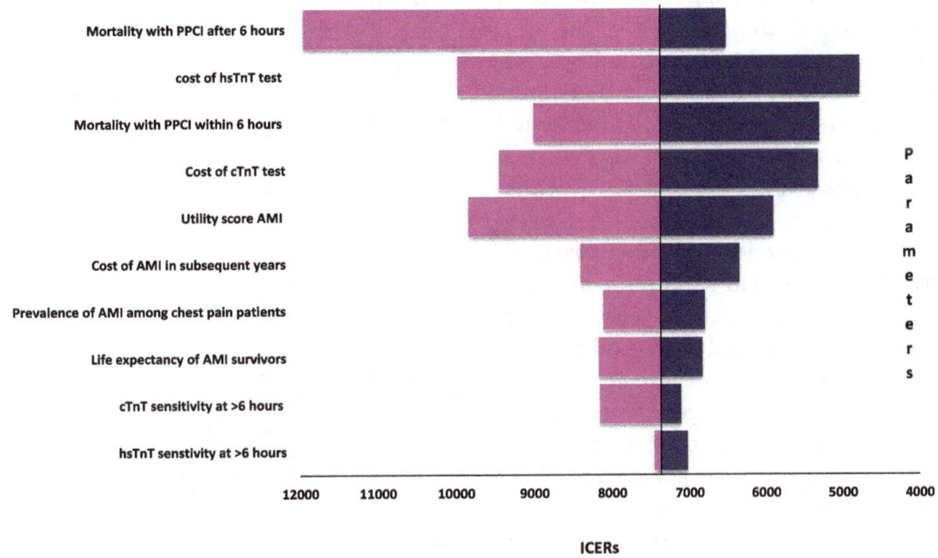

Figure 3 One way sensitivity analysis: Tornado diagram.

shows top ten model parameters influencing the model results (ICER).

Discussion

This modelling study assessed the cost effectiveness of two biomarker strategies for the early diagnosis of AMI i.e. hsTnT and the combination of hsTnT and H-FABP. Economic and clinical consequences of using these new tests instead of conventional cTnT test were extrapolated by decision modelling. Our findings suggested that hsTnT is a cost effective tool to diagnose AMI at the Emergency Department in patients presenting with chest pain. Use of hsTnT diagnostic assay resulted in gain of additional QALYs compared with the existing 4thgeneration diagnostic cTnT test. A combination strategy of performing the 5thgeneration hsTnT and H-FABP assays simultaneously did not bring any additional benefit and even incurred higher costs.

This study was performed with a health care payer's perspective. The societal perspective for this study was not considered because the average age of AMI patients in The Netherlands is 66.7 years [28]. Therefore, productivity loss in this age group may not be significant and impact of this effect was not weighed or included. Indirect costs associated with time spent by family members for the care of these patients are also difficult to estimate for the societal perspective.

A potential limitation of this study is that the probabilities of clinical outcomes in our model are derived from diagnostic accuracy estimates for hsTnT and H-FABP from a single cohort with relatively small number of patients from Bad Nauheim Acute Coronary Syndrome II Registry, Germany. However, in sensitivity analysis our test accuracy data was varied between full ranges of confidence interval (CI) limits to test the robustness of the model. Application of the net monetary benefit (NMB) framework revealed the dominance of hsTnT strategy showing highest net monetary benefit for it. Furthermore, a recently published meta-analysis [29] for diagnostic accuracy of cTnT and hsTnT at the time of patient's presentation to the emergency department has similar accuracy figures as our source article by Bongaerts et al. [17].

This study shares the general limitations of economic modelling. Complex medical practice is difficult to transform into a decision tree model. This applies to our model as well. All test positive patients will not undergo PPCI in real life situation. Repeated biomarker testing, clinical judgment and ECG findings play a crucial role in decision making on invasive intervention. Our decision tree model attempts to reflect the true clinical practice as closely as possible and the model's robustness has been rigorously tested for changes in clinical and economic variables. All the model assumptions and uncertainties were addressed by performing one way sensitivity analysis and state-of-the-art Probabilistic Sensitivity Analysis. PSA is one of the most sophisticated methods to address uncertainty allowed systematic propagation of uncertainty in all model parameters and offered a statistical interpretation of the joint distribution of incremental costs and effects. The model outcomes (expected costs and QALYs of the strategies) were based on the results of the probabilistic sensitivity analysis (PSA) with 1,000 simulations. The results of our study are in line and are comparable to the recently published National Institute for Health Research (NIHR) UK, document showing the value of hsTnT based early diagnosis of AMI. This document also concludes that there is currently insufficient evidence to support routine use of alternative biomarkers alongside troponin [30].

Our estimation of post PPCI mortality is based on averaged mortality figures reported by Rathore et al. and covers the 15–240 min delay from diagnosis to PPCI after arrival to hospital [3]. The study by Rathore et al. [3] shows that more than 80% of patients underwent a PPCI within 120 minutes of hospital arrival, implying that the applied average mortality rate in our model may be an overestimation. Lower mortality rate will shift ICER more in favour of hsTnT and would make hsTnT even more cost effective.

Our model conforms to the principles of good practice for decision analytic models with use of transparent data and modelling technique as per the guidelines laid by the international society for pharmacoeconomics and outcome research (ISPOR) task force [31]. Strength of this model is its potential transferability as model inputs can be adapted to a new setting easily. Inter- or intra-country variations in costs, prevalence of AMI and therapeutic intervention outcomes caused by availability and accessibility of health care can be incorporated into the model. Using cost effectiveness threshold from WHO-CHOICE (world health organization – CHOosing Interventions that are Cost Effective) project for ceiling ratio in a particular country, cost effectiveness analysis can be performed for that country [32].

The newly introduced hsTnT biomarker assay significantly contributes to the early diagnosis of AMI and appears to be a promising diagnostic intervention for AMI. Although a multi-marker approach using hsTnT and H-FABP may allow an early rule out of the disease but economic modelling of cost and consequences for this combination predicts its inferiority to hsTnT alone. Moreover, in a non ST elevation AMI patients study by Giannitsis et al. showed that a doubling of the hs-TnT concentration within 3 hours with the second concentration above the 99th percentile value is associated with a positive predictive value for AMI of 100% and a negative predicting value of 88% [33]. This indicates that with the hsTnT assay within 3 hours instead of the 6 hours examined in this study, a definitive outcome can be obtained.

Conclusions

This economic evaluation concludes that hsTnT assay is a cost effective alternative for the diagnosis of AMI to the existing diagnostic marker assay in clinical practice. Combination of two biomarkers, hsTnT and H-FABP for the diagnosis of AMI does not bring any added advantage. Future replacement of cTnT with hsTnT in clinical practice is expected to save substantial health care costs and to improve Health Related Qulaity of Life among AMI patients. However, data for hsTnT and its combination with other biomarkers from further research is needed to support and strengthen the results of this modelling study.

Abbreviations

ACS: Acute coronary syndrome; AMI: Acute myocardial infarction; ECG: Electrocardiogram; cTnT: Cardiac troponin; hsTnT: High-sensitive troponin; H-FABP: Heart type fatty acid binding protein; PPCI: Primary percutaneous coronary intervention; MUMC: Maastricht university medical centre; LYG: Life year gained; QALY: Quality adjusted life years; CEA: Cost effectiveness analysis; CUA: Cost utility analysis; PSA: Probabilistic sensitivity analysis; CI: Confidence interval; NMB: Net monetary benefit; ICER: Incremental cost effectiveness ratio; CEAC: Cost-effectiveness acceptability curve; CHOICE: CHOosing interventions that are cost effective.

Competing interest

The authors declare that they have no competing interests.

Authors' contributions

Conceived and designed the economic evaluation: AV and JLS. Data: BWCB and EALB. Wrote the paper: AV, JLS, EALB. Critical revision of the manuscript: KBJMC, PJN, LH and MDV. Final approval of the manuscript for publication: JLS and EALB. All authors read and approved the final manuscript.

Acknowledgments

We hereby acknowledge Mr Mat Rousch, senior technician at pathology Department MUMC for his contribution in time and motion study to determine the costs of experimental assays, and Mr Vincent Kleijnen from the Department of Clinical Chemistry for performing the hsTnT assays.

Author details

[1]Department of Clinical Epidemiology and Medical Technology Assessment (KEMTA), Maastricht University Medical Centre, PO Box 5800, Maastricht 6202 AZ, The Netherlands. [2]School for Public Health and Primary Care (CAPHRI), Maastricht University, Maastricht, The Netherlands. [3]Institute of Health Policy and Management, Erasmus University Rotterdam, Rotterdam, The Netherlands. [4]iMTA - Institute of Technology Assessment, Erasmus University Rotterdam, Rotterdam, The Netherlands. [5]Department of Pathology, Cardiovascular Research Institute Maastricht (CARIM), Maastricht University Medical Centre, Maastricht, The Netherlands. [6]Cardiology Center Netherlands, Utrecht, The Netherlands. [7]Department of Clinical Chemistry, Maastricht University, Maastricht, The Netherlands. [8]Department of Epidemiology, Maastricht University, Maastricht, The Netherlands.

References

1. Boersma E, Maas AC, Deckers JW, Simoons ML: **Early thrombolytic treatment in acute myocardial infarction: reappraisal of the golden hour.** *Lancet* 1996, **348**(9030):771–775.
2. Forberg JL, Henriksen LS, Edenbrandt L, Ekelund U: **Direct hospital costs of chest pain patients attending the emergency department: a retrospective study.** *BMC Emerg Med* 2006, **6:**6.
3. Rathore SS, Curtis JP, Chen J, Wang Y, Nallamothu BK, Epstein AJ, Krumholz HM: **Association of door-to-balloon time and mortality in patients admitted to hospital with ST elevation myocardial infarction: national cohort study.** *BMJ* 2009, **338:**b1807.
4. Thygesen K, Alpert JS, White HD, Jaffe AS, Apple FS, Galvani M, Katus HA, Newby LK, Ravkilde J, Chaitman B, Clemmensen PM, Dellborg M, Hod H, Porela P, Underwood R, Bax JJ, Beller GA, Bonow R, Van der Wall EE, Bassand JP, Wijns W, Ferguson TB, Steg PG, Uretsky BF, Williams DO, Armstrong PW, Antman EM, Fox KA, Hamm CW, Ohman EM, *et al*: **Universal definition of myocardial infarction.** *Circulation* 2007, **116**(22):2634–2653.
5. Pope JH, Selker HP: **Acute coronary syndromes in the emergency department: diagnostic characteristics, tests, and challenges.** *Cardiol Clin* 2005, **23**(4):423–451. v-vi.
6. Menown IB, Mackenzie G, Adgey AA: **Optimizing the initial 12-lead electrocardiographic diagnosis of acute myocardial infarction.** *Eur Heart J* 2000, **21**(4):275–283.
7. Reichlin T, Hochholzer W, Bassetti S, Steuer S, Stelzig C, Hartwiger S, Biedert S, Schaub N, Buerge C, Potocki M, Noveanu M, Breidthardt T, Twerenbold R, Winkler K, Bingisser R, Mueller C: **Early diagnosis of myocardial infarction with sensitive cardiac troponin assays.** *N Engl J Med* 2009, **361**(9):858–867.

8. Kontos MC, Schmidt KL, McCue M, Rossiter LF, Jurgensen M, Nicholson CS, Jesse RL, Ornato JP, Tatum JL: **A comprehensive strategy for the evaluation and triage of the chest pain patient: a cost comparison study.** *J Nucl Cardiol* 2003, **10**(3):284–290.
9. Mingels AM, Joosen IA, Versteylen MO, Laufer EM, Winkens MH, Wildberger JE, Van Dieijen-Visser MP, Hofstra L: **High-sensitivity cardiac troponin T: risk stratification tool in patients with symptoms of chest discomfort.** *PLoS One* 2012, **7**(4):e35059.
10. Keller T, Zeller T, Peetz D, Tzikas S, Roth A, Czyz E, Bickel C, Baldus S, Warnholtz A, Frohlich M, Sinning CR, Eleftheriadis MS, Wild PS, Schnabel RB, Lubos E, Jachmann N, Genth-Zotz S, Post F, Nicaud V, Tiret L, Lackner KJ, Munzel TF, Blankenberg S: **Sensitive troponin I assay in early diagnosis of acute myocardial infarction.** *N Engl J Med* 2009, **361**(9):868–877.
11. Pelsers MM, Hermens WT, Glatz JF: **Fatty acid-binding proteins as plasma markers of tissue injury.** *Clin Chim Acta* 2005, **352**(1–2):15–35.
12. Mad P, Domanovits H, Fazelnia C, Stiassny K, Russmuller G, Cseh A, Sodeck G, Binder T, Christ G, Szekeres T, Laggner A, Herkner H: **Human heart-type fatty-acid-binding protein as a point-of-care test in the early diagnosis of acute myocardial infarction.** *QJM* 2007, **100**(4):203–210.
13. McCann CJ, Glover BM, Menown IB, Moore MJ, McEneny J, Owens CG, Smith B, Sharpe PC, Young IS, Adgey JA: **Novel biomarkers in early diagnosis of acute myocardial infarction compared with cardiac troponin T.** *Eur Heart J* 2008, **29**(23):2843–2850.
14. Kukreja N, Onuma Y, Garcia-Garcia H, Daemen J, Van Domburg R, Serruys PW: **Primary Percutaneous Coronary Intervention for Acute Myocardial Infarction / CLINICAL PERSPECTIVE.** *Circ Cardiovasc Interv* 2008, **1**(2):103–110.
15. Tiemann O: **Variations in hospitalisation costs for acute myocardial infarction - a comparison across Europe.** *Health Econ* 2008, **17**(1 Suppl):S33–S45.
16. Selmer R, Halvorsen S, Myhre KI, Wisloff TF, Kristiansen IS: **Cost-effectiveness of primary percutaneous coronary intervention versus thrombolytic therapy for acute myocardial infarction.** *Scand Cardiovasc J* 2005, **39**(5):276–285.
17. Brenda WC Bongaerts MW, Mat R, Stefanie D, van Dieijen-Visser MP, Jan FC G, Anil V, Severens HL, Kitty BJM C, Nelemans PJ, Erik AL B: **High-sensitivity Troponin T Advances the Diagnosis of Acute Myocardial Infarction.** *PLoS One* 2013, Resubmitted after revision.
18. Anderson HV, Shaw RE, Brindis RG, McKay CR, Klein LW, Krone RJ, Ho KK, Rumsfeld JS, Smith SC Jr, Weintraub WS: **Risk-adjusted mortality analysis of percutaneous coronary interventions by American College of Cardiology/American Heart Association guidelines recommendations.** *Am J Cardiol* 2007, **99**(2):189–196.
19. Sullivan PW, Slejko JF, Sculpher MJ, Ghushchyan V: **Catalogue of EQ-5D Scores for the United Kingdom.** *Med Decis Making* 2011, **31**(6):800–804.
20. Pope JH, Aufderheide TP, Ruthazer R, Woolard RH, Feldman JA, Beshansky JR, Griffith JL, Selker HP: **Missed diagnoses of acute cardiac ischemia in the emergency department.** *N Engl J Med* 2000, **342**(16):1163–1170.
21. *Standaard prijslijst overige zorgproducten academisch ziekenhuis Maastricht per 1-7-2013.* [http://wiki.mumc.nl/sites/wiki/files/passantentarieflijst_per_1-7-2013_ovp.pdf]
22. Thurston SJ, Heeg B, De Charro F, Van Hout B: **Cost-effectiveness of clopidogrel in STEMI patients in the Netherlands: a model based on the CLARITY trial.** *Curr Med Res Opin* 2010, **26**(3):641–651.
23. *Consumer prices; European harmonised price index.* [http://statline.cbs.nl/StatWeb/publication/?DM=SLEN&PA=80087ENG&D1=0&D2=0&D3=38,51,64,77,90,103,l&LA=EN&HDR=G1,T&STB=G2&VW=T accessed on 12 Jan 2012]
24. *Guidelines for pharmacoeconomic research, updated version.* [http://www.ispor.org/peguidelines/source/HTAGuidelinesNLupdated2006.pdf accessed on 15 Nov 2011]
25. Drummond MF, Sculpher MJ, Torrance GW: *Methods for the economic evaluation of health care programmes.* Oxford: Oxford University Press; 2005.
26. Briggs AH, Claxton K, Sculpher MJ: *Decision modelling for health economic evaluation.* Oxford: Oxford University Press; 2006.
27. Fenwick E, Marshall DA, Levy AR, Nichol G: **Using and interpreting cost-effectiveness acceptability curves: an example using data from a trial of management strategies for atrial fibrillation.** *BMC Health Serv Res* 2006, **6**:52.
28. Koek HL, De Bruin A, Gast A, Gevers E, Kardaun JW, Reitsma JB, Grobbee DE, Bots ML: **Incidence of first acute myocardial infarction in the Netherlands.** *Neth J Med* 2007, **65**(11):434–441.
29. Thokala P, Goodacre SW, Collinson PO, Stevens JW, Mills NL, Newby DE, Morris F, Kendall J, Stevenson MD: **Cost-effectiveness of presentation versus delayed troponin testing for acute myocardial infarction.** *Heart* 2012, **98**(20):1498–1503.
30. Goodacre S, Thokala P, Carroll C, Stevens JW, Leaviss J, Al Khalaf M, Collinson P, Morris F, Evans P, Wang J: **Systematic review, meta-analysis and economic modelling of diagnostic strategies for suspected acute coronary syndrome.** *Health Technol Assess* 2013, **17**(1):1–188. v-vi.
31. Weinstein MC, O'Brien B, Hornberger J, Jackson J, Johannesson M, McCabe C, Luce BR: **Principles of good practice for decision analytic modeling in health-care evaluation: report of the ISPOR Task Force on Good Research Practices–Modeling Studies.** *Value Health* 2003, **6**(1):9–17.
32. *CHOosing Interventions that are Cost Effective (WHO-CHOICE): Cost-effectiveness thresholds.* [http://www.who.int/choice/costs/CER_thresholds/en/index.html accessed on 12 Dec 2011]
33. Giannitsis E, Becker M, Kurz K, Hess G, Zdunek D, Katus HA: **High-sensitivity cardiac troponin T for early prediction of evolving non-ST-segment elevation myocardial infarction in patients with suspected acute coronary syndrome and negative troponin results on admission.** *Clin Chem* 2010, **56**(4):642–650.

15

Myocardial infarction, symptomatic third degree atrioventricular block and pulmonary embolism caused by thalidomide

Shengyu Zhang[1], Jing Yang[2], Xiaofeng Jin[2] and Shuyang Zhang[2*]

Abstract

Background: Thalidomide has been reported to cause numerous thromboembolic events. Deep vein thrombosis and pulmonary embolism are more common. It can also cause bradycardia and even total atrioventricular block. Rarely, it causes coronary artery spasm and even myocardial infarction. But almost simultaneous onset of myocardial infarction, third degree atrioventricular block and pulmonary embolism in one patient has not been reported so far.

Case presentation: A 53-year old man presented because of chest pain, nausea and then syncope for several minutes. Previous medical history included neurodermitis for which thalidomide was given and hypercholesterolemia with simvastatin taking. The patient didn't exhibit any other established risk factors for coronary artery disease. Electrocardiography showed sinus rhythm with third degree atrioventricular block and complete right bundle branch block, and precordial leads ST segment elevation. The diagnosis of acute coronary syndrome was suspected, but further coronary angiography demonstrated no flow-limiting lesions in coronary arteries, and temporary pacemaker was implanted. After admission, low SpO_2 and elevated D-dimer level was mentioned. Further computed tomography pulmonary angiography revealed pulmonary embolism. Thalidomide was thought to be the cause of hypercoagulability and coronary spasm, so it was ceased immediately. Therapeutic low molecule weight heparin was initiated and then switched to warfarin with appropriate INR, and nifedipine was described for coronary spasm. The patient's symptoms completely relived and SpO_2 recovered, and atrioventricular block had disappeared during hospitalization with pacemaker removed.

Conclusion: This is the very first case in which myocardial infarction, third degree atrioventricular block and pulmonary embolism almost simultaneously developed. We should be ware that anti-thrombotic prophylaxis, which needs further investigation for optimal drug and dosage, may be beneficial in thalidomide therapy. And it is also important to monitor patients taking thalidomide for signs and symptoms of bradycardia or higher degree atrioventricular block.

Keywords: Thalidomide, Myocardial infarction, Third degree atrioventricular block, Pulmonary embolism

Background

Oral immunomodulatory drugs, namely thalidomide and its analogues (lenalidomide and pomalidomide), presently play a crucial role in the treatment of multiple myeloma (MM) and other diseases such as Crohn's disease, refractory aphthous ulcer in HIV and dermatologic conditions [1]. As it is cautiously being reintroduced into clinical use, new adverse effects are being described. Trials have reported numerous thromboembolic events attributed to thalidomide therapy, especially in multiple myeloma patients; deep vein thrombosis (DVT) and pulmonary embolism (PE) are more common, but occasional arterial thrombotic events have also been reported [1]; it also can cause bradycardia [2–4] and even total atrioventricular block (AVB) (the only case ever

* Correspondence: shuyangzhang103@126.com
[2]Department of Cardiology, Peking Union Medical College Hospital, Chinese Academy of Medical Sciences, Beijing, China
Full list of author information is available at the end of the article

reported) [5]. Even Rarely, thalidomide can caused coronary artery spasm [5] and myocardial infarction (MI).

Herein we report the first case taking thalidomide with almost simultaneous onset of MI, third degree AVB and PE.

Case presentation

A 53-year old man presented in the emergency room because of suddenly onset of chest pain, nausea and then syncope for several minutes. Previous medical history included neurodermitis for which ebastine and ketotifen were given but proven ineffective, so thalidomide (150 mg/d) therapy was initiated 2 weeks before; medical history also included hypercholesterolemia and simvastatin taking. No other medication including corticosteroids was reported and electrocardiography (ECG) in the past was almost normal (Fig. 1a). The patient did not exhibit any other established risk factors for coronary artery disease, such as obesity, diabetes, hypertension or family history, with the exception of current smoking. Physical examination on admission revealed a heart rate of 47 bpm, blood pressure of 96/61 mmHg and normal SpO_2 (98 % without oxygen). The 12-lead ECG showed sinus rhythm with a first-degree AV block and complete right bundle branch block (CRBBB), and I, aVL, V2-4 leads ST segment elevation (Fig. 1b); about 1 h later repeated ECG showed third-degree AV block but no ST-T dynamic change (Fig. 1c). So the diagnosis of acute coronary syndrome was suspected. The treatment of aspirin and clopidogrel was initiated for anti-platelet after which patient's chest pain relieved partially, but intravenous nitroglycerin was avoided because of relatively low blood pressure and slow heart rate. 1 h after presentation, emergency coronary angiography was conducted and demonstrated no flow-limiting lesions in coronary arteries except minor atherosclerosis (Fig. 2), and meanwhile temporary pacemaker was implanted (Fig. 1d). Hours later the patient was admitted into cardiac care unit, blood tests showed LDL-C level 2.23 mmol/L and cardiac troponin I (cTnI) level elevated significantly (maximum 50.83 μg/L reached at 24 h after symptoms onset, normal upper limit was 0.04 μg/L; Fig. 3). And echocardiography only showed hypokinesis of middle and inferior segment of anterior wall with normal ejaculation fraction (EF) of 53 %, without tricuspid regurgitation or pulmonary hypertension, and no evidence of left or right-sided heart thrombi or right-left shunt was found; ^{99m}Tc-MIBI myocardial perfusion single photon emission computed tomography showed reduced perfusion in the middle anterior wall of left ventricle; and further cardiac magnetic resonance imaging (MRI) showed thinning of apical anterior wall of left ventricle and subendocardial late gadolinium enhancement (Fig. 4). So it was likely that acute coronary event had happened. In CCU we continued aspirin for anti-platelet, but 2 days later patient's SpO_2 fell to 95 % at 10 L/min oxygen with reservoir mask, and D-dimer level elevated significantly (3.06 mg/L, normal range within 0.55 mg/L). Further ultrasound examination found no thrombi in deep veins of both lower limbs, but computed tomography pulmonary angiography (CTPA) revealed scattered embolism of subsegmental pulmonary arteries of both sides (Fig. 5). Tests for hypercoagulability was ordered and demonstrated normal coagulation parameters (also including factor V Leiden mutation and levels of protein C, protein S and anti-thrombin III), normal homocysteine level, negative anti-nuclear antibodies, anti-cardiolipin antibodies, lupus anticoagulant and tumor markers. So thalidomide was thought to be the cause of hypercoagulability, and this medication was ceased immediately; therapeutic low molecule weight heparin was initiated and then switched to warfarin with a target INR of 2 ~ 3, and nifedipine was given for coronary spasm. The patient reported no symptoms after therapy modification and SpO_2 rose up to normal (97 % without oxygen) gradually, and third degree AV block also disappeared during hospitalization with temporary pacemaker removed (Fig. 1e). After discharge, patient was followed up over a period of 12 months, and warfarin was continued for 3 months with appropriate INR. No further recurrences of chronotropic or ischemic cardiac symptoms were reported.

Discussion

The severe teratogenic side effects of thalidomide led to its well-publicized withdrawal in the 1970s. Thalidomide appears to have several immunomodulatory properties, including suppression of TNF-α production, down-regulation of cell-surface adhesion molecules involved in leukocyte migration, decreasing circulating helper T cell to suppressor T-cell ratio, and inhibition of IFN-γ, and more roles recognized including inhibition of angiogenesis as well as anti-fibrotic and anti-oncogenic properties [6]. Therefore thalidomide is being used in an increasing number of diseases nowadays.

Thalidomide is associated with higher risk of thromboembolism, both venous and arterial. Potential mechanisms have been explored: serum levels of the anticoagulant pathway cofactor thrombomodulin transiently dropped during the first month of thalidomide therapy, with gradual recovery over the following two months [7]; patients with MM treated with thalidomide had extremely high levels of von Willebrand factor antigen and factor VIII, factors known to be associated with an increased risk of thrombotic events in the general population [8]. But the reason for thromboembolism in the non-MM setting remains undefined. As noted in our patient, MI and PE had developed almost simultaneously. A reasonable explanation for PE is

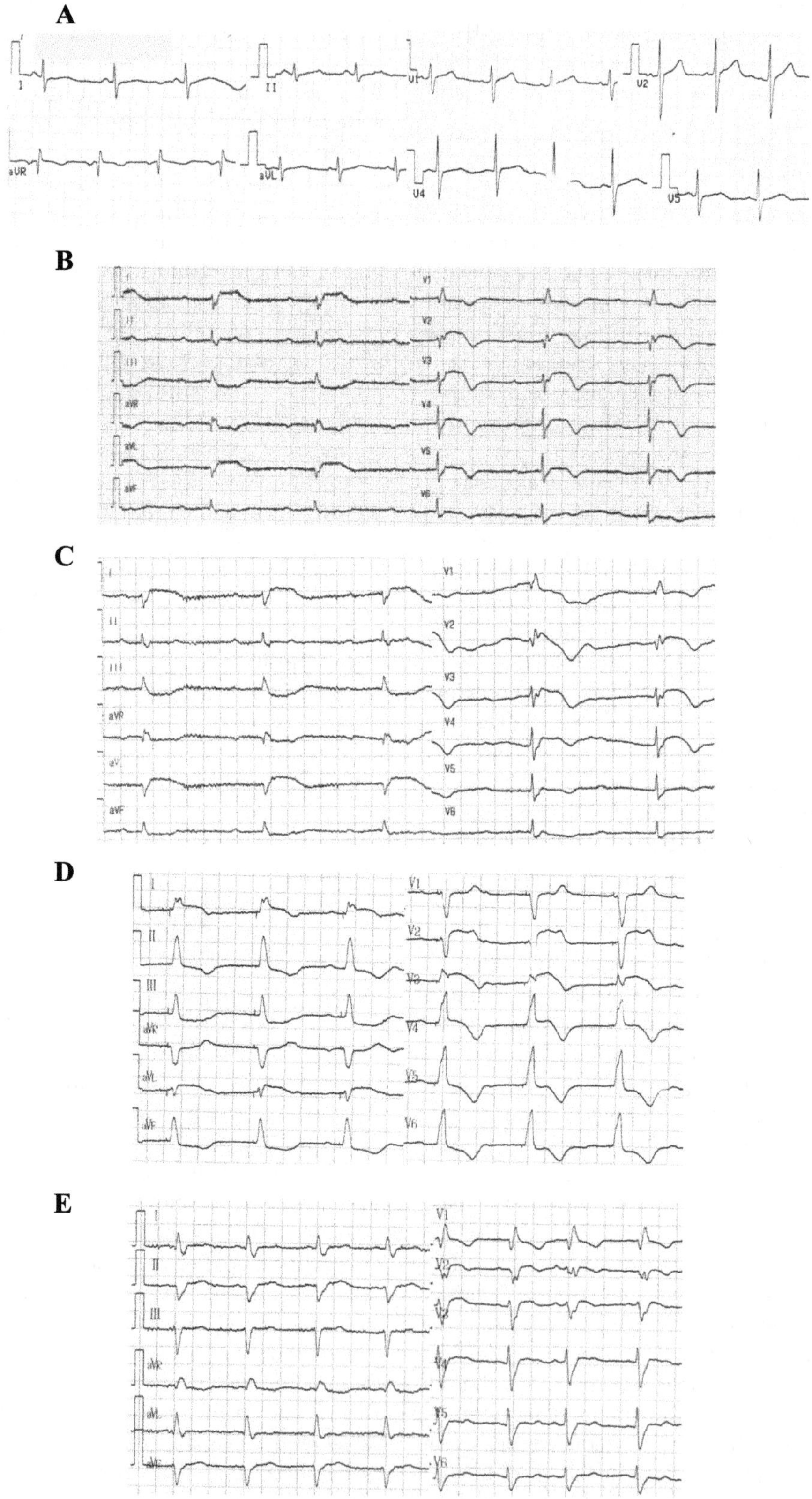

Fig. 1 Electrocardiography development. **a** Almost normal ECG shows no conduction block. **b** ECG indicates first-degree AV block and CRBBB with precordial leads ST segment elevation. **c** ECG indicates third-degree AV block with precordial leads ST segment elevation. **d** ECG shows right ventricular stimulation of temporary pacemaker and elevated ST segment restoring (after emergency coronary angiography). **e** ECG indicates third-degree AV block disappeared and pacemaker removed, but CRBBB was left over

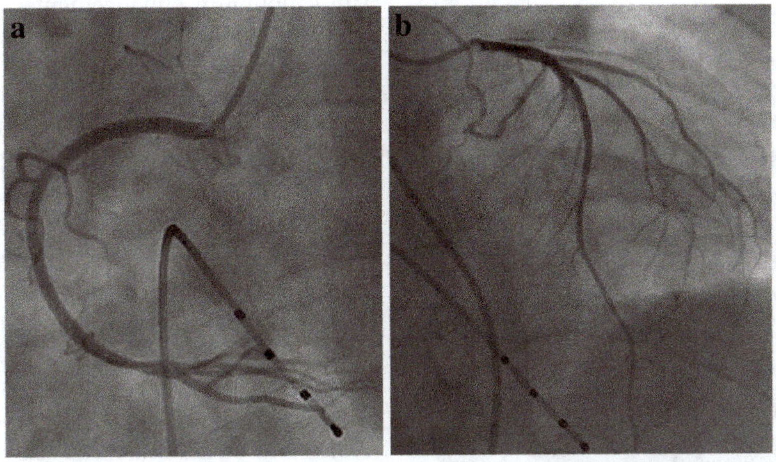

Fig. 2 Coronary angiography. Emergency coronary angiography revealed no flow-limiting lesions. **a** For view of right coronary artery. **b** For view of left anterior descending artery and left circumflex artery

hypercoagulability induced by thalidomide caused grand thrombotic events in venous system. Because no right-left shunt was found in heart, paradoxical embolism of coronary artery from venous thrombi was not likely. Because coronary angiography demonstrated no flow-limiting lesions or thrombus in major coronary arteries, it probably was the coronary spasm that caused myocardial infarction [9], which had been reported as a rare complication of thalidomide therapy (only one case in the past) [2] and maybe further ergonovine provocation test was needed to ensure the existence of it. The precise mechanism that caused spasm remains undefined, and someone believed thalidomide could cause vasoconstriction through endothelial disruption [2]. And the ST segment elevation was persistent even though no obvious coronary spasm observed during angiography, probably because of acute myocardial infarction (likely ST elevated myocardial infarction) caused by coronary spasm. Another possible cause for MI was thrombus formed in coronary artery and needed to be confirmed by coronary angiography. Often

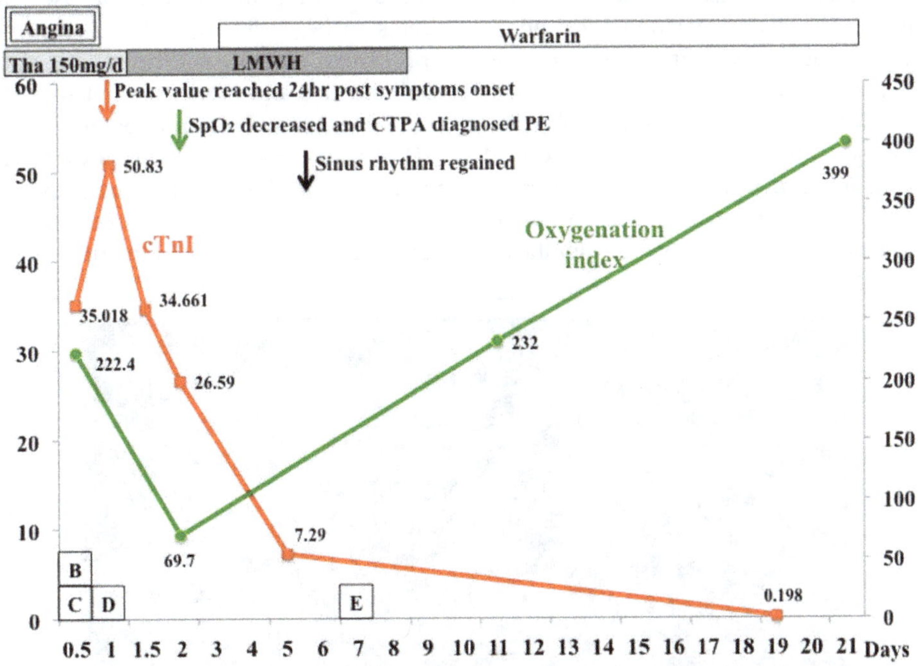

Fig. 3 Clinical course. The solid red line indicates the cTnI level (μg/L). The solid green line indicates the oxygenation index (a ratio of the partial pressure of arterial oxygen to the fraction of inspired oxygen). Horizontal axis indicates time (days) after symptoms onset. *b, c, d* in textboxes indicates different ECG (for Fig. 1b, c, d and e, respectively). Tha = thalidomide. cTnI = cardiac troponin I

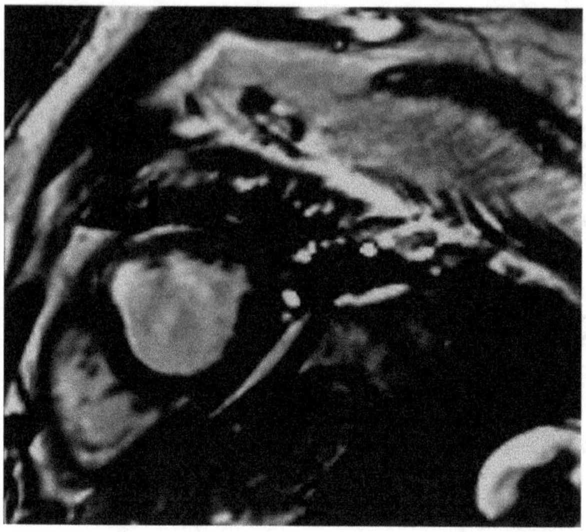

Fig. 4 Cardiac magnetic resonance imaging. Cardiac MRI revealed thinning of apical anterior wall of left ventricle and subendocardial late gadolinium enhancement (*arrow*); estimated left ventricular EF was 44.3 %

thrombosis is formed at atherosclerotic site and seen during angiography, but may resolve spontaneously leaving almost no residual lesions. So this cause could not be completely ruled out.

Meanwhile Takotsubo cardiomyopathy was also considered as an important differential diagnosis, for chest pain symptoms, precordial leads ST segment elevation and negative result of coronary angiography. But we believed that Takotsubo cardiomyopathy stood a less possibility. The reasons were as follows: first, there was no risk factors such like stress trigger, sepsis or pheochromocytoma; second, cTnI elevated so obviously (above 1, 000 multiple of normal upper limit) [10] and dropped slowly, and the ratio between peak cTnI and EF measured at admission was 95.9 (much higher than cut-off value of ≤60) [11]; third, cardiac MRI showed significant late gadolinium enhancement of subendocardial area in anterior wall [12, 13]. But further follow-up was needed (such as echocardiography and cardiac MRI) to provide more evidence.

Cardiac adverse effects associated with thalidomide also include bradycardia [2–4]. The mechanism for this remains unclear although interference with autonomic nervous system has been suggested, with parasympathetic over activity caused by inhibition of TNF-α by thalidomide in the dorsal motor neurons of valgus nerve [4]. Despite a few reports of thalidomide-induced bradycardia, only one case of total AV-block have been published so far. Hinterseer M et al. [5] had reported the first case taking thalidomide developed third degree AV block, and thalidomide was ceased immediately but ECG didn't regain sinus rhythm until 2 months later during which a permanent pacemaker was implanted. Our patient's ECG also didn't regained sinus rhythm until 3 days after thalidomide discontinuation. The mechanisms of additional long lasting effects of thalidomide (half-life period 4–7 h) on conduction system are not clear, but may base on stimulation of immune responses similar to myocarditis. It also informs us that if bradycardia or high grade AV block happens in patients taking thalidomide, maybe the ECG will be monitored for several days even up to a week before the decision of permanent pacemaker implantation.

Since high risk of thromboembolism, there are guidelines issued for antithrombotic prophylaxis in cancer clinical setting for thalidomide use [14]. Because there seems to be a similar and well-documented risk in the non-cancer setting, antithrombotic prophylaxis may be also effective and beneficial, but needs further investigation for optimal drug and dosage.

It is also important to monitor patients taking thalidomide for signs and symptoms of bradycardia or higher degree AV block, especially in those with concomitant medications affecting cardiac conduction

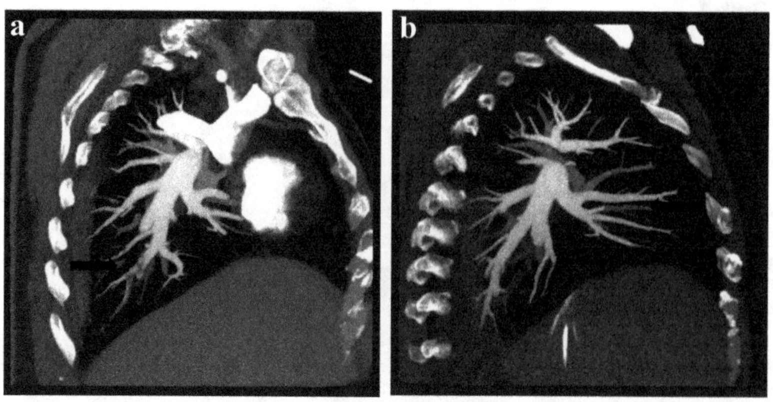

Fig. 5 Computed tomography pulmonary angiography. CTPA revealed scatter embolism of subsegmental pulmonary arteries of both sides. **a**, **b** curved sheet reconstruction showed the emboli (*arrows*)

system [3]. Early detection of conduction delay might help to modify therapy before symptomatic clinical events occur.

Conclusion

This is the very first case in which myocardial infarction, third degree atrioventricular block and pulmonary embolism almost simultaneously developed. We should be ware that anti-thrombotic prophylaxis, which needs further investigation for optimal drug and dosage, may be beneficial in thalidomide therapy. And it is also important to monitor patients taking thalidomide for signs and symptoms of bradycardia or higher degree atrioventricular block.

Consent

Written informed consent was obtained from the patient for publication of this Case report and any accompanying images. A copy of the written consent is available for review by the Editor of this journal.

Abbreviations

AVB: atrioventricular block; CRBBB: complete right bundle branch block; cTnI: cardiac troponin I; CTPA: computed tomography pulmonary angiography; DVT: deep venous thrombus; ECG: electrocardiography; EF: ejaculation fraction; MI: myocardial infarction; MM: multiple myeloma; MRI: magnetic resonance imaging; PE: pulmonary embolism; Tha: thalidomide.

Competing interests

The authors declare that they have no competing interests.

Authors' contributions

SZ collected the data, image and all information needed and wrote the manuscript. JY directed the medical care throughout patient's admission. XJ conducted the coronary angiography and advised the antithrombotic therapy. SZ supervised all the diagnostic and therapeutic measuers. All authors read and approved the final manuscript.

Author details

[1]Department of Internal Medicine, Peking Union Medical College Hospital, Chinese Academy of Medical Sciences, Beijing, China. [2]Department of Cardiology, Peking Union Medical College Hospital, Chinese Academy of Medical Sciences, Beijing, China.

References

1. Palumbo A, Palladino C. Venous and arterial thrombotic risks with thalidomide: evidence and practical guidance. Ther Adv Drug Saf. 2012;3: 255–66.
2. Ali A, Hothi SS, Thompson A, Malik N. Negative chronotropic effects and coronary ischaemic abnormalities following thalidomide therapy. Cardiology. 2013;125:34–7.
3. Lopez-de la Cruz I, Aguayo-Gonzalez A, Lopez-Karpovitch X. Thalidomide-associated bradycardia in patients with hematologic diseases: a single institution experience. Rev Invest Clin. 2006;58:424–31.
4. Fahdi IE, Gaddam V, Saucedo JF, Kishan CV, Vyas K, Deneke MG, et al. Bradycardia during therapy for multiple myeloma with thalidomide. Am J Cardiol. 2004;93:1052–5.
5. Hinterseer M, Becker A, Kaab S, Lang N, Nabauer M, Steinbeck G. Thalidomide-induced symptomatic third-degree atrioventricular block. Clin Res Cardiol. 2006;95:474–6.
6. Matthews SJ, McCoy C. Thalidomide: a review of approved and investigational uses. Clin Ther. 2003;25:342–95.
7. Corso A, Lorenzi A, Terulla V, Airo F, Varettoni M, Mangiacavalli S, et al. Modification of thrombomodulin plasma levels in refractory myeloma patients during treatment with thalidomide and dexamethasone. Ann Hematol. 2004;83:588–91.
8. Minnema MC, Fijnheer R, De Groot PG, Lokhorst HM. Extremely high levels of von willebrand factor antigen and of procoagulant factor viii found in multiple myeloma patients are associated with activity status but not with thalidomide treatment. J Thromb Haemost. 2003;1:445–9.
9. Kardasz I, De Caterina R. Myocardial infarction with normal coronary arteries: a conundrum with multiple aetiologies and variable prognosis: an update. J Intern Med. 2007;261:330–48.
10. Komamura K, Fukui M, Iwasaku T, Hirotani S, Masuyama T. Takotsubo cardiomyopathy: pathophysiology, diagnosis and treatment. World J Cardiol. 2014;6:602–9.
11. Novo G, Giambanco S, Bonomo V, Sutera MR, Giambanco F, Rotolo A, et al. Troponin i/ejection fraction ratio: a new index to differentiate takotsubo cardiomyopathy from myocardial infarction. Int J Cardiol. 2015;180:255–7.
12. Eitel I, von Knobelsdorff-Brenkenhoff F, Bernhardt P, Carbone I, Muellerleile K, Aldrovandi A, et al. Clinical characteristics and cardiovascular magnetic resonance findings in stress (takotsubo) cardiomyopathy. JAMA. 2011;306:277–86.
13. Kohan AA, Levy Yeyati E, De Stefano L, Dragonetti L, Pietrani M, Perez de Arenaza D, et al. Usefulness of MRI in takotsubo cardiomyopathy: a review of the literature. Cardiovasc Diagn Ther. 2014;4:138–46.
14. Farge D, Debourdeau P, Beckers M, Baglin C, Bauersachs RM, Brenner B, et al. International clinical practice guidelines for the treatment and prophylaxis of venous thromboembolism in patients with cancer. J Thromb Haemost. 2013;11:56–70.

16

Acute effects of using an electronic nicotine-delivery device (electronic cigarette) on myocardial function: comparison with the effects of regular cigarettes

Konstantinos E Farsalinos*, Dimitris Tsiapras, Stamatis Kyrzopoulos, Maria Savvopoulou and Vassilis Voudris

Abstract

Background: Electronic cigarettes have been developed and marketed in recent years as smoking substitutes. However, no studies have evaluated their effects on the cardiovascular system. The purpose of this study was to examine the immediate effects of electronic cigarette use on left ventricular (LV) function, compared to the well-documented acute adverse effects of smoking.

Methods: Echocardiographic examinations were performed in 36 healthy heavy smokers (SM, age 36 ± 5 years) before and after smoking 1 cigarette and in 40 electronic cigarette users (ECIG, age 35 ± 5 years) before and after using the device with "medium-strength" nicotine concentration (11 mg/ml) for 7 minutes. Mitral flow diastolic velocities (E, A), their ratio (E/A), deceleration time (DT), isovolumetric relaxation time (IVRT) and corrected-to-heart rate IVRT (IVRTc) were measured. Mitral annulus systolic (Sm), and diastolic (Em, Am) velocities were estimated. Myocardial performance index was calculated from Doppler flow (MPI) and tissue Doppler (MPIt). Longitudinal deformation measurements of global strain (GS), systolic (SRs) and diastolic (SRe, SRa) strain rate were also performed.

Results: Baseline measurements were similar in both groups. In SM, IVRT and IVRTc were prolonged, Em and SRe were decreased, and both MPI and MPIt were elevated after smoking. In ECIG, no differences were observed after device use. Comparing after-use measurements, ECIG had higher Em ($P = 0.032$) and SRe ($P = 0.022$), and lower IVRTc ($P = 0.011$), MPI ($P = 0.001$) and MPIt ($P = 0.019$). The observed differences were significant even after adjusting for changes in heart rate and blood pressure.

Conclusions: Although acute smoking causes a delay in myocardial relaxation, electronic cigarette use has no immediate effects. Electronic cigarettes' role in tobacco harm reduction should be studied intensively in order to determine whether switching to electronic cigarette use may have long-term beneficial effects on smokers' health.

Keywords: Electronic cigarette, Smoking, Myocardial function, Diastolic function, Tobacco harm reduction, Nicotine

* Correspondence: kfarsalinos@gmail.com
Department of Cardiology, Onassis Cardiac Surgery Center, Sygrou 356, Kallithea 17674, Greece

Background

Smoking is a major risk factor for cardiovascular disease [1,2]. Although several pharmaceutical products are available for smoking cessation, long term quit-rates are relatively low [3]. Therefore, tobacco harm reduction strategy and products have been developed, with the main goal to reduce the amount of harmful substances administered to the human body.

Electronic cigarettes have been introduced to the market in recent years as an alternative-to-smoking habit. They consist of a battery-part, a cartridge containing liquid and an electrical resistance that is heated by activation of the battery and evaporates the liquid. The liquid usually contains glycerol, propylene glycol, water, nicotine and a variety of flavours that the user can choose. By using this device, nicotine is delivered to the upper and lower respiratory tract without any combustion involved. Millions of people are using electronic cigarettes worldwide; however, lack of clinical research has raised global debate, controversy and serious public health concerns [4].

Several studies have shown that, even in healthy smokers, acute smoking inhalation has significant adverse effects on left ventricular (LV) myocardial function that can be detected by echocardiography [5-7]. No study has ever evaluated the effects of electronic cigarette use on cardiac function; thus, the purpose of the current study was to investigate the acute effects of using an electronic cigarette ad lib for 7 minutes on haemodynamic parameters and myocardial function, compared to the effects of smoking a tobacco cigarette.

Methods

Study sample

The study sample consisted of consecutive healthy subjects visiting our hospital for routine examinations that volunteered to participate. All participants were asymptomatic, had normal physical examination and resting electrocardiogram and were not taking any medications. Smokers (group SM) were included if they were smoking for at least 5 years and were consuming at least 15 cigarettes per day. The reason for including only heavy smokers was that a study examining the characteristics of electronic cigarette consumers showed that most electronic cigarette users were formerly heavy smokers [8]. Electronic cigarette users (group ECIG) were included if they had quit smoking and were using electronic cigarettes with nicotine-containing liquid for at least 1 month, according to self-report. To avoid potential compensatory effects from using lower nicotine-containing liquid, participants were included if they were daily consumers of similar "strength" liquids (9-12 mg/ml nicotine concentration) to that used in the study (11 mg/ml). Exclusion criteria were: presence of any major risk factor for cardiovascular disease (i.e. diabetes, hypertension, hyperlipidemia and family history of premature coronary artery disease), history of endocrine disorders, body-mass index > 30 kg/m2 and more than occasional alcohol intake. Additional exclusion criteria were derived from the echocardiography studies: elevated LV mass index (>115 g/m2 for males and > 95 g/m2 for females), abnormal LV function (LV ejection fraction < 55%) and more than mild valve regurgitation.

In total, 81 subjects were eligible to participate. Three smokers did not present for the scheduled evaluation. One electronic cigarette user was excluded because of moderate aortic regurgitation and ascending aorta dilatation due to bicuspid aortic valve. One smoker was excluded due to mildly depressed ejection fraction and hypokinesia of LV lateral wall. The final study sample consisted of 76 subjects, 40 electronic cigarette users (3 females) and 36 smokers (3 females). Written informed consent was obtained from all subjects for participation in the study, and the protocol was approved by the ethics committee of Onassis Cardiac Surgery Center.

Materials

All smokers were asked to use one commercially-available tobacco cigarette of the same nicotine (1.0 mg), tar (10 mg) and carbon monoxide (10 mg) yields. Electronic cigarette users were asked to use a commercially-available device with liquid containing 11 mg/ml nicotine concentration. The device used was an eGo-T battery (Nobacco, Athens, Greece) with an eGo-C atomiser (Alter Ego, Athens, Greece). It is considered a "second-generation" device. Unlike cigarette-like devices which consist of a small battery and a polyfil-containing atomiser (commonly called "cartomiser"), the electronic cigarette used in this study is a multi-piece system (Figure 1). It consists of a 650 mAh rechargeable lithium battery, delivering 3.5 volts to the atomiser (measured by a volt-meter), and an atomiser consisting of 4 parts: the tank which stores the liquid (capacity of approximately 1.1 ml), the atomiser body, the atomiser head which includes the resistance, and the atomiser cap. It is a manually-activated device, by pressing a button; it does not produce any vapour when not activated by the user.

The electronic cigarette liquid used in the study contained 11 mg/ml nicotine and is considered "medium strength" according to manufacturer's report (USA Mix Med, formerly known as MLB-Med, Nobacco, Athens, Greece). It is sold in 20 ml bottles. It was the only liquid tested by an independent laboratory (National Center for Scientific Research "Demokritos", mass spectrometry and dioxin analysis laboratory) at the time of study initiation [9]. According to the laboratory report, the contents were: propylene glycol (α -propylene glycol or 1,2-propanediol) in a concentration > 60%, linalool (3,7-dimethylocta-1, 6-dien-3-ol) in a concentration < 5%, nicotine (<10%), tobacco essence (<5%), and methyl vanillin (4-hydroxy-

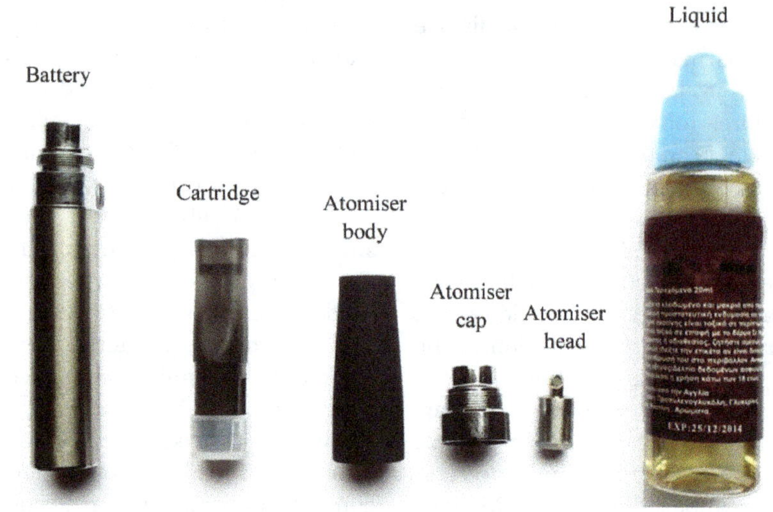

Figure 1 Electronic cigarette device and liquid used in the study.

3-methoxybenzaldehyde) at < 1%. No tobacco-specific nitrosamines or polycyclic aromatic hydrocarbons were detected.

For every participant, a new cartridge and atomiser head was used. One of the researchers filled the cartridge with 1 ml of liquid; subsequently it was positioned in the atomiser and the participant started using it. The battery was fully charged before being used by each subject.

Study protocol

Participants presented to the echocardiographic laboratory after fasting and refraining from alcohol and caffeine consumption for 4 hours; they were also asked to refrain from smoking and electronic cigarette use for 4 hours before the study.

Participants were allowed to rest for 5 minutes before initiating the echocardiographic examination. A baseline echocardiographic examination was performed in smokers, who were then transferred to a room next to the echocardiography laboratory and smoked 1 tobacco cigarette. For electronic cigarette users, after the baseline echocardiogram they were asked to use the electronic cigarette device ad lib for 7 minutes in another room which was not used by smokers, to avoid environmental exposure to smoke. Subsequently, all participants returned to the echocardiography laboratory and, after 5 minutes of rest, a second echocardiogram was performed in both groups.

Heart rate and BP were measured before and during each echocardiographic examination. The Brinkman index was calculated (product of number of cigarettes smoked daily and years of smoking) according to participants' self-report. Echocardiograms were performed using a commercially available system (Vivid 7, GE Vingmed, Horten, Norway). Studies were digitally recorded on hard disk for offline analysis using dedicated software (Echopac, GE Medical Systems, Horten, Norway) by a single, blinded to the protocol, experienced echocardiographer. Reported values represent the average of 3 consecutive beats.

Two-dimensional echocardiographic measurements

The echocardiographic examinations were performed according to recent guidelines [9]. LV dimensions, septal and posterior wall thickness were measured from standard 2-dimensional images at parasternal long-axis view. LV mass was indexed to body-surface area. Ejection fraction was evaluated from the apical four and two-chamber views using the Simpson's rule [10]. Left atrial (LA) antero-posterior diameter was also measured.

Doppler flow and tissue Doppler velocity measurements

From transmitral flow measurements, peak early (E) and late (A) velocities, their ratio (E/A) and E wave deceleration time (DT) were estimated. Ejection time was estimated by recording LV outflow tract velocity. By simultaneously recording aortic and mitral flows using continuous-wave Doppler the isovolumetric relaxation time (IVRT) was measured, and was then corrected to heart rate by dividing it with the square root of R-R interval (IVRTc).

Pulsed-wave Doppler tissue velocities were measured by placing a 1.5 mm sample volume at the lateral, septal, anterior and inferior insertion sites of the mitral leaflets. Systolic (Sm), early diastolic (Em) and late diastolic (Am) peak velocities were measured and averaged from the 4 sites. The ratio of early-to-late annular velocity (Em/Am) and early mitral flow to early diastolic mitral annular velocity (E/Em) were also determined.

Myocardial performance index was measured by two methods (Figure 2): using Doppler flow velocity

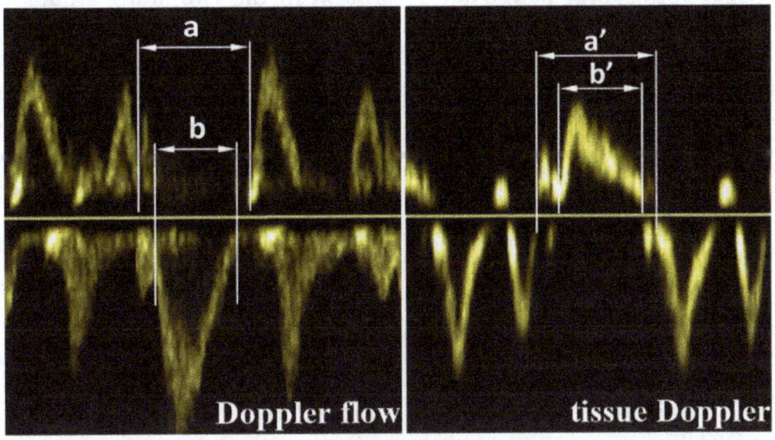

Figure 2 Myocardial performance index, measured by two methods: (1) Doppler flow velocity measurements of mitral inflow and left ventricular outflow tract; the index was derived by the formula: MPI = (a-b)/b, and (2) Pulsed-wave tissue Doppler measurements of mitral annulus velocity; the index was derived from the formula: MPIt = (a'-b')/b'.

measurements as described by Tei et al. [11] (MPI) and using pulsed-wave tissue Doppler measurements of mitral annulus velocities (MPIt) [12].

To check for reproducibility of measurements, the intraobserver mean percent error (the absolute difference between two measurements divided by their mean) was calculated from 10 randomly selected studies 15 days later, analyzed by the same blinded echocardiographer who performed all measurements. The results were 5.1 ± 2.9% for IVRT, 3.5 ± 2.5% for MPI, 3.6 ± 2.2% for MPIt and 2.6 ± 1.9% for Em.

Longitudinal deformation measurements

Longitudinal deformation measurements were performed by analyzing two-dimensional echocardiographic images using the method of speckle tracking echocardiography [13]. End-diastole was defined as the peak of the R wave on the electrocardiographic trace; end-systole (aortic valve closure) was defined from pulsed-wave Doppler tracing at the LV outflow tract as the end of systolic forward flow. Subjects with inadequate tracking of more than one LV segment in each view were excluded from the analysis. By averaging segmental values in all views, end-systolic global strain (GS) was measured. Global peak longitudinal systolic (SRs), early diastolic (SRe) and late diastolic (SRa) strain rate were measured. The intraobserver mean percent error of longitudinal deformation measurements in our laboratory was 3.1 ± 1.5% for GS, 3.6 ± 1.8% for SRs, 3.9 ± 1.9% for SRe and 3.6 ± 2.0% for SRa.

Statistical analysis

The Kolmogorov-Smirnov tests were applied to assess the normality of data; all parameters were normally distributed except from daily cigarette consumption. Continuous variables were expressed as mean ± SD or median (interquartile range). Categorical variables were expressed as number (percentage). Inter-group comparisons of baseline characteristics data were made by unpaired Student's t-test and Mann–Whitney test; Fisher's exact test was used for categorical variables.

Repeated measurements analysis of variance (ANOVA) was used in order to evaluate changes in parameters before and after smoking one cigarette or using the electronic cigarette device (before-use and after-use measurements). Changes in echocardiographic and deformation parameters that were significantly different between the two study groups from analysis of variance were further analyzed using linear regression analyses, in order to find if the effect of smoking was significant after adjusting for changes in heart rate and systolic BP. For every parameter, a different linear regression analysis was performed. Change (Δ) in parameter was the dependent variable; group (SM vs. ECIG) and change in heart rate and systolic BP were the independent variables. All P values reported are two-tailed. Statistical significance was set at 0.05 and analyses were conducted using SPSS statistical software (version 18.0, SPSS Inc., Chicago, USA).

A repeated measures ANOVA power analysis was conducted. For this design, 76 participants (40 in the smokers group and 36 in the electronic cigarette users group) achieved a power of 0.90 for the between-subjects main effect at an effect size of 0.30; a power of 0.90 for the within-subjects main effect at an effect size of 0.15; and a power of 0.90 for the interaction effect at an effect size of 0.15.

Results

Both groups had similar baseline characteristics (Table 1). Electronic cigarette users had quit smoking for 97 ± 50 days and were using electronic cigarettes for 100 ±

Table 1 Baseline characteristics of the study population

Characteristic	Smokers (n = 36)	Electronic cigarette users (n = 40)	P-value
Males n (%)	32 (88.9)	36 (90)	1.000[a]
Age (years)	36 ± 5	35 ± 5	0.764
Body mass index (kg/m^2)	24.8 ± 2.3	25.3 ± 2.4	0.304
Body surface area (m^2)	2.03 ± 0.15	2.00 ± 0.18	0.322
Smoking duration (years)	16 ± 5	17 ± 5	0.571
Cigarette consumption (n/d)[b]	20 (20–26)	30 (20–35)	0.004[c]
Brinkman index	371 ± 132	493 ± 228	0.005
Electronic cigarette use duration[d]		6 ± 4	
Systolic BP (mmHg)	123.0 ± 9.8	123.9 ± 8.6	0.653
Diastolic BP (mmHg)	75.8 ± 5.6	75.6 ± 6.1	0.834
Heart rate (beats/m)	67.5 ± 7.9	67.1 ± 10.3	0.841
Pressure-rate product	8308 ± 1235	8312 ± 1363	0.989
Glucose (mmol/l)	4.51 ± 0.34	4.44 ± 0.35	0.410
Total cholesterol (mmol/l)	4.85 ± 0.21	4.77 ± 0.30	0.177
LDL cholesterol (mmol/l)	2.99 ± 0.23	2.91 ± 0.26	0.175
HDL cholesterol (mmol/l)	1.38 ± 0.15	1.38 ± 0.18	0.943
Triglycerides (mmol/l)	1.05 ± 0.14	1.04 ± 0.18	0.693
Ejection fraction (%)	63 ± 5	62 ± 4	0.463
LA diameter (mm)	35 ± 4	34 ± 3	0.359
LV mass index (g/m^2)	64 ± 10	65 ± 13	0.663

BP, blood pressure, LVEDV, left ventricular end-diastolic volume; LVESV, left ventricular end-systolic volume; LDL, low-density lipoprotein; HDL, high-density lipoprotein; LA, left atrium.
[a]Fisher's exact test; [b]Values expressed as median (interquartile range); [c]Mann-Whitney test; [d]Duration expressed in months.

49 days. They had higher lifetime smoking exposure, with Brinkman index 33% higher compared to smokers, due to higher daily cigarette consumption when they were smokers.

Changes in haemodynamic, Doppler echocardiography and longitudinal deformation measurements for the study groups are presented in Tables 2 and 3. Baseline measurements were similar between groups for all parameters.

After-use values of systolic BP, heart rate and pressure-rate product were elevated in the SM group but not in the ECIG group (Table 2). The overall change from baseline was significantly different between the two groups. In contrast, diastolic BP increased equally in both groups.

From Doppler flow echocardiographic measurements (Table 2), E velocity and DT remained unchanged after use in both groups. A velocity was increased and E/A was decreased in SM, but the overall change was not significantly different between the two groups ($P = 0.317$ and $P = 0.053$, respectively). IVRT, IVRTc and MPI were increased after smoking one cigarette in the SM group, and the degree of change was significantly different between the two study groups ($P = 0.001$, $P < 0.001$ and $P = 0.001$ respectively). The after-use levels of IVRTc and MPI were greater in SM compared to ECIG, as was shown by the between-groups analysis.

Concerning Doppler tissue velocity measurements (Table 3), Sm and Am remained unchanged after use in both groups. However, Em was significantly reduced in SM group after smoking. It was lower when compared to ECIG after using the device, and the degree of change was significantly different between the two groups ($P < 0.001$). Em/Am was reduced and E/Em was increased in SM, but the difference of the overall change between the two groups was statistically significant for Em/Am only ($P = 0.011$). MPIt increased after smoking in SM; the degree of change was significantly different between the two groups ($P < 0.001$), with after-use levels being significantly higher in SM compared to ECIG ($P = 0.019$).

Longitudinal deformation measurements (Table 3) were feasible in 37 electronic cigarette users and 34 smokers. No difference in GS, SRs and SRa was observed in ECIG and SM after use. However, SRe was significantly reduced in SM post-smoking, with the degree of change being statistically significant between groups ($P < 0.001$).

The results of multiple linear regression analyses are displayed in Table 4. Even after adjusting for changes in systolic BP and heart rate, changes in IVRT, IVRTc, MPI, Em, MPIt and SRe were significantly higher in SM group.

Discussion

This is the first study to examine the acute effects of electronic cigarette use on myocardial function. No adverse effects on LV myocardial function were observed after using electronic cigarette with nicotine-containing liquid for 7 minutes. On the contrary, significant changes in diastolic function parameters were found after smoking 1 tobacco cigarette.

The acute adverse effects of smoking on myocardial relaxation were originally observed in coronary artery disease patients [14], with acute impairment of coronary vasomotion implicated as the main cause [15]. Such effects on diastolic function are also detected in healthy smokers [5-7] Cigarette smoke contains significant amounts of free radicals, promoting oxidative stress and inflammation [16] At the cellular level, decreased function of myocardial mitochondria [17] and DNA damage [18] has been observed. These mechanisms may be implicated in delaying myocardial relaxation from acute use and promoting atherosclerosis and cardiovascular disease from chronic use. In this study, several parameters commonly used for evaluating diastolic function [19] and longitudinal deformation measurements which are considered more sensitive in detecting pathology [20] were significantly altered after smoking inhalation.

Electronic cigarettes were invented in 2003, but awareness and use has significantly increased over the past

Table 2 Haemodynamic and Doppler flow measurements in electronic cigarette users (ECIG, n = 40) and smokers (SM, n = 36), before and after device and cigarette use respectively

Parameter	Before use	After use	Change	P-value[a]	P-value[b]
Systolic BP (mmHg)					
ECIG	123.9 ± 8.6	124.6 ± 9.9	0.7 ± 4.6	0.374	< 0.001
SM	123.0 ± 9.8	129.6 ± 9.2	6.6 ± 5.2	< 0.001	
P-value[c]	0.653	0.025			
Diastolic BP (mmHg)					
ECIG	75.6 ± 6.1	78.5 ± 5.9	3.0 ± 3.6	< 0.001	0.079
SM	75.8 ± 5.6	80.2 ± 5.8	4.4 ± 3.3	< 0.001	
P-value[c]	0.834	0.209			
Heart rate (beats/m)					
ECIG	67.1 ± 10.3	67.5 ± 10.6	0.4 ± 4.8	0.649	< 0.001
SM	67.5 ± 7.9	73.5 ± 6.8	5.9 ± 4.7	< 0.001	
P-value[c]	0.841	0.005			
Pressure-rate product					
ECIG	8312 ± 1363	8397 ± 1462	84 ± 708	0.456	< 0.001
SM	8308 ± 1235	9556 ± 1084	1248 ± 840	< 0.001	
P-value[c]	0.989	< 0.001			
E (cm/s)					
ECIG	70.1 ± 12.5	71.4 ± 13.2	1.2 ± 5.0	0.130	0.132
SM	72.9 ± 8.5	72.2 ± 10.2	−0.6 ± 6.1	0.565	
P-value[c]	0.268	0.756			
A (cm/s)					
ECIG	51.1 ± 10.2	52.7 ± 9.8	1.6 ± 5.6	0.083	0.317
SM	50.4 ± 8.8	53.3 ± 9.1	2.9 ± 5.7	0.007	
P-value[c]	0.774	0.764			
E/A					
ECIG	1.41 ± 0.29	1.37 ± 0.26	−0.03 ± 0.14	0.171	0.053
SM	1.49 ± 0.32	1.39 ± 0.30	−0.10 ± 0.16	0.001	
P-value[c]	0.235	0.809			
DT (ms)					
ECIG	173 ± 11	174 ± 14	1 ± 8	0.581	0.570
SM	170 ± 16	172 ± 16	3 ± 10	0.086	
P-value[c]	0.448	0.719			
IVRT (ms)					
ECIG	74.6 ± 9.5	73.6 ± 9.9	−1.0 ± 5.7	0.275	0.001
SM	73.0 ± 8.7	77.7 ± 13.5	5.6 ± 9.2	< 0.001	
P-value[c]	0.450	0.132			
IVRTc (ms)					
ECIG	78.9 ± 11.8	77.7 ± 11.6	−1.2 ± 6.9	0.286	< 0.001
SM	77.3 ± 10.1	86.1 ± 16.4	10.4 ± 10.1	< 0.001	
P-value[c]	0.524	0.011			

Table 2 Haemodynamic and Doppler flow measurements in electronic cigarette users (ECIG, n = 40) and smokers (SM, n = 36), before and after device and cigarette use respectively *(Continued)*

MPI					
ECIG	0.39 ± 0.07	0.38 ± 0.06	−0.01 ± 0.04	0.330	0.001
SM	0.40 ± 0.05	0.43 ± 0.06	0.03 ± 0.04	0.002	
P-value[c]	0.355	0.001			

BP, blood pressure; E, mitral flow early diastolic velocity; A, mitral flow late diastolic velocity; DT, deceleration time of early mitral flow; IVRT, isovolumetric relaxation time; IVRTc, IVRT corrected to heart rate; MPI, myocardial performance index estimated by Doppler flow echocardiography.
[a]P-value for time effect.
[b]Repeated measurements ANOVA. Effects reported are significant differences between the two groups in the degree of change in each particular variable.
[c]P-value for group effect.

3 years [21]. They do not contain tobacco and their use does not involve combustion. However, lack of research on their health effects has generated significant controversy over their safety. FDA and WHO issued public statements in 2009, expressing concern and recommending that electronic cigarette use should be avoided. WHO has specifically asked for studies to be performed before regulation or even ban is imposed. Cahn and Siegel summarized the results of 16 studies evaluating the chemical composition of liquids used for electronic cigarettes [22]. Nitrosamines were found in only two of the studies, at levels similar to those present in nicotine patch; a recent review indicated that the levels of nitrosamines in electronic cigarettes were up to 1800 times lower compared to tobacco cigarettes [23]. The main constituents, besides nicotine, were propylene glycol and glycerine, which are also present in tobacco cigarettes; however, the combustion process from smoking leads to production of acrolein, acetaldehyde and formaldehyde, which promote oxidative stress and have cardiotoxic properties [24]. In electronic cigarettes, such chemicals may be formed from the heating process during liquid evaporation; however, the levels found were lower compared to tobacco cigarettes by orders of magnitude [25]. This may explain the results from laboratory studies, in which electronic cigarette vapour was significantly less cytotoxic compared to cigarette smoke on cultured cells [26,27]. Cardiotoxic substances like nitrosamines, heavy metals and polycyclic aromatic hydrocarbons were not detected in the liquid used in this study [9]. These parameters may explain the differences in diastolic function observed between smokers and electronic cigarette users after smoking and device use. Moreover, a study evaluating the effects of smoking compared to nicotine delivered by gum showed that nicotine alone did not cause acute changes in diastolic function [28]. It seems that nicotine absorption rate is lower from electronic compared to tobacco cigarette use [29], even when using new-generation devices [30]; the difference in haemodynamic response between the two groups may be attributed to this. However, haemodynamic parameters cannot explain the differences in diastolic function parameters, since linear regression analyses revealed that changes in Doppler and deformation parameters were associated with cigarette smoking even after adjusting for changes in systolic BP and heart rate.

From a public health perspective, epidemiological studies have shown that tobacco harm reduction strategy and products may be promising regarding cardiovascular disease risk reduction [31]. Electronic cigarettes are unique since they are the only products that do not contain tobacco, while they mimic the act of smoking and provide motor and sensory stimulation. Thus, they may deal with both the chemical (nicotine delivery) and behavioural components of cigarette addiction [22] and studies indicate that they may be effective in promoting smoking cessation [32,33]. This study provides the first clinical evidence that electronic cigarettes have less acute adverse effects on myocardial function when compared to tobacco cigarettes.

Some limitations apply to this study. A small sample size was studied, and examination focused only on immediate effects. The results do not indicate that electronic cigarettes are absolutely safe for the cardiovascular system. Other parameters known to be adversely affected by acute smoking, such as coronary microvascular and endothelial function or vascular distensibility, were not examined. Moreover, the parameters examined are affected mainly by heart rate changes. Although heart rate was not included as a covariate in the repeated-measures ANOVA, the linear regression analysis showed that changes in diastolic function were significantly different between groups independently of the changes in heart rate and systolic BP. This can be explained by the small difference in post-use heart rate between groups of only 6 beats per minute. Studies on long-term effects are necessary; however, more time of use is needed before any such studies are published since electronic cigarettes were introduced to the market in recent years and there is a substantial delay between smoking initiation and development of clinically-evident disease. We asked subjects to use the electronic cigarette for 7 minutes. It is unknown whether more time of use could have had a different impact. However, timing was based on the approximate time of smoking 1 regular

Table 3 Tissue Doppler velocity and longitudinal deformation measurements in electronic cigarette users (ECIG, n = 40) and smokers (SM, n = 36), before and after device and cigarette use respectively*

Parameter	Before use	After use	Change	P-value[a]	P-value[b]
Sm (cm/s)					
ECIG	9.7 ± 1.6	9.9 ± 1.6	0.2 ± 0.7	0.171	0.613
SM	9.7 ± 1.4	9.7 ± 1.5	−0.8 ± 1.1	0.571	
P-value[c]	0.896	0.723			
Em (cm/s)					
ECIG	12.7 ± 1.9	12.9 ± 2.1	0.2 ± 0.7	0.095	< 0.001
SM	12.8 ± 2.1	11.9 ± 1.5	−0.7 ± 1.4	< 0.001	
P-value[c]	0.892	0.032			
Am (cm/s)					
ECIG	9.7 ± 1.7	9.9 ± 1.6	0.2 ± 0.8	0.122	0.441
SM	9.3 ± 1.2	9.4 ± 1.3	0.1 ± 0.6	0.801	
P-value[c]	0.212	0.099			
Em/Am					
ECIG	1.34 ± 0.29	1.33 ± 0.28	−0.01 ± 0.13	0.540	0.011
SM	1.40 ± 0.28	1.30 ± 0.24	−0.08 ± 0.13	0.004	
P-value[c]	0.408	0.655			
E/Em					
ECIG	5.60 ± 1.04	5.61 ± 1.11	0.01 ± 0.47	0.869	0.052
SM	5.83 ± 0.95	6.10 ± 0.98	0.29 ± 0.74	0.021	
P-value[c]	0.311	0.044			
MPIt					
ECIG	0.48 ± 0.08	0.47 ± 0.09	−0.01 ± 0.04	0.080	< 0.001
SM	0.49 ± 0.06	0.52 ± 0.07	0.03 ± 0.05	0.004	
P-value[c]	0.654	0.019			
GS (%)					
ECIG	−21.1 ± 1.9	−21.5 ± 1.6	−0.4 ± 1.2	0.059	0.087
SM	−21.0 ± 2.6	−20.7 ± 3.1	0.2 ± 1.7	0.441	
P-value[c]	0.769	0.192			
SRs (s^{-1})					
ECIG	−1.13 ± 0.10	−1.14 ± 0.11	−0.01 ± 0.07	0.362	0.613
SM	−1.08 ± 0.13	−1.10 ± 0.13	−0.2 ± 0.1	0.150	
P-value[c]	0.059	0.115			
SRe (s^{-1})					
ECIG	1.47 ± 0.25	1.49 ± 0.23	0.01 ± 0.08	0.347	< 0.001
SM	1.43 ± 0.25	1.35 ± 0.24	−0.08 ± 0.12	< 0.001	
P-value[c]	0.493	0.022			
SRa (s^{-1})					
ECIG	0.88 ± 0.20	0.89 ± 0.18	0.01 ± 0.08	0.462	0.441
SM	0.86 ± 0.14	0.88 ± 0.14	0.03 ± 0.09	0.111	
P-value[c]	0.536	0.796			

*Longitudinal deformation measurements were performed in 37 electronic cigarette users and 34 smokers.
Sm, mitral annulus systolic velocity; Em, mitral annulus early diastolic velocity; Am, mitral annulus late diastolic velocity; MPIt, myocardial performance index estimated by tissue Doppler echocardiography; GS, global longitudinal strain; SRs, peak systolic strain rate; SRe, peak early diastolic strain rate; SRa, peak late diastolic strain rate.
[a]P-value for time effect.
[b]Repeated measurements ANOVA. Effects reported are significant differences between the two groups in the degree of change in each particular variable.
[c]P-value for group effect.

Table 4 Results from linear regression analyses for the effect of group (smokers vs. electronic cigarette users) on changes (Δ) of Doppler echocardiography measurements, after adjusting for changes in systolic blood pressure and heart rate

Dependent variable	β*	SE**	P-value
ΔIVRT (ms)	4.64	2.12	0.032
ΔIVRTc (ms)	5.46	2.34	0.022
ΔMPI	0.03	0.01	0.013
ΔEm (cm/s)	−0.87	0.25	0.001
ΔMPIt	0.04	0.01	0.001
ΔSRe (s^{-1})	−0.06	0.03	0.039

*Regression coefficient for the comparison of SM group to ECIG group, adjusted for changes in systolic blood pressure and heart rate.
**Standard Error.

cigarette; in fact, it took smokers 5 minutes to smoke one cigarette while electronic cigarette users were asked to use the device for a longer time. Additionally, experienced users were examined, who use the device more intensively than novice users [34]. Unfortunately, there are no other means of comparing electronic with tobacco cigarette use. Although plasma nicotine levels were not measured, the haemodynamic response observed suggests that the nicotine delivery rate from electronic cigarettes is lower and slower compared to tobacco cigarettes. This has been validated by studies performed recently [30,35]. The results of this study are not necessarily applicable to all liquids available in the market. If non-pharmaceutical grade nicotine is used, several tobacco impurities may be present and inhaled by the user. The same applies for other liquid constituents [21]. Finally, although all subjects were considered healthy based on history taking, clinical examination, resting ECG and echocardiogram, it cannot be excluded that some subjects may suffer from subclinical coronary artery disease. However, there was no indication to perform any additional examinations in the study population.

Conclusions

Although acute smoking inhalation caused a delay in LV myocardial relaxation in smokers, electronic cigarette use was found to have no such immediate effects in daily users of the device. This short-term beneficial profile of electronic cigarette compared to smoking, although not conclusive about its overall health-effects as a tobacco harm reduction product, provides the first evidence about the cardiovascular effects of this device. Since awareness and use of electronic cigarettes are continuously rising, more studies are urgently needed, focusing on the pathophysiological mechanisms of disease where smoking is implicated and ultimately on long-term effects. Such studies will provide additional scientific data to public health authorities so that they decide on the regulatory status of this product.

Competing interests
After this study was completed, the authors have performed studies using funds provided to the institution by e-cigarette companies.

Authors' contributions
KF was responsible for study conception and design. KF, DT and MS were responsible for data collection. SK was responsible for off-line measurements of echocardiographic parameters. KF, DT and VV were responsible for statistical analysis and interpretation. KF, DT and VV drafted the manuscript. All authors read and approved the manuscript.

Funding
This research received no specific grant from any funding agency in the public, commercial, or not-for-profit sectors.

References

1. Ockene IS, Miller NH: **Cigarette smoking, cardiovascular disease, and stroke: a statement for healthcare professionals from the American Heart Association.** *Circulation* 1997, **96**(9):3243–3247.
2. Merry AH, Boer JM, Schouten LJ, Feskens EJ, Verschuren WM, Gorgels AP, van den Brandt PA: **Smoking, alcohol consumption, physical activity, and family history and the risks of acute myocardial infarction and unstable angina pectoris: a prospective cohort study.** *BMC Cardiovasc Disord* 2011, **11**:13.
3. Rigotti NA, Pipe AL, Benowitz NL, Arteaga C, Garza D, Tonstad S: **Efficacy and safety of varenicline for smoking cessation in patients with cardiovascular disease: a randomized trial.** *Circulation* 2010, **121**(2):221–229.
4. Cobb NK, Byron MJ, Abrams DB, Shields PG: **Novel nicotine delivery systems and public health: the rise of the "e-cigarette".** *Am J Public Health* 2010, **100**(12):2340–2342.
5. Lichodziejewska B, Kurnicka K, Grudzka K, Malysz J, Ciurzynski M, Liszewska-Pfejfer D: **Chronic and acute effects of smoking on left and right ventricular relaxation in young healthy smokers.** *Chest* 2007, **131**(4):1142–1148.
6. Karakaya O, Barutcu I, Esen AM, Kaya D, Turkmen M, Melek M, Onrat E, Esen OB, Celik A, Kilit C, Saglam M, Kirma C: **Acute smoking-induced alterations in Doppler echocardiographic measurements in chronic smokers.** *Tex Heart Inst J* 2006, **33**(2):134–138.
7. Farsalinos K, Tsiapras D, Kyrzopoulos S, Voudris V: **Acute and chronic effects of smoking on myocardial function in healthy heavy smokers: a study of Doppler flow, Doppler tissue velocity, and two-dimensional speckle tracking echocardiography.** *Echocardiography* 2013, 30(3):285–292.
8. Farsalinos KE, Romagna G, Tsiapras D, Kyrzopoulos S, Voudris V: **Evaluating nicotine levels selection and patterns of electronic cigarette use in a group of "vapers" who had achieved complete substitution of smoking.** *Subst Abuse* 2013, **7**:139–146.
9. Leontiadis L: *Results of Chemical Analyses in NOBACCO Electronic Cigarette Refills.* Athens: Mass Spectrometry and Dioxin Analysis Laboratory, National Centre for Scientific Research "Demokritos"; 2009. accessed 11 December 2012.
10. Lang RM, Bierig M, Devereux RB, Flachskampf FA, Foster E, Pellikka PA, Picard MH, Roman MJ, Seward J, Shanewise J, Solomon S, Spencer KT, St John Sutton M, Stewart W, American Society of Echocardiography's Nomenclature and Standards Committee; Task Force on Chamber Quantification; American College of Cardiology Echocardiography Committee; American Heart Association; European Association of Echocardiography, European Society of Cardiology: **Recommendations for chamber quantification.** *Eur J Echocardiogr* 2006, **7**(2):79–108.
11. Tei C, Ling LH, Hodge DO, Bailey KR, Oh JK, Rodeheffer RJ, Tajik AJ, Seward JB: **New index of combined systolic and diastolic myocardial performance: a simple and reproducible measure of cardiac function: a study in normals and dilated cardiomyopathy.** *J Cardiol* 1995, **26**(6):357–366.
12. Gaibazzi N, Petrucci N, Ziacchi V: **Left ventricle myocardial performance index derived either by conventional method or mitral annulus tissue-Doppler: a comparison study in healthy subjects and subjects with heart failure.** *J Am Soc Echocardiogr* 2005, **18**(12):1270–1276.
13. Amundsen BH, Helle-Valle T, Edvardsen T, Torp H, Crosby J, Lyseggen E, Støylen A, Ihlen H, Lima JA, Smiseth OA, Slørdahl SA: **Noninvasive myocardial strain measurement by speckle tracking echocardiography:**

validation against sonomicrometry and tagged magnetic resonance imaging. *J Am Coll Cardiol* 2006, **47**(4):789–793.
14. Kyriakides ZS, Kremastinos DT, Rentoukas E, Mavrogheni S, Kremastinos DI, Toutouzas P: **Acute effects of cigarette smoking on left ventricular diastolic function.** *Eur Heart J* 1992, **13**(6):743–748.
15. Deanfield JE, Shea MJ, Wilson RA, Horlock P, de Landsheere CM, Selwyn AP: **Direct effects of smoking on the heart: Silent ischemic disturbances of coronary flow.** *Am J Cardiol* 1986, **57**(13):1005–1009.
16. Ambrose JA, Barua RS: **The pathophysiology of cigarette smoking and cardiovascular disease: an update.** *J Am Coll Cardiol* 2004, **43**(10):1731–1737.
17. Gvozdjáková A, Bada V, Sány L, Kucharská J, Krutý F, Bozek P, Trstanský L, Gvozdják J: **Smoke cardiomyopathy: disturbance of oxidative processes in myocardial mitochondria.** *Cardiovasc Res* 1984, **18**(4):229–232.
18. Izzotti A, D'Agostini F, Balansky R, Degan P, Pennisi TM, Steele VE, De Flora S: **Exposure of mice to cigarette smoke and/or light causes DNA alterations in heart and aorta.** *Mutat Res* 2008, **644**(1–2):38–42.
19. Nagueh SF, Appleton CP, Gillebert TC, Marino PN, Oh JK, Smiseth OA, Waggoner AD, Flachskampf FA, Pellikka PA, Evangelisa A: **Recommendations for the evaluation of left ventricular diastolic function by echocardiography.** *Eur J Echocardiogr* 2009, **10**(2):165–193.
20. Korinek J, Wang J, Sengupta PP, Miyazaki C, Kjaergaard J, McMahon E, Abraham TP, Belohlavek M: **Two-dimensional strain–a Doppler-independent ultrasound method for quantitation of regional deformation: validation in vitro and in vivo.** *J Am Soc Echocardiogr* 2005, **18**(12):1247–1253.
21. Pearson JL, Richardson A, Niaura RS, Vallone DM, Abrams DB: **E-cigarette awareness, use, and harm perceptions in US adults.** *Am J Public Health* 2012, **102**(9):1758–1766.
22. Cahn Z, Siegel M: **Electronic cigarettes as a harm reduction strategy for tobacco control: a step forward of a repeat of past mistakes?** *J Public Health Policy* 2011, **32**(1):16–31.
23. Farsalinos KE, Polosa R: **Safety evaluation and risk assessment of electronic cigarettes as tobacco cigarette substitutes: a systematic review.** *Ther Adv Drug Safety* 2014, **5**(2):67–86.
24. Luo J, Hill BG, Gu Y, Cai J, Srivastava S, Bhatnagar A, Prabhu SD: **Mechanisms of acrolein-induced myocardial dysfunction: implications for environmental and endogenous aldehyde exposure.** *Am J Physiol Heart Circ Physiol* 2007, **293**(6):H3673–H3684.
25. Goniewicz ML, Knysak J, Gawron M, Kosmider L, Sobczak A, Kurek J, Prokopowicz A, Jablonska-Czapla M, Rosik-Dulewska C, Havel C, Jacob P III, Benowitz N: **Levels of selected carcinogens and toxicants in vapour from electronic cigarettes.** *Tob Control* 2013, Mar 6. [Epub ahead of print].
26. Romagna G, Allifranchini E, Bocchietto E, Todeschi S, Esposito M, Farsalinos KE: **Cytotoxicity evaluation of electronic cigarette vapor extract on cultured mammalian fibroblasts (ClearStream-LIFE): comparison with tobacco cigarette smoke extract.** *Inhal Toxicol* 2013, **25**(6):354–361.
27. Farsalinos KE, Romagna G, Allifranchini E, Ripamonti E, Bocchietto E, Todeschi S, Tsiapras D, Kyrzopoulos S, Voudris V: **Comparison of the cytotoxic potential of cigarette smoke and electronic cigarette vapour extract on cultured myocardial cells.** *Int J Environ Res Public Health* 2013, **10**(10):5146–5162.
28. Gembala MI, Ghanem F, Mann CA, Sorrell VL: **Acute changes in left ventricular diastolic function: cigarette smoking versus nicotine gum.** *Clin Cardiol* 2006, **29**(2):61–64.
29. Bullen C, McRobbie H, Thornley S, Glover M, Lin R, Laugesen M: **Effects of an electronic nicotine delivery device (e cigarette) on desire to smoke and withdrawal, user preferences and nicotine delivery: randomised cross-over trial.** *Tob Control* 2010, **19**(2):98–103.
30. Farsalinos KE, Spyrou A, Tsimopoulou K, Stefopoulos C, Romagna G, Voudris V: **Nicotine absorption from electronic cigarette use: comparison between first and new-generation devices.** *Sci Rep* 2014, **4**:4133.
31. Janzon E, Hedblad B: **Swedish snuff and incidence of cardiovascular disease: a population-based cohort study.** *BMC Cardiovasc Disord* 2009, **9**:21.
32. Siegel MB, Tanwar KL, Wood KS: **Electronic cigarettes as smoking-cessation tool: results of an online survey.** *Am J Prev Med* 2011, **40**(4):472–475.
33. Caponnetto P, Campagna D, Cibella F, Morjaria JB, Caruso M, Russo C, Polosa R: **Efficiency and safety of an electronic cigarette (ECLAT) as tobacco cigarettes substitute: a prospective 12-month randomized control design study.** *PLoS One* 2013, **8**(6):e66317.
34. McQueen A, Tower S, Sumner W: **Interviews with "vapers": implications for future research with electronic cigarettes.** *Nicotine Tob Res* 2011, **13**(9):860 867.

17

Neighborhood socioeconomic characteristics and statin medication in patients with myocardial infarction

Per-Ola Forsberg, Xinjun Li* and Kristina Sundquist

Abstract

Background: Coronary heart disease (CHD) and myocardial infarction (MI) are associated with neighborhood-level socioeconomic status (SES). Statins are important drugs for secondary prevention of MI. However, no study has determined whether neighborhood-level SES is associated with statin medication in MI patients. We aimed to determine whether there is a difference in statin medication rate in MI patients across different levels of neighborhood SES.

Methods: All patients in Sweden, diagnosed with incident MI from January 1st, 2000 until December 31st 2010, were followed ($n = 116{,}840$). Of these, 89.7 % received statin medication. Data were analyzed by multilevel logistic regression, with individual-level characteristics (age, marital status, family income, educational attainment, country of origin, urban/rural status and comorbidities/chronic conditions related to MI) as covariates.

Results: Low neighborhood-level SES was significantly associated with low statin medication rate (Odds Ratio 0.80). In the full model, which took into account individual-level socioeconomic characteristics and MI comorbidities, the odds no longer remained significant.

Conclusions: Individual-level approaches may be most important in health care policies regarding statin medication in MI patients.

Keywords: Myocardial infarction, Neighborhood deprivation, Socioeconomic status, Statins

Background

Coronary heart disease (CHD) and in particular myocardial infarction (MI) is a major cause of morbidity, mortality and health expense worldwide [1]. Up to 70 % of CHD incidence can be explained by individual-level sociodemographic characteristics (age, sex, socioeconomic status (SES)); health behaviors (smoking, physical inactivity, poor diet); and metabolic risk factors (hypertension, diabetes, hypercholesterolemia) [2]. Today, CHD prevention includes both primary and secondary prevention with lifestyle changes as well as medical treatment of risk factors, primarily hypertension, diabetes, and hypercholesterolemia. HMG CoA-reductase inhibitors, or statins, are a class of cholesterol lowering drugs that are widely used in this context, in particular for secondary prevention of MI [3]. Statins reduce both mortality and morbidity for CHD patients [4].

Although individual-level sociodemographic characteristics, such as low individual SES, are important risk factors for CHD incidence, recent work has also shown that low neighborhood SES is associated with an increased risk of CHD, after adjustment for individual SES [5–9].

However, no study has examined whether neighborhood SES is associated with statin medication rates, after taking individual socioeconomic factors into account. Such studies are important because if there are differences in statin medication by certain neighborhood-level characteristics, interventions will need to target such neighborhoods.

* Correspondence: Xinjun.li@med.lu.se
Center for Primary Health Care Research, Clinical Research Centre (CRC), Lund University, building 28, floor 11, Jan Waldenströms gata 35, SE-205 02 Malmö, Sweden

Sweden is a suitable setting for such a study because it is a country which has universal health coverage for all residents and good availability of health-related resources [10]. It is therefore possible to examine whether statin medication patterns differ, by both individual and neighborhood level SES, in a country that has almost equal availability of health care.

The aim of this study is to determine whether the statin medication rates for MI patients differ across neighborhoods with different levels of neighborhood SES, after taking individual factors into account.

Methods

All data were linked by the personal Swedish identification number, which was replaced by a serial number in the dataset in order to maintain anonymity for all individuals. Health care data were retrieved from nationwide Swedish in-patient as well as out-patient specialist care; the latter in order to increase the number of cases as well as generalizability of findings. The Swedish Hospital Discharge Register contains nationwide hospital main and secondary discharge diagnoses encoded in the International Classification of Diseases (ICD) format. The tenth revision (ICD-10) has been in use since 1997 [11]. The diagnoses in the Hospital Discharge Register have a positive predictive value between 85 and 95 %, and the validity of many cardiovascular diseases are even higher; e.g., MI, angina pectoris and atrial fibrillation have a positive predictive value of > 95 % [11–13]. Since 2000, the proportion of missing primary diagnoses has been only 0.5–0.9 % [11].

Inclusion criteria was MI registered as the main diagnosis in the Hospital Discharge Register or Outpatient Register within the study interval (2000 to 2010) using ICD-10 codes I21, I22, and I23. Only patients who previously had no CHD were included. This was achieved by excluding patients with a recorded main or secondary diagnosis of CHD (ICD-10 I20-I25) during a 3-year period, i.e., from 1997 to 1999, before study start. Patients, who died between 1 January 2000 and 30 June 2005, were excluded as medication data was not available for this time period. Also, all patients who died within one month of MI diagnosis were excluded, as we assumed that some of them might not have had a chance to pick up the medication. Patients above 80 years of age were excluded as the proportion of patients aged 80+ with statin medication was low.

Outcome (dependent) variable

The outcome variable of medication of statins was defined according to the ATC code C10AA for the Medication Register.

The statins (HMG CoA reductase inhibitors, code C10AA) included were:

C10AA01 Simvastatin
C10AA02 Lovastatin
C10AA03 Pravastatin
C10AA04 Fluvastatin
C10AA05 Atorvastatin
C10AA06 Cerivastatin
C10AA07 Rosuvastatin
C10AA08 Pitavastatin

Individual-level variables

The individual-level variables used in models were sex, age at the start of the study, marital status, family income, education level, country of origin, urban/rural status, and chronic conditions related to MI (comorbidities) [14–16].

Sex: Male or female.

Age was assessed at start of follow-up. Age was used as a continuous variable in the models.

Marital status: Individuals were classified as married/cohabitating or widowed/divorced/never married.

Family income by quartile: Information on family income in 2001 came from the Total Population Register, provided by Statistics Sweden. Income was categorized into quartiles: low income, middle-low income, middle-high income, and high income. The income was divided by the number of people in the family. A weighted system was also used; small children were given lower weights than adolescents since the costs of living for a small child are lower than those for an adolescent.

Education level was classified as completion of compulsory school or less (≤9 years), vocational high school or some theoretical high school (10–12 years), and completed theoretical high school and/or college (>12 years).

Country of origin: Born in: 1) Sweden (reference), 2) Finland, 3) Western countries, 4) Eastern European countries, 5) Middle Eastern countries, or 6) other countries. *Urban/rural status*: Residence in major cities (Stockholm, Gothenburg or Malmö), southern or northern Sweden.

Chronic conditions related to MI–comorbidities were defined as the first diagnosis (main or additional diagnosis) ten years before the study and during the follow-up period of: 1) chronic lower respiratory diseases (ICD-9: 490–496; ICD-10: J40-J49), 2) alcoholism and alcohol-related liver disease (ICD-9: 291, 303, and 571; ICD-10: F10 and K70), 3) hypertension (ICD-9: 401–405; ICD-10: I10-I19), and 4) diabetes mellitus (ICD-9: 250; ICD-10: E10-E14).

Neighborhood-level socioeconomic status (SES)

The home addresses of all Swedish individuals have been geocoded to small geographical units that have boundaries defined by homogeneous types of buildings. These neighborhood areas, developed by Statistics Sweden, are called small areas for market statistics (SAMS) and have an average of 1000 people each. SAMS were used as proxies for neighborhoods, as in previous research [7, 17]. A summary index was calculated to characterize neighborhood-level SES [5]. The neighborhood index was based on information on men and women aged 20–64, who lived in the neighborhood, because people in this age group are the most socioeconomically active. In other words, as a population group they have a stronger impact on the socioeconomic structure of the neighborhood than children, younger men/women and retirees. The neighborhood index was based on four items: low education level (<10 years of formal education), low income (income from all sources, including that from interest and dividends, defined as less than 50 % of the median individual income), unemployment (excluding full-time students, those completing compulsory military service, and early retirees) and receipt of social welfare. The index was categorized into the following three groups: low neighborhood SES (more than 1 SD below the mean), middle neighborhood SES (within 1 SD of the mean), and high neighborhood SES (more than 1 SD above the mean) [5]. The neighborhood SES index in the year 2000 was used in the models.

Statistical methods

Multilevel (hierarchical) logistic regression models were used to estimate odds ratios (OR) for statin medication rates for different levels of neighborhood SES. The analyses were performed using MLwiN version 2.27. The first model only included neighborhood-level SES to determine the crude odds of statin medication by level of neighborhood SES (Model 1). The second model also included the individual-level characteristics age and sex (Model 2). The third model added family income, marital status, country of origin, educational attainment and urban/rural status (Model 3). Last, a full model was created which also included hospitalization due to chronic lower respiratory disease, alcoholism and related liver disease, type 2 diabetes mellitus or hypertension (Model 4, not shown in tables).

Random effects

The between-neighborhood variance was estimated with a random intercept. It was regarded to be significant if it was more than 1.96 times the size of the standard error, in accordance with the precedent set in previous studies [18–20].

We computed the intraclass correlation (ICC)—that is, the intra-neighborhood correlation—in order to estimate to what extent the individual chance of statin medication for individuals, within the same SAMS, was similar compared with individuals in other SAMS areas. The ICC expresses the proportion of the total variance that is at the neighborhood level. The ICC in multilevel logistic regression can be estimated by different procedures. We applied the latent variable method [21] as exemplified by:

$$ICC = \frac{V_n}{V_n + \pi^2/3}$$

where Vn is the variance between neighborhoods and $\pi^2/3$ is the variance between individuals.

The proportion of the second level variance explained by the different variables was calculated as:

$$V_{EXPLAINED} = \frac{V_0 - V_1}{V_0} \times 100,$$

where Vo is the age adjusted variance in the initial model and V_1 is the second level variance in the different models.

First order interactions between neighborhood deprivation and individual-level characteristics for statin medication in MI patients were also analyzed.

For comparison, we also calculated logistic regression models using the SAS statistical package (version 9.3; SAS Institute, Cary, NC, USA).

Results

Table 1 shows the distribution of the study population and number of patients receiving statins by neighborhood-level SES. For statin medication, the number (No) of patients receiving statins as well as the share of patients on statin medication within each patient group (%) is presented. Of the 116,840 patients with MI included in this study, 104,766 (89.7 %) received statins during the study period. Of the total population, 19 %, 62 %, and 19 % lived in high, middle, and low SES neighborhoods, respectively. Age-standardized statin medication rates was 90.6 % in neighborhoods with high SES; 89.7 % in neighborhoods with middle SES; and 88.6 % in neighborhoods with low SES. This slight difference in statin medication rate by neighborhood-level SES was observed across all individual-level variables, as shown in Table 1.

Table 2 shows the age-adjusted ORs for each covariate. Patients with low family income had significantly lower odds of statin medication (OR 0.49) compared to patients with high family income. Low educational attainment was also associated with lower odds of statin medication (OR 0.71) compared to patients with high educational attainment.

Table 3 shows the results of the different multilevel logistic regression models. In the crude model (Model 1), the odds of statin medication were lower for patients living in neighborhoods with low SES. The OR for statin medication in patients with MI living in neighborhoods with low compared to high neighborhood-level SES was 0.80 (95 % confidence interval (CI) 0.75–0.86). In Model 2, neighborhood-level SES remained significantly associated with statin

Table 1 Distribution of study population (patients with myocardial infarction, MI), number of statin medication events, and age-standardized rates by neighborhood socioeconomic status (SES)

	Population	Distribution	Statin medication		Neighborhood SES		
		(%)	No.	%	High	Middle	Low
Total population (%)	116,840				22,172 (19 %)	72,655 (62 %)	22,013 (19 %)
Statin medication			104,766	89.7	90.6	89.7	88.6
Sex							
Men	80,351	68.8	73,223	91.1	91.8	90.6	89.0
Women	36,489	31.2	31,543	86.4	87.5	87.6	87.4
Age (years)							
< 50	18,623	15.9	17,185	92.3	92.1	92.5	91.7
50–59	34,009	29.1	32,147	94.5	95.1	94.6	93.6
60–69	40,034	34.3	36,786	91.9	92.3	92.1	90.8
70–79	24,174	20.7	18,648	77.1	78.6	77.4	74.8
Educational attainment							
≤ 9	55,061	47.1	47,813	86.8	89.5	88.9	87.9
10–12	31,699	27.1	29,147	91.9	91.2	91.2	89.5
> 12	30,080	25.7	27,806	92.4	92.2	91.3	89.9
Marital status							
Married/cohabiting	71,108	60.9	64,923	91.3	91.6	91.4	91.0
Never married, widowed, or divorced	45,732	39.1	39,843	87.1	88.4	87.1	85.9
Family income							
Low income	29,298	25.1	25,201	86.0	88.1	87.7	87.5
Middle–low income	29,175	25.0	25,538	87.5	89.1	89.1	87.2
Middle–high income	29,202	25.0	26,812	91.8	90.8	91.0	90.5
High income	29,165	25.0	27,215	93.3	92.1	91.6	91.7
Country of origin							
Sweden	99,947	85.5	89,581	89.6	90.6	89.8	88.5
Finland	5113	4.4	4568	89.3	90.4	88.2	87.0
Western countries	1379	1.2	1235	89.6	91.2	88.9	90.6
Eastern European countries	2500	2.1	2310	92.4	90.7	90.6	89.8
Middle Eastern countries	2469	2.1	2287	92.6	88.1	88.9	90.1
Others	5432	4.6	4785	88.1	89.3	88.4	86.5
Urban/rural status							
Large cities	52,572	45.0	46,829	89.1	90.1	89.0	87.6
Southern Sweden	41,907	35.9	38,125	91.0	92.2	90.9	90.4
Northern Sweden	22,361	19.1	19,812	88.6	89.5	88.7	87.7

medication after adjustment for age and sex (OR 0.80, 95 % CI 0.75–0.86).

However, in the third model, after adding individual-level sociodemographic variables, the ORs no longer remained significant. The fourth model also included the variables for comorbidities, which did not change the ORs further, and the results are therefore not shown.

The between-neighborhood variance was significant in all models. The explained variance was 6 % in Model 1, indicating that the neighborhood variable explained only a small proportion of the total variance, and increased to 23 % in Model 2 and 39 % in Model 3.

The ICC was low, varying between 1.6 and 2.4 % in the different models, indicating that the clustering within neighborhoods was low.

Analyzing first order interactions between neighborhood SES and individual-level characteristics for statin medication in MI patients showed significant interactions

Table 2 Odds ratios (OR) and 95 % confidence intervals (CI) for statin medication in patients with myocardial infarction; Results of multi-level logistic regression models for each variable, adjusted for age

	OR	95 % CI		Variance (S.E.)	*Explained variance (%)*	*Intra class correlation*
Neighborhood-level Socioeconomic status (SES, ref. High)				0.068 (0.011)	22	0.020
Middle	0.93	0.88	0.98			
Low	0.79	0.74	0.84			
Sex (ref. Female)	1.39	1.34	1.45	0.072 (0.011)	17	0.021
Family income (ref. High income)				0.077 (0.011)	11	0.023
Low income	0.49	0.47	0.52			
Middle-low income	0.59	0.56	0.63			
Milddle-high income	0.84	0.79	0.89			
Marital status (ref. Married/ co-habiting)				0.060 (0.011)	31	0.018
Never married, widowed, or divorced	0.59	0.57	0.62			
Country of origin (ref. Born in Sweden)				0.075 (0.011)	14	0.022
Finland	0.90	0.82	0.99			
Western countries	1.06	0.89	1.26			
Eastern European countries	1.10	0.94	1.28			
Middle eastern countries	0.99	0.84	1.16			
Others	0.80	0.74	0.88			
Educational attainment (ref. > 12 years)				0.075 (0.011)	14	0.022
≤ 9 years	0.71	0.67	0.74			
10–12 years	0.92	0.87	0.98			
Urban/rural status (ref. large cities)				0.059 (0.011)	32	0.018
Southern Sweden	1.28	1.22	1.34			
Northern Sweden	0.98	0.93	1.03			

between neighborhood level SES and education level only. The results of this analysis are shown in Additional file 1: Table S1.

Discussion

The present study shows that MI patients living in low SES neighborhoods had 20 % lower odds of statin medication compared to those living in middle and high SES neighborhoods. However, the odds no longer remained significant after adjusting for the individual-level sociodemographic characteristics and comorbidities. To the best of our knowledge, the potential influence of neighborhood SES on statin use in MI patients has not been examined previously.

Previous studies have shown that statin medication rates in CHD patients may vary due to individual-level factors such as the patients' age and comorbidities. In addition, low individual-level SES may affect medication patterns negatively [22–25] and it has been shown that when a larger proportion of the medication costs are required from the patients, statin utilization decreases, in particular for less regularly compliant patients [26]. Individuals in neighborhoods with low SES are likely to have small financial margins [27], which might affect their willingness to pay for prescribed drugs. The findings of the present study indicate that the lower odds of statin medication in MI patients living in deprived neighborhoods may be explained by individual-level socioeconomic factors. This could imply that the neighborhood in itself does not affect statin medication in this patient group.

Although the present study was unable to detect a neighborhood effect on statin medication in CHD patients, previous studies have shown that neighborhood-level deprivation is a strong predictor for CHD incidence and fatality from CHD after adjusting for individual-level

Table 3 Odds ratios (OR) and 95 % confidence intervals (CI) for statin medication in patients with myocardial infarction; Results of multi-level logistic regression models

	Model 1			Model 2			Model 3			
	OR	95 % CI		OR	95 % CI		OR	95 % CI		
Neighborhood-level socioeconomic status (SES, ref. High)										
Middle	0.90	0.86	0.95	0.94	0.89	0.99	1.07	1.01	1.13	0.016
Low	0.80	0.75	0.86	0.80	0.75	0.86	1.03	0.96	1.10	0.368
Age (years)				0.95	0.95	0.95	0.96	0.96	0.96	<0.001
Sex (ref. Female)				1.39	1.33	1.44	1.23	1.19	1.29	<0.001
Family income (ref. High income)										
Low income							0.49	0.46	0.52	<0.001
Middle-low income							0.62	0.58	0.65	<0.001
Milddle-high income							0.83	0.78	0.89	<0.001
Marital status (ref. Married/co-habiting)										
Never married, widowed, or divorced							0.61	0.58	0.63	<0.001
Country of origin (ref. Born in Sweden)										
Finland							1.02	0.93	1.12	0.689
Western countries							1.07	0.89	1.27	0.484
Eastern European countries							1.33	1.14	1.55	<0.001
Middle eastern countries							1.33	1.13	1.56	<0.001
Others							0.92	0.84	1.00	0.046
Educational attainment (ref. > 12 years)										
≤ 9 years							0.89	0.84	0.94	<0.001
10–12 years							1.13	1.06	1.21	<0.001
Urban/rural status (ref. large cities)										
Southern Sweden							1.30	1.24	1.37	<0.001
Northern Sweden							1.02	0.97	1.08	0.424
Variance (S.E.)	0.082 (0.011)			0.067 (0.011)			0.053 (0.011)			
Explained variance (%)	6			23			39			
Intra class correlation	0.024			0.020			0.016			

Model 1. Crude model; Model 2: Adjusted for age and sex; Model 3: Adjusted for age, sex, and individual socioeconomic variables

sociodemographic characteristics [5]. In addition, a recent study of ours has shown that neighborhood-level deprivation affects prescription patterns of statins in patients with atrial fibrillation, after adjusting for individual-level factors [28]. Adults with atrial fibrillation living in high SES neighborhoods were more often prescribed statins (men and women, OR 1.23) compared to their counterparts residing in middle SES neighborhoods [28]. It is unclear why neighborhood-level deprivation affects statin medication for patients with atrial fibrillation, but not for the MI patients in the present study.

One possible explanation could be that statin medication after MI is initiated almost exclusively at the hospital, i.e., in immediate relation to the event, whereas statin medication, for other reasons, might be initiated at a local health care center where the potential neighborhood effects may be stronger than in hospitals that cover a wider geographic area. Previous research has shown that prescription patterns among doctors working in local health care centers may be affected by neighborhood SES [29]. Additionally, individuals living in more affluent neighborhoods may be better informed as patients, irrespective of individual-level SES.

Finally, differences in medication patterns may in some cases be explained by "medication deserts", where pharmacies in low SES neighborhoods may have lower availability of drugs [30]. In Sweden, with universal health care and good availability of drugs, this is unlikely a problem.

The results of the current study, including all MI patients in Sweden during the study period, show that statin medication rates for these patients are generally high. Of the 116,840 patients with MI, 89.7 % received statins. For comparison, 89 and 88 % of patients were treated with statins according to Italian data from the REAL registry [31] and French data from the FAST-MI registry [32], respectively.

In the US, several studies of statin medication for CHD patients have shown medication rates of about 60-70 % [33–35]. However, those studies only included a sub-set of MI patients, and the authors of one of the studies that reported high medication rates explained their findings as a result of only including highly motivated medical practices [36]. It has previously been shown that in countries without universal health insurance, lack of individual health insurance is associated with lower likelihood of being treated with a statin [35, 36]. It is also possible that availability of generic statins will result in lower costs for the patients and improved compliance. The high statin medication rates in this study indicates that universal health care may improve statin medication for MI patients, which could be an argument in support of providing universal health care to the entire population.

Limitations and strengths

Our study has some limitations. Residual confounding may exist as socioeconomic measures only represent proxies for individual-level status. However, as the lower odds of statin medication in those MI patients living in deprived neighborhoods no longer remained significant after the statistical adjustments, it is likely that our socioeconomic measures are relatively good proxies of individual-level socioeconomic status. Another limitation is that we did not account for mobility, i.e., move to a different neighborhood during the follow-up period. However, we have previously checked the mobility in this age group and found it to be low. In addition, the follow-up period was relatively short, which implies that most people likely remained in their neighborhood during the study period.

This study has also, however, several strengths. The large cohort, which included practically all patients diagnosed with MI in Sweden during the study period, increases the generalizability of our results as very little data is missing. Another strength is the use of personal identification numbers, which made it possible to link health care data to socioeconomic data as well as following individuals in different national registers. A further strength is the use of the Hospital Discharge Register, which has high validity, especially for cardiovascular disorders [11–13]. Finally, the use of multilevel modeling helped us to separate neighborhood-level and individual-level effects and allowed for consideration of both random and fixed effects.

Conclusion

Neighborhood-level SES was modestly associated with statin medication rates in MI patients and this association was no longer significant after adjusting for individual-level sociodemographic factors. These findings raise important clinical and public health concerns, and indicate that individual-level approaches may be most important in health care policies regarding statin medication in MI patients.

Highlight

- This is the first study to determine whether neighborhood socioeconomic status is associated with statin medication rates in myocardial infarction (MI) patients.
- Low neighborhood-level socioeconomic status was significantly associated with lower statin medication rates (odds ratio 0.80).
- After adjustment for individual-level socioeconomic characteristics and comorbidities, this association was no longer significant.
- Individual-level approaches may be most important in health care policies regarding statin medication in MI patients.

Abbreviations

CHD, Coronary heart disease; ICC, intraclass correlation; ICD, International Classification of Diseases; MI, myocardial infarction; OR, Odds ratio; SES, socioeconomic status

Acknowledgements

This work was supported by the Swedish Research Council to Kristina Sundquist and the National Heart, Lung, And Blood Institute of the National Institutes of Health under Award Number R01HL116381 to Kristina Sundquist. The content is solely the responsibility of the authors and does not necessarily represent the official views of the National Institutes of Health.

Funding

The funding sources had no role in the design, conduct, or analysis of the study or in the decision to submit the manuscript for publication.

Authors' contributions

All authors contributed to the conception and design of the study; KS contributed to the acquisition of data; XL contributed to the analysis and interpretation of data; POF drafted the manuscript; and all authors revised it critically and approved the final version. All authors had full access to all of the data (including statistical reports and tables) and take responsibility for the integrity of the data and the accuracy of their analysis.

Competing interests

The authors declare that they have no competing interests.

References

1. Mozaffarian D, Benjamin EJ, Go AS, Arnett DK, Blaha MJ, Cushman M, et al. Heart disease and stroke statistics–2015 update: a report from the American Heart Association. Circulation. 2015;131:e29–322.
2. Lynch JW, Kaplan GA, Cohen RD, Tuomilehto J, Salonen JT. Do cardiovascular risk factors explain the relation between socioeconomic status, risk of all-cause mortality, cardiovascular mortality, and acute myocardial infarction? Am J Epidemiol. 1996;144:934–42.
3. Taylor F, Huffman MD, Macedo AF, Moore TH, Burke M, Davey Smith G, et al. Statins for the primary prevention of cardiovascular disease. Cochrane Database Syst Rev. 2013;1:Cd004816.

4. Group Scandinavian Simvastatin Survival Study. Randomised trial of cholesterol lowering in 4444 patients with coronary heart disease: the Scandinavian Simvastatin Survival Study (4S). Lancet. 1994;344:1383–9.
5. Winkleby M, Sundquist K, Cubbin C. Inequities in CHD incidence and case fatality by neighborhood deprivation. Am J Prev Med. 2007;32:97–106.
6. Sundquist K, Winkleby M, Ahlen H, Johansson SE. Neighborhood socioeconomic environment and incidence of coronary heart disease: a follow-up study of 25,319 women and men in Sweden. Am J Epidemiol. 2004;159:655–62.
7. Cubbin C, Sundquist K, Ahlen H, Johansson SE, Winkleby MA, Sundquist J. Neighborhood deprivation and cardiovascular disease risk factors: protective and harmful effects. Scand J Public Health. 2006;34:228–37.
8. Sundquist K, Malmstrom M, Johansson SE. Neighbourhood deprivation and incidence of coronary heart disease: a multilevel study of 2.6 million women and men in Sweden. J Epidemiol Community Health. 2004;58:71–7.
9. Sundquist K, Li X. Coronary heart disease risks in first- and second-generation immigrants in Sweden: a follow-up study. J Intern Med. 2006; 259:418–27.
10. Kawakami N, Winkleby M, Skog L, Szulkin R, Sundquist K. Differences in neighborhood accessibility to health-related resources: a nationwide comparison between deprived and affluent neighborhoods in Sweden. Health Place. 2011;17:132–9.
11. Ludvigsson JF, Andersson E, Ekbom A, Feychting M, Kim JL, Reuterwall C, et al. External review and validation of the Swedish national inpatient register. BMC Public Health. 2011;11:450.
12. Ingelsson E, Arnlov J, Sundstrom J, Lind L. The validity of a diagnosis of heart failure in a hospital discharge register. Eur J Heart Fail. 2005;7:787–91.
13. Nilsson AC, Spetz CL, Carsjo K, Nightingale R, Smedby B. Reliability of the hospital registry. The diagnostic data are better than their reputation. Lakartidningen. 1994;91(598):603–5.
14. Zöller B, Li X, Sundquist J, Sundquist K. Neighborhood deprivation and hospitalization for venous thromboembolism in Sweden. J Thromb Thrombolysis. 2012;34:374–82.
15. Zöller B, Li X, Sundquist J, Sundquist K. Neighbourhood deprivation and hospitalization for atrial fibrillation in Sweden. Europace. 2013;15:1119–27.
16. Li X, Sjöstedt C, Sundquist K, Zöller B, Sundquist J. Neighborhood deprivation and childhood autism: a nationwide study from Sweden. J Psychiatr Res. 2014;53:187–92.
17. Sundquist J, Johansson SE, Yang M, Sundquist K. Low linking social capital as a predictor of coronary heart disease in Sweden: a cohort study of 2.8 million people. Soc Sci Med. 2006;62:954–63.
18. Johnell K, Lindstrom M, Melander A, Sundquist J, Eriksson C, Merlo J. Anxiolytic-hypnotic drug use associated with trust, social participation, and the miniaturization of community: a multilevel analysis. Soc Sci Med. 2006;62:1205–14.
19. Johnell K, Lindstrom M, Sundquist J, Eriksson C, Merlo J. Individual characteristics, area social participation, and primary non-concordance with medication: a multilevel analysis. BMC Public Health. 2006;6:52.
20. Sundquist K, Theobald H, Yang M, Li X, Johansson SE, Sundquist J. Neighborhood violent crime and unemployment increase the risk of coronary heart disease: A multilevel study in an urban setting. Soc Sci Med. 2006;62:2061–71.
21. Snijders PTABB, Bosker TABSRJ, Bosker PRJ. Multilevel analysis: an introduction to basic and advanced multilevel modeling: SAGE. 1999.
22. Brooks JM, Cook EA, Chapman CG, Kulchaitanaroaj P, Chrischilles EA, Welch S, et al. Geographic variation in statin use for complex acute myocardial infarction patients: evidence of effective care? Med Care. 2014;52 Suppl 3:S37–44.
23. Reid FD, Cook DG, Whincup PH. Use of statins in the secondary prevention of coronary heart disease: is treatment equitable? Heart. 2002;88:15–9.
24. Headen Jr AE, Masia NA, Axelsen KJ. Effects of medicaid access restrictions on statin utilisation for patients treated by physicians practising in poor and minority neighbourhoods. PharmacoEconomics. 2006;24 Suppl 3:41–53.
25. Tuppin P, Ricci-Renaud P, de Peretti C, Fagot-Campagna A, Alla F, Danchin N, et al. Frequency of cardiovascular diseases and risk factors treated in France according to social deprivation and residence in an overseas territory. Int J Cardiol. 2014;173:430 5.
26. Thiebaud P, Patel BV, Nichol MB. The demand for statin: the effect of copay on utilization and compliance. Health Econ. 2008;17:83–97.
27. Carlsson A, Starrin B, Gigante B, Leander K, Hellenius M-L, de Faire U. Financial stress in late adulthood and diverse risks of incident cardiovascular disease and all-cause mortality in women and men. BMC Public Health. 2014;14:17.
28. Carlsson AC, Wändell P, Gasevic D, Sundquist J, Sundquist K. Neighborhood deprivation and warfarin, aspirin and statin prescription - A cohort study of men and women treated for atrial fibrillation in Swedish primary care. Int J Cardiol. 2015;187:547–52.
29. Pimenta E, Stowasser M. Uncontrolled hypertension: beyond pharmacological treatment. Hypertens Res. 2009;32:729–31.
30. Amstislavski P, Matthews A, Sheffield S, Maroko A, Weedon J. Medication deserts: survey of neighborhood disparities in availability of prescription medications. Int J Health Geogr. 2012;11:48.
31. Campo G, Guastaroba P, Marzocchi A, Santarelli A, Varani E, Vignali L, et al. Impact of COPD on long-term outcome after ST-segment elevation myocardial infarction receiving primary percutaneous coronary intervention. Chest. 2013;144:750–7.
32. Hanssen M, Cottin Y, Khalife K, Hammer L, Goldstein P, Puymirat E, et al. French registry on acute ST-elevation and non ST-elevation myocardial infarction 2010. FAST-MI 2010. Heart. 2012;98:699–705.
33. Johansen ME, Green LA, Sen A, Kircher S, Richardson CR. Cardiovascular risk and statin use in the United States. Ann Fam Med. 2014;12:215–23.
34. Goff DC, Gu L, Cantley LK, Sheedy DJ, Cohen SJ. Quality of care for secondary prevention for patients with coronary heart disease: results of the Hastening the Effective Application of Research through Technology (HEART) trial. Am Heart J. 2003;146:1045–51.
35. Johansen ME, Hefner JL, Foraker RE. Antiplatelet and statin use in US patients with coronary artery disease categorized by race/ethnicity and gender, 2003 to 2012. Am J Cardiol. 2015;115:1507–12.
36. Arnold SV, Spertus JA, Tang F, Krumholz HM, Borden WB, Farmer SA, et al. Statin use in outpatients with obstructive coronary artery disease. Circulation. 2011;124:2405–10.

18

Financial burden of survivors of medically-managed myocardial infarction and its association with selected social determinants and quality of life in a lower middle income country

P. K. B. Mahesh[1*], M. W. Gunathunga[2], S. Jayasinghe[3], S. M. Arnold[1], D. S. V. Mallawarachchi[4], S. K. Perera[5] and U. A. D. Wijesinghe[6]

Abstract

Background: Burden from ischemic heart disease is rising in Sri Lanka due to the demographic and epidemiological transitions. Documented literature is scarce on quality of life, financial burden and its determinants in relation to myocardial infarction (MI). This study was done to describe the financial burden among the survivors of MI managed only with drugs (i.e. those who did not undergo Percutaneous Coronary Intervention or Coronary Artery Bypass Graft) and its association with selected social determinants (SDHs) and quality of life (QOL).

Methods: A cross sectional study was done among MI survivors in 13 hospitals in the premier province of Sri Lanka. Out of 336 participants recruited at hospital stay, 270 responded through a self-administered questionnaire at 1 month post discharge. Questionnaire included sections on financial burden, selected SDHs and on QOL measured by the EQ-5D-3 L QOL tool. Presence of financial burden was determined using an operational definition. Associations were tested with Mann–Whitney-U test, Chi square test and Spearman-correlation-coefficient at 5% significant level.

Results: Around 40% ($n = 116$) had to seek financial support for out-of-pocket expenditure. Nearly 5% ($n = 6$) of previously employed participants had lost their job. Of the employed respondents ($n = 139$, 51.5%), 29% ($n = 85$) had limited physical activity and 40% ($n = 115$) had limitations of employment time. Of the respondents, 15.4% had to apply for a loan, 7.8% had to sell a property, 19.1% had an income loss and 33.8% had to restrict usual expenses. Financial burden was not significantly associated with gender ($p = 0.146$), ethnicity ($p = 0.068$), highest education ($p = 0.184$) and area of residence ($p = 0.369$). Influence of income ($p = 0.001$), social support ($p = 0.002$) and the health infrastructure ($p < 0.001$) were significantly associated with the occurrence of a financial burden. In the group with a financial burden, the index score ($p = 0.002$) and VAS score ($p < 0.001$) of EQ-5D-3 L were significantly lower.

Conclusions: Financial burden is common among survivors of medically-managed occurring irrespective of the gender, ethnicity, education and the area. It is influenced significantly by the income, level of social support and the level of health infrastructure. The financial burden is influencing the post-discharge-1-month QOL.

Keywords: Myocardial infarction, financial burden, Quality of life, Social Determinants of Health, EQ-5D-3 L, STEMI, NSTEMI

* Correspondence: buddhikamaheshpk@gmail.com; rdhs.cb@healthdept.wp.gov.lk
[1]Office of Regional Director of Health Services, Colombo, Sri Lanka
Full list of author information is available at the end of the article

Background

Chronic Non Communicable Diseases (NCDs) impose a severe threat for lower and middle income countries with Sri Lanka being a no exception [1–3]. Cardiovascular diseases are a category with high global disease burden falling under the chronic NCDs [4–6]. Among cardiovascular diseases, myocardial infarction (MI) is a main acute critical events endangering the lives of affected people and decreasing the quality of life [7–9].

It has been shown that chronic NCDs potentially make all people vulnerable to a financial risk and this risk is more in poorer people [2, 10–12]. The magnitude of Catastrophic Health Expenditure (CHE) is significantly associated with many social factors [13, 14]. It is acknowledged that health cannot be improved without addressing the Social Determinants of Health (SDHs) [15]. The WHO Commission on Social Determinants of Health (CSDH) has introduced the CSDH conceptual framework for action on SDHs [14, 16].

Literature from the South Asian region shows that, in some occasions a significant amount of total household expenditure is spent for healthcare payments [3, 10, 17]. Making the situation worse, when a critical event is experienced on top of chronic NCDs, more financial burden is resulted. In relation to critical illnesses, the similar findings have been highlighted in the global literature [18–22].

In MI, patients are managed as in-ward patients and are later followed up at out-patient ambulatory clinics. Even though the state services provide free-of-charge care in Sri Lanka, there are instances patients have to experience out-of-pocket expenditure and indirect costs [2]. When concomitant comorbid conditions are found the financial burden for concomitant coronary heart disease is even higher [13].

Exploring the financial burden of the survivors of MI provides the true scenario on aspects like equity in healthcare. The evaluation of the associations between SDHs with the financial burden, provide scientific hints for the prioritization of families that need potential financial support. Furthermore the evaluation of the association of the financial burden with QOL would reveal the impact of the disease on their lifestyle as a whole. In relation to the association between financial burden and social determinants, comprehensive literature is not commonly found globally [23]. In relation to the lower middle income countries like Sri Lanka, the documented literature on these aspects is rarer. This study was done to bridge this gap with the aim of describing the financial burden faced by the survivors of MI who were medically managed [i.e. without Percutaneous Coronary Intervention (PCI) or Coronary Artery Bypass Graft (CABG)] and its association with selected social determinants and quality of life.

Methods

The study included two cross sectional data collections in 13 government hospitals, in the Western Province of Sri Lanka. Study population included the patients who were admitted to the above settings with the diagnosis of MI. Inclusion criteria included the criteria for the diagnosis of MI Category A of the 2008–2009 revisions of the World Health Organization's diagnostic criteria [24]. These included: at least one value of increased level of cardiac biomarkers (preferably troponin) with at least one of the following; development of pathological Q waves, symptoms of ischemia, ECG changes (new ST-T changes or new left bundle branch block) and imaging evidence [24]. The demarcation of STEMI and NSTEMI were done based on European Society for Cardiology guidelines [25]. Participants with duration of stay less than 48 h, participants who underwent invasive interventions (i.e. PCI or CABG) and with known pre-MI physical or mental disabilities which would potentially reduce the quality of life were excluded.

All patients who satisfy the above criteria who were admitted to the mentioned 13 settings within the Western province were selected as eligible for the study. Sample size was calculated with the formula $n = z^2 \times p\ (1\text{-}p)^2/d^2$ getting the expected prevalence of financial burden based on documented literature [20, 21, 23, 26]. It was calculated that a minimal number of 235 records would be needed at data analysis stage. With an assumed response rate of 70%, the minimum sample size needed to be recruited at the data collection stage was 336. Data collection started simultaneously in all the study settings on 1st of January 2015 and continued until the sample size was in March 2015.

Data collection was done by the investigators and seven trained data collectors who were medically qualified graduates prior to their medical internship. Data collectors daily visited the medical wards that were respectively allocated to them out of the study settings. They verified the inclusion criteria of the patients who had been diagnosed with MI by the ward staff. A self-administered questionnaire was given to the participants with a stamped envelope addressed to the principal investigator. The contact details were obtained and a reminder was given at the completion of 28 days.

The questionnaire consisted of three sections; data on the post-discharge 1 month QOL, financial burden and the social determinants. The post-discharge 1-month QOL was assessed using the EQ-5D-3 L generic QOL tool. The financial burden section included the questions formed with the literature review and expert guidance. The questions were based on the operational definition of "a situation in which the participant has experienced an actual or potential financial loss and is worried about it". Four structural SDHs (i.e. gender, ethnicity, income and highest education level) and three intermediate SDHs (place of living, social support and level of health infrastructure) were selected as contextually relevant and as influencing the financial burden [15, 16].

Gender, Ethnicity and residence were coded as categorical variables. Place of living was categorized as "urban" or "rural" according to the "concepts and definitions" of the department of census and statistics [27]. Income, highest educational level, level of social support and health infrastructure were noted as quantitative variables. For measuring the social support a modified tool was used with a maximum score of 10, based on the set of questions used by Mallawarachchi in 2007 (Table 1) [28, 29].

Following literature review and expert opinions, a judgmentally validated tool was used for quantifying the level of health infrastructure with a maximum score of 5 (Table 2) [29]. The consulted expert panel included local specialists from the fields of medicine, primary-care and community medicine.

The severity of illness of MI was described with the Thrombolysis in Myocardial Infarction (TIMI) risk score [30]. For NSTEMI it was calculated by allocating a score out of seven; four of which was related to the past medical history and three for the clinical presentation [31]. For STEMI, the score was out of maximum 14; four of which was given for the past medical history, eight for the examinations and two for presentation [32]. The higher the TIMI score, the worse the severity of the disease.

Data was entered into a pre-designed sheet in Statistical package for Social Sciences (SPSS version 20). Demographic factors and several aspects of financial burden were elaborated using descriptive statistics. The group with financial burden was defined as at least having one of the phenomena mentioned in Table 3. The association between the presence of financial burden and the SDHS in categorical form was evaluated by the chi square test. The score of the SDHs which were in quantitative form and the QOL scores were non-normally distributed when assessed by Q-Q plots and Kolmogorov–Smirnov test. Hence non-parametric tests were used in analyzing their associations. Mann Whitney U test was used for analysis of associations of financial burden with numerically-measured SDHs and with QOL. The same test was used to analyze for the association between QOL and the type of MI. Spearman correlation coefficient was used to describe the association between QOL versus TIMI risk score and left ventricular ejection fraction prior to hospital discharge.

Informed written consent was obtained similar to methods used by Hofhuis et al. in 2007 [33]. Data collections were done without disturbing the patient management processes. Ethical clearance was obtained and administrative permissions were obtained prior to the initiation of data collection.

Table 1 Scoring method of the tool to assess the level of social support

Question	Score
Availability of someone to call	1
Availability of someone to talk to	1
Availability of someone to encourage	1
Availability of someone to help in daily activities	1
Availability of someone to help in house keeping	1
Availability of someone to take to the doctor	1
Availability of someone to provide financial assistance	1
Availability of someone to provide a vehicle	1
Availability of someone to give information about the disease	1
Availability of help from any institution/ group	1
Total	10

Table 2 Scoring method for the tool for quantifying the health infrastructure

Domain	Scores and criteria	
i. Distance to the nearest pharmacy	< 1km 0.5	> 1 km 0
ii. Distance to the nearest place a doctor can be consulted	< 1km 1	> 1 km 0
iii. Distance to the nearest hospital	< 1km 1	> 1 km 0
iv. Distance to the nearest hospital with specialist care	< 1km 1	> 1 km 0
v. Availability of a healthcare personnel for health advices/ clarifications	Yes 1	No 0
vi. Ownership of vehicles	Yes 0.25	No 0
vii. Condition of roads	Does not cause delays 0.25	Cause delays 0

Results

The median (IQR) of the age distribution of the recruited study sample was 62.0 (54.0–70.0). Out of the recruited participants 270 either posted back the questionnaire or gave the responses over the phone with

Table 3 Financial burden experienced by the study population

Burden	Yes N (%)	No N (%)	Not mentioned N (%)
Had to apply for a loan	45 (15.4)	209 (71.3)	16 (13.3)
Had to sell a property	23 (7.8)	222 (75.8)	25 (16.4)
Had a potential income loss	56 (19.1)	192 (65.5)	22 (15.4)
Had to restricted other expenses	99 (33.8)	154 (52.6)	17 (13.6)

a general response rate of 80.8%. The non-responders had either died following the hospital admission or could not be contacted. The analysis of the characteristics of responders and non-responders showed that the non-response bias is unlikely [34, 35].

Out of the respondents 65 were with a STEMI and 205 were with NSTEMI. The median (IQR) age was 58 (51–67) years. Male to female ratio was 7:3with 186 males and 84 females. The median (IQR) TIMI score for the STEMI group was 3 (3 to 5) and for NSTEMI was 2 (2 to 4). All recruited STEMI patients were given streptokinase as the intravenous fibrinolytic therapy and NSTEMI patients received parenteral anticoagulant therapy.

Out of the responders, 139 (51.5%) had been employed by 1 month of hospital discharge. Around 31% ($n = 85$) of the employees stated that they had a limitation of physical activity and around 43% ($n = 115$) had to limit the employment time due to the effects of the MI. Nearly 5% ($n = 6$) of those who were not employed by one month had lost their previously engaged job due to the illness.

Around 43% ($n = 116$) have stated that they had to request the financial support from a third party due to the illness. Around 86% ($n = 231$) need to have someone to accompany him or her for any form of further medical management following hospital discharge. Out of these companions, around 60% are engaged in a daytime job and they had to limit some portion of their working time for accompanying the participant.

Table 3 summarizes the financial burden experienced by the participants in relation to four selected questions. Out of the respondents, 137 (50.7%) had experienced at least one of the four occurrences mentioned.

The Table 4 shows that the group without financial burden has better figures for the education level, income, level of social support and the level of health infrastructure. When analyzed by the non-parametric Mann Whitney U test the latter three show a statistically significant difference between the two groups.

The SDHs mentioned in Table 5 which are gender, ethnicity and place of living do not show a statistically significant different association between the two groups.

The QOL at post-discharge 1 month, shows a significant difference between the two groups in relation to both the index value ($p = 0.002$) and the Visual Analogue Scale (VAS) value ($p < 0.001$) (Table 6) of the EQ-5D-3 L QOL tool.

EQ-5D index value did not show a significant association with the TIMI risk score for the STEMI group ($p = 0.075$) nor with the NSTEMI group ($p = 0.058$). Similarly the EQ-5D VAS values too, did not show a statistically significant association between STEMI ($p = 0.35$) or NSTEMI groups ($p = 0.364$). Furthermore in a subgroup analysis of approximately one fourth of the participants, the left ventricular ejection fraction prior to hospital discharge did not show a significant association with either the EQ-5D-index score ($p = 0.222$) or the EQ-5D-VAS score ($p = 0.693$). Neither the EQ-5D index score ($p = 0.392$) nor the EQ-5D-VAS ($p = 0.125$) showed a statistically significant difference between STEMI and NSTEMI groups.

Discussion

The study shows that a substantial number of MI survivors had experienced a financial burden. Furthermore, the financial burden experienced by them has a significant association with three SDHs and with the post-discharge QOL at one month. The Sri Lankan health financing system involves two main sources: general taxation and out-of-pocket household spending [2]. Private insurance is a supplementary-optional method. Since the uptake of insurance is weak, there is a potential for out-of-pocket expenditures to be incurred by patients with MI. Higher magnitude of Out of Pocket expenditure is a major restriction in the country's path towards achieving Universal Health Coverage. It not only leads to impoverishment, but also restricts access to medical care.

Table 4 Association between financial burden and selected social determinants

Social determinant	Financial burden category	Mean (SD)	Median (IQR)	Significance of difference[a]
Education level	With burden	8.09 (3.91)	9.00 (5.00–11.00)	$p = 0.184$
	No burden	8.65 (4.15)	10.0 (5.50–11.00)	
Income	With burden	2.20 (1.32)	2.00 (1.00–3.00)	$p = 0.001$[b]
	No burden	2.69 (1.31)	3.00 (2.00–4.00)	
Social support	With burden	7.03 (2.13)	7.00 (6.00–9.00)	$p = 0.002$[b]
	No burden	7.83 (1.79)	8.00 (7.00–9.00)	
Health infrastructure	With burden	1.86 (1.26)	1.50 (0.75–2.75)	$p < 0.001$[b]
	No burden	3.28 (1.04)	3.25 (2.50–4.13)	

[a]Analyzed by the Mann–Whitney U test
[b]significant at 5% level

Table 5 Association between financial burden and selected social determinants

Selected SDH	Yes N (%)	No N (%)	Total N (%)	Significance of difference[a]
Gender				
-Male	98	85	183 (100)	p value = 0.146
-Female	36	46	82 (100)	
Ethnicity				
-Sinhala	117	100	217 (100)	p value = 0.068
-Others	18	28	46 (100)	
Area				
-Urban	79	70	149 (100)	p value = 0.369
-Rural	35	40	75 (100)	

[a]Analyzed by the chi-square test

The financial burden summarized in Table 3 needs to be interpreted while recognizing the presence of co-morbid conditions. Some participants, who were previously unaware about the presence of co-morbidities, had them detected during the current admission. Managing these co-morbidities would have worsened the financial burden. For example if a drug becomes temporarily out-of-stock in the hospital pharmacy, the patient would need to purchase it from a private pharmacy.

Following one month of the hospital discharge, 51.5% mentioned that they were working. A quicker return to work may have been necessitated by the economic burden as documented in global literature too [18]. The employed participants had to face some limitations in activities and had to compromise some aspects of the lifestyle comparable to the global literature [23]. The financial restraints are major concerns of the survivors of chronic illnesses as documented in the global literature [18, 20, 21, 23, 36]. Similarly the present study shows that in a lower-middle-income country these concerns remain the same. These results indicate that the economic consequences are multi-faceted and have a negative impact on the lifestyles. These issues are not usually captured by the routine health information systems.

The associations between SDHs in Tables 5 and 6 suggest that the gender (p = 0.146), ethnicity (p = 0.068), highest education (p = 0.184) and the area of residence (p = 0.369) are not significantly associated with the financial burden. Hence the findings can be generalized irrespective of the gender, ethnicity or place of living. The influence of income (p = 0.001), social support (p = 0.002) and the health infrastructure ($p < 0.001$) were noted as statistically significant. This fact strengthens the available scientific literature which shows the association between financial burden versus the SDHs [13, 14, 16]. When these SDHs were unfavorable, the financial burden was seemingly worse.

When the pre-event income is low, the presence of a financial burden following the MI is more likely. This would have been resulted by the lack of savings. A better level of social support minimizes the risk of the occurrence of financial burden. This may not be only due to the mere financial inputs and would be due to the other factors like knowledge sharing as well. Similarly a better health infrastructure would have a protective effect preventing the MI survivors going into financial burden.

The EQ-5D-3 L QOL tool has been developed by EuroQol group. It consist of EQ-5D descriptive system as well as EQ-5D VAS [37, 38]. It focuses on the day of the measurement of the QOL. It has been validated in previous studies in Sri Lanka [29, 39]. The minimum time taken for the completion and the relative simplicity make it a suitable QOL tool to be used to measure the one month post-hospital discharge QOL of MI survivors. The results revealed a significantly lower QOL in relation to both components (index score and VAS) among the group which was with a financial burden (Table 6). It points towards the importance of financial interventions in improving the QOL of MI survivors.

MI has significant negative consequences for the sufferers in relation to physical, emotional and social dimensions. Globally it is shown that the QOL of the coronary patients anyhow is significantly impaired following the illness [7, 40–42]. Measuring QOL of cardiac patients provide the opportunity of reflecting the success of the management in the patient's point of view [43].

This is an era that the whole world is concerned about the equity issues in relation to health financing. Different income inequality measures are available in the literature such as; Gini coefficient, Atkinson index, generalized-entropy index, Kakwani index [44–46]. It is timely that

Table 6 Association between financial burden and the quality of life

QOL	Financial burden category	Mean (SD)	Median (IQR)	Significance of difference[a]
EQ-5D index value	With burden	0.486 (0.38)	0.516 (0.49–0.73)	$p = 0.002^b$
	No burden	0.671 (0.19)	0.585 (0.52–0.85)	
EQ-5D VAS value	With burden	60.97 (21.46)	60.0 (50.00–77.50)	$p < 0.001^b$
	No burden	71.56 (15.39)	70.0 (60.00–80.00)	

[a]Analyzed by Mann Whiney U test
[b]significant at 5% level

lower-middle-income countries like Sri Lanka encourage more scientific literature on these regards. This further provides evidence on actual necessity of health-economic reforms like social insurance systems and guided donations.

There were several limitations of the study. The financial burden was in categorical form and the quantification with a monetary value was not done. It was the best possible option as exploring quantification evidence could not be possible especially when the respondent is not exposed to a face-to-face interview. Secondly the out-of-pocket expenditure in some patients may be due to the temporary scarcities of certain medicines in particular hospitals requiring the patient to purchase them. This should be considered in interpreting the results. Thirdly the present study only recruited the medically-managed survivors of MI. This was due to the fact that at the time of data collection, there was no uniform financial-supporting system for all the MI patients who were managed with invasive interventions. Hence the exclusion of these patients enabled the applicability of the findings for the medically-managed patients in relation to the financial-burden, even if the policies related to surgical interventions change from time to time. However, since the mode of management may influence the post-discharge QOL, the findings of the present study on the QOL too, should not be generalized to the survivors of MI who underwent an invasive intervention. Since the study did not have an objective of describing any incidence-related parameter, the total participants who were screened for eligibility was not documented. Finally the left ventricular ejection fraction analysis was done for only one fourth of the respondents. This should be concerned in interpreting its associations.

Conclusions

The survivors of MI who are medically-managed, have to face financial burden due to the out-of-pocket expenditure as well as due to the limitations the illness imposes on their occupations. This burden occurs irrespective of the gender, ethnicity, education and the place of residence. It is influenced significantly by the income, level of social support and the level of health infrastructure. The financial burden is influencing the post-discharge 1 month QOL of the medically-managed MI survivors. More research should be encouraged in these regards and the evidences must be coupled with health reforms to mitigate the impact of financial burden due to illness.

Abbreviations

CABG: Coronary Artery Bypass Graft; CHE: Catastrophic Health Expenditure; CSDH: Commission on Social Determinants of Health; EQ-5D-3 L: EuroQol-five-dimensional-3-level questionnaire; MI: myocardial infarction; NCDs: Non Communicable Diseases; NSTEMI: Non- ST elevation myocardial infarction; PCI: Percutaneous Coronary Intervention; QOL: quality of life; SDHs: social determinants; STEMI: ST elevation myocardial infarction; TIMI risk score: Thrombolysis in Myocardial Infarction (TIMI) risk score; VAS: Visual Analogue Scale

Acknowledgements

Authors like to acknowledge the EuroQOL group for providing the Sinhalaese translation of the EQ-5D-3 L questionnaire (Registration ID:6554) and the UK-TTO dataset free of charge.

Funding

The study was self-funded and was not funded by a third party.

Authors' contributions

All authors were involved in the planning of the research study. PKBM was the principal investigator and involved in getting ethics permissions, data collection, data analysis and writing of the manuscript. MWG, SJ, SMA and DSVM were involved in data analysis, data interpretation and writing of the manuscript. SKP and UADW were involved in data collection, data entering, interpretation of data and in writing the manuscript. All authors went through the final manuscript. All authors read and approved the final manuscript.

Competing interests

The authors declare that they have no competing interests.

Author details

[1]Office of Regional Director of Health Services, Colombo, Sri Lanka. [2]Department of Community Medicine, Faculty of Medicine, University of Colombo, Colombo, Sri Lanka. [3]Department of Clinical Medicine, Faculty of Medicine, University of Colombo, Colombo, Sri Lanka. [4]Non Communicable Disease Unit, Ministry of Health, Colombo, Sri Lanka. [5]Post Graduate Institute of Medicine, University of Colombo, Colombo, Sri Lanka. [6]Cardiology Unit, National Hospital Sri Lanka, Colombo, Sri Lanka.

References

1. WHO. Global Status Report on Non Communicable Diseases. Geneva: World Health Organization; 2014. http://apps.who.int/iris/bitstream/10665/148114/1/9789241564854_eng.pdf
2. Engelgau M, Okamoto K, Navaratne KV, Gopalan S. Prevention and Control of Selected Chronic NCDs in Sri Lanka: Policy Options and Action. Health, Nutrition and Population Family. Human Development Network. Washington: World Bank; 2010. http://hdl.handle.net/10986/13607.
3. Joseph N. Assessment of Economic Impact Among In-Patients with Non-Communicable Diseases in a Private Tertiary Care Hospital in Southern India. J Clin Diagn Res. 2016; doi:10.7860/JCDR/2016/19426.8059.
4. Moran AE, Forouzanfar MH, Roth GA, et al. The Global Burden of Ischemic Heart Disease in 1990 and 2010: The Global Burden of Disease 2010 Study. Circulation. 2014;129(14):1493–501. doi:10.1161/CIRCULATIONAHA.113.004046.
5. Sanchis-Gomar F, Perez-Quilis C, Leischik R, Lucia A. Epidemiology of coronary heart disease and acute coronary syndrome. Ann Transl Med. 2016;4(13):256. 10.21037/atm.2016.06.33.
6. Schlatter RP, Hirakata VN, Polanczyk CA. Estimating the direct costs of ischemic heart disease: evidence from a teaching hospital in BRAZIL, a retrospective cohort study. BMC Cardiovasc Disord. 2017;17(1):180. doi:10.1186/s12872-017-0615-1.
7. Mahesh PKB, Gunathunga MW, Jayasinghe S, Arnold SM, Haniffa R, De Silva AP. Pre-event quality of life and its influence on the post-event quality of life among patients with ST elevation and non-ST elevation myocardial infarctions of a premier province of Sri Lanka. Health Qual Life Outcomes. 2017;15(1):154. doi:10.1186/s12955-017-0730-9.
8. Medagama A, Bandara R, De Silva C, Galgomuwa MP. Management of acute coronary syndromes in a developing country; time for a paradigm shift? an

observational study. BMC Cardiovasc Disord. 2015;15(1):133. doi:10.1186/s12872-015-0125-y.

9. Anderson JL, Morrow DA. Acute Myocardial Infarction. N Engl J Med. 2017; 376(21):2053–64. doi:10.1056/NEJMra1606915.
10. Pankaj SN, Kanchan M. Economic Effect of Coronary Heart Disease on Households – A study in Mumbai. Int J Med Public Heal. 2016;6(4):184–8. doi:10.5530/ijmedph.2016.4.8.
11. Dhaliwal KK, King-Shier K, Manns BJ, Hemmelgarn BR, Stone JA, Campbell DJT. Exploring the impact of financial barriers on secondary prevention of heart disease. BMC Cardiovasc Disord. 2017;17(1):61. doi: 10.1186/s12872-017-0495-4.
12. Campbell DJT, Manns BJ, Weaver RG, Hemmelgarn BR, King-Shier KM, Sanmartin C. Financial barriers and adverse clinical outcomes among patients with cardiovascular-related chronic diseases: a cohort study. BMC Med. 2017;15(1):33. doi:10.1186/s12916-017-0788-6.
13. Wang Q, Liu H, Lu ZX, Luo Q, Liu JA. Role of the new rural cooperative medical system in alleviating catastrophic medical payments for hypertension, stroke and coronary heart disease in poor rural areas of China. BMC Public Health. 2014;14(1):907. doi:10.1186/1471-2458-14-907.
14. Daivadanam M, Thankappan KR, Sarma PS, Harikrishnan S. Catastrophic health expenditure & coping strategies associated with acute coronary syndrome in Kerala, India. Indian J Med Res. 2012;136(4):585–92. http://www.ncbi.nlm.nih.gov/pmc/articles/PMC3516025/
15. CSDH. Closing the gap in a generation, Closing Gap Gener Heal Equity Through Action Soc Determ Heal Final Rep Comm Soc Determ Heal; 2008. p. 246. doi:10.1080/17441692.2010.514617.
16. Krumeich A, Meershoek A. Health in global context; beyond the social determinants of health? Glob Health Action. 2014;7(SUPP.1) doi:10.3402/gha.v7.23506.
17. Jaspers L, Colpani V, Chaker L, et al. The global impact of non-communicable diseases on households and impoverishment: a systematic review. Eur J Epidemiol. 2015;30(3):163–88. doi:10.1007/s10654-014-9983-3.
18. Herridge MS, Cheung AM, Tansey CM, et al. One-year outcomes in survivors of the acute respiratory distress syndrome. N Engl J Med. 2003;348(8):683–93. doi:10.1056/NEJMoa022450.
19. Griffiths JA, Barber VS, Cuthbertson BH, Young JD. A national survey of intensive care follow-up clinics. Anaesthesia. 2006;61(10):950–5. doi:10.1111/j.1365-2044.2006.04792.x.
20. Swoboda SM, Lipsett PA. Impact of a prolonged surgical critical illness on patients' families. Am J Crit Care. 2002;11(5):459–66.
21. Covinsky KE, Goldman L, Cook EF, et al. The impact of serious illness on patients' families. SUPPORT Investigators. Study to Understand Prognoses and Preferences for Outcomes and Risks of Treatment. JAMA. 1994;272(23): 1839–44. doi:10.1001/jama.272.23.1839.
22. Campbell DJT, King-Shier K, Hemmelgarn BR, et al. Self-reported financial barriers to care among patients with cardiovascularrelated chronic conditions. Heal Rep. 2014;25(5):3–12.
23. Griffiths J, Hatch RA, Bishop J, et al. An exploration of social and economic outcome and associated health-related quality of life after critical illness in general intensive care unit survivors: a 12-month follow-up study. Crit Care. 2013;17(3):R100. doi:10.1186/cc12745.
24. Mendis S, Thygesen K, Kuulasmaa K, et al. World Health Organization definition of myocardial infarction: 2008–09 revision. Int J Epidemiol. 2011;40(1):139–46. doi:10.1093/ije/dyq165.
25. Steg PG, James SK, Atar D, et al. ESC Guidelines for the management of acute myocardial infarction in patients presenting with ST-segment elevation: The Task Force on the management of ST-segment elevation acute myocardial infarction of the European Society of Cardiology (ESC). Eur Heart J. 2012;33(20):2569–619. doi:10.1093/eurheartj/ehs215.
26. Suresh K, Chandrashekara S. Sample size estimation and power analysis for clinical research studies. J Hum Reprod Sci. 2012;5(1):7. doi:10.4103/0974-1208.97779.
27. Department of Census and Statistics. Sri Lanka Census on Population and Housing. 2012. http://www.statistics.gov.lk/PopHouSat/CPH2011/index.php?fileName=FinalPopulation&gp=Activities&tpl=3.
28. Mallawarachchi DSV. Quality of Life of Stroke Patients Presenting to Selected Hospitals in the Colombo District and the Possibility of Common Mental Disorders among the Principal Informal Caregivers. MD thesis in Community Medicine. Colombo: Post Graduate Institute of Medicine; 2007.
29. Mahesh PKB, Gunathunga MW, Jayasinghe S. Influence of social determinants on the disease-outcome, financial burden and quality of life after a critical illness due to chronic Non Communicable Diseases, among patients treated at government hospitals in the Western province of Sri Lanka. MD thesis in Community Medicine. Colombo: Post Graduate Institute of Medicine; 2015.
30. Hudzik B, Lekston A, Gasior M. Risk Prediction in Acute Myocardial Infarction. J Am Coll Cardiol. 2016;68(25):2918–9. doi:10.1016/j.jacc.2016.08.078.
31. Numasawa Y, Kohsaka S, Miyata H, et al. Use of Thrombolysis in Myocardial Infarction Risk Score to predict bleeding complications in patients with unstable angina and non-ST elevation myocardial infarction undergoing percutaneous coronary intervention. Cardiovasc Interv Ther. 2013;28(3):242–9. doi:10.1007/s12928-013-0162-3.
32. Silveira DS, Jaeger CP, Hatschbach L, Manenti ERF. Validation of TIMI Risk Score for STEMI. Int J Cardiovasc Sci. 2016; doi:10.5935/2359-4802.20160034.
33. Hofhuis JG, Spronk PE, van Stel HF, Schrijvers AJ, Bakker J. Quality of life before intensive care unit admission is a predictor of survival. Crit Care. 2007;11(4):R78. doi:10.1186/cc5970.
34. Wittwer R, Hubrich S. Nonresponse in Household Surveys: A Survey of Nonrespondents from the Repeated Cross-sectional Study "Mobility in Cities – SrV" in Germany. Transp Res Procedia. 2015;11:66–84. doi:10.1016/j.trpro.2015.12.007.
35. Johnson TP. Response Rates and Nonresponse Errors in Surveys. JAMA. 2012;307(17):1805. doi:10.1001/jama.2012.3532.
36. Panos RJ, Krywkowski-Mohn SM, Sherman SN, Lach LA. Patient Reported Determinants of Health: A Qualitative Analysis of Veterans with Chronic Obstructive Pulmonary Disease. COPD. 2013;10:333–47. doi:10.3109/15412555.2012.752805.
37. Reenen M, Oppe M. EQ-5D-3L User Guide. EuroQol Research Foundation: Netherland; 2015.
38. Gusi N, Olivares PR, Rajendram R. The EQ-5D Health-Related Quality of Life Questionnaire. In: Handbook of Disease Burdens and Quality of Life Measures. New York: Springer; 2010. p. 87–99. doi:10.1007/978-0-387-78665-0_5.
39. Kularatna S, Whitty JA, Johnson NW, Jayasinghe R, Scuffham PA. EQ-5D-3L Derived Population Norms for Health Related Quality of Life in Sri Lanka. PLoS One. 2014;9(11):e108434. doi:10.1371/journal.pone.0108434.
40. Duenas M, Salazar A, Ojeda B, Failde I. Health Related Quality of Life in Coronary Patients. In: Recent Advances in Cardiovascular Risk Factors. Prof. Mehnaz Atiq (Ed.), InTech. 2012. doi:10.5772/31903.
41. Höfer S, Doering S, Rumpold G, Oldridge N, Benzer W. Determinants of health-related quality of life in patients with coronary artery disease. Eur J Cardiovasc Prev Rehabil. 2006;13(3):398–406. http://www.ncbi.nlm.nih.gov/pubmed/16926670
42. Failde II, Soto MM. Changes in health related quality of life 3 months after an acute coronary syndrome. BMC Public Health. 2006;6(1):18. doi:10.1186/1471-2458-6-18.
43. Fayers PM, Machin D. Quality of Life: The Assessment, Analysis and Interpretation of Patient-Reported Outcomes: Second Edition. ISBN 9780470024515. Chichester: Wiley; 2007.
44. Kondo N, Sembajwe G, Kawachi I, van Dam RM, Subramanian SV, Yamagata Z. Income inequality, mortality, and self rated health: meta-analysis of multilevel studies. BMJ. 2009;339:b4471. doi:10.1136/bmj.b4471.
45. De Maio FG. Income inequality measures. J Epidemiol Community Health. 2007;61(10):849–52. doi:10.1136/jech.2006.052969.
46. Haghparast-Bidgoli H, Pulkki-Brännström A-M, Lafort Y, et al. Inequity in costs of seeking sexual and reproductive health services in India and Kenya. Int J Equity Health. 2015;14(1):84. doi:10.1186/s12939-015-0216-5.

19

Relationship key factor of inflammation and the development of complications in the late period of myocardial infarction in patients with visceral obesity

Olga Gruzdeva[1], Evgenya Uchasova[1*], Yulia Dyleva[1], Olga Akbasheva[2], Vera Matveeva[1], Victoria Karetnikova[1], Alexander Kokov[1] and Olga Barbarash[1]

Abstract

Background: Cytokines play an significant role in regulating non-specific inflammatory response involved in many pathological processes. The current study tested the hypothesis that myocardial infarction in patients with obesity can lead to increased production of proinflammatory cytokines and unfavorable course of the pathological process.

Methods: The study recruited 232 male patients with ST-elevated myocardial infarction. The mean age of the patients was 58.7 (52.2-69.9) years. All the patients were assigned to two groups according to the computed tomography findings: 1 ($n = 160$) patients with visceral obesity (VO), and 2 ($n = 72$) patients without VO. Interleukins were measured in blood serum on days 1 and 12 after MI.

Results: All patients with MI demonstrated elevated levels of proinflammatory markers and reduced anti-inflammatory markers in the in-hospital period. The results suggested that among all studied inflammatory markers IL-6 (OR 1.9; 95% CI (1.6–2.8) and CRP (OR 1.3; 95% CI (1.1–1.8) were closely related to VO. One year after MI adverse cardiovascular outcome frequently occurred in patients with VO. There were two cardiac deaths (3.1%), 6 cases (9.3%) of recurrent MI, 19 cases (29.6%) of repeated hospitalizations for unstable angina, whereas only 2 patients without VO (6.6%) were hospitalized for unstable angina. The results of the logistic regression analysis demonstrated that IL-6, IL-12, and IL-10 had the highest predictive value for occurrence of adverse cardiovascular events in patients with VO.

Conclusion: Cytokine profile in MI patients with VO is characterized by an imbalance caused by elevated pro-inflammatory interleukins and decreased anti-inflammatory interleukins. Obesity in patients was associated with a marked increase in IL-6 and CRP levels.

Background

Cytokines play an significant role in regulating non-specific inflammatory response involved in many pathological processes [1]. Pro-inflammatory (TNF-α, IL-1β, IL-6, IL-8 and IL-12) and anti-inflammatory (IL-10) cytokines defines adaptive course of inflammation. An imbalance in the can lead to chronic inflammation. Chronic inflammation is a key factor in the initiation and progression of atherosclerosis that ultimately results in the destabilization of atherosclerotic plaques, coronary artery thrombosis, myocardial infarction (MI) [1]. Obesity-induced adipose tissue inflammation is considered to be an independent risk factor for cardiovascular disease (CVD), which is the leading cause of death and disability among working-age people in developed countries [2]. Cytokines are produced mainly by immune system cells and adipocytes [3]. The expression of the anti-inflammatory cytokines is stimulated in adipose tissue of healthy subjects, while large quantities of pro-inflammatory cytokine are secreted in patients with CVD [4]. The current study tested the

* Correspondence: evg.uchasova@yandex.ru
[1]Federal State Budgetary Institution "Research Institute for Complex Issues of Cardiovascular Disease", Kemerovo, Russia
Full list of author information is available at the end of the article

hypothesis that myocardial infarction in patients with obesity can lead to increased production of proinflammatory cytokines and unfavorable course of the pathological process.

Purpose

To study the relationships between key inflammatory factors and complications in the late post myocardial infarction period in patients with visceral obesity.

Methods

The study recruited 232 male patients with MI. Acute MI was diagnosed according to the 2007 Russian National Cardiology Society guidelines and ESC/ACCF/AHA/WHF based on clinical (presence of typical pain lasting longer than 15 min), electrocardiographic (ST-segment elevation of 0.1 mW in two or more contiguous leads), echocardiographic and biochemical signs (elevated creatine phosphokinase, creatine phosphokinase-MB, troponin T levels(>0,1 ng/ml).

The exclusion criteria were as follows: age <50 or >80 years, the presence of T2DM, and a prior history of pronounced renal failure (glomerular filtration rate <30 mL/min). Also excluded from the study were excluded HIV-infected patients, and cancer patients with known pathology [5].

All patients provided written informed consent prior to their participation in the study.

The mean age of the patients was 58.7 (52.2–69.9) years.

All the patients underwent multi-slice computed tomography (CT) using a Lightspeed VCT 64 (General Electric, Fairfield, CT, USA) to measure abdominal adipose tissue. Visceral adipose tissue (VAT) and subcutaneous adipose tissue (SAT) areas as well as the ratio of VAT to SAT were measured. Two diagnostic criteria (the proposed method L. Sjoestrom) were used to confirm visceral obesity (VO): VAT area >130 cm^2 and the ratio of VAT to SAT ≥0.4 [6].

All the patients were assigned to two groups according to the CT findings: Group 1 ($n = 160$) patients with VO, and Group 2 ($n = 72$) patients without VO.

The clinical and demographic data are shown in Table 1. All the patients underwent primary percutaneous coronary intervention of the infarct-related artery as a reperfusion therapy. The control group included 30 males without diagnosed CVD and comparable in age and sex with the patients included in the study (aged 58.42 (52.2–61.1) years). The CT findings demonstrated that none of the control subjects suffered from VO (VAT area was 110.0 [104.0–128.0] cm^2 and the VAT/SAT ratio 0.35 [0.2–0.39]).

Blood sampling and biochemical assays

The serum of each patient was separated from blood by centrifugation at 3 000 × g for 20 min and stored at −70 °C. Proinflammatory markers were measured in blood serum on days 1 and 12 after MI. Serum concentrations of interleukins (IL-1β, IL-6, IL-8, IL-10 IL-12 and TNF-α,) were determined with ELISA using the Monobind ELISA test systems (USA). C-reactive protein (CRP) levels were measured using a standard Thermo Fisher Scientific test system (Thermo Fisher Scientific Oy, Vantaa, Finland) in a Konelab 30i biochemistry analyzer (Thermo Fisher Scientific Oy).

Statistical analysis

Statistical analysis was performed using Statistica 6.1 (InstallShield Software Corp., Chicago, IL, USA) and SPSS 17.0 for Windows (SPSS Inc., Chicago, IL, USA). The Kolmogorov–Smirnov test was used to assess the distribution of two data sets. Results are presented as median (Me) and 25 and 75% quartiles Me (Q1;Q3). The statistical analysis was performed using the nonparametric Mann–Whitney test for skewed distributions. Stepwise logistic regression and a receiver operating characteristic (ROC) curve with the area under the curve (AUC) measurement were used to determine the most informative VO parameters, the hazard ratio (HR) and the confidence interval (95%). P values <0.05 were considered statistically significant.

Results

All patients with MI demonstrated elevated levels of proinflammatory markers (TNF-α, IL1β, IL6, IL8, IL12, CRP) and reduced anti-inflammatory (IL-10) markers in the in-hospital period. However, these changes were more pronounced during the whole follow-up period in the presence of VO (Table 2).

TNF-α and IL-1β are the first line cytokines that are produced in response to inflammatory stimuli. The production and secretion of cytokines may not be predominantly caused by myocardial ischemia-reperfusion injury, but also by macrophages infiltrating adipose tissue, and adipocytes. Thus, statistically significant increase in the levels of TNF-α and IL-1β was found in patients with VO on days 1 and 12 after MI (Table 2). TNF-α and IL-1β levels in patients with VO on day 1 after MI was 1.2- and 1.6-fold higher compared to patients without excess VO. On day 12, there was a 1.4-fold increase in TNF-α levels compared to the values obtained on day 1. However, IL-1β levels did not change significantly. Patients without VO reported no significant differences in the levels of cytokines compared to the levels in the control group during the study.

On day 1, IL-12 levels were relatively elevated in patients with VO (a 2.1-fold increase), and without VO

Table 1 Baseline clinical characteristics of patients

Variable	Patients with visceral obesity, $n = 160$	Patients without visceral obesity, $n = 72$	p
Men	58 (54;69)	57 (50;67)	0.92
Arterial hypertension, n (%)	160 (100.0)	60 (83.3)	0.05
Current smoking	65 (40.6)	39 (54.2)	0.46
Family history of IHD	105 (65.6)	24 (33.3)	0.04
Family history of T2DM	35 (21.9)	8 (11.1)	0.04
Features history			
Angina prior to myocardial infarction	85 (53.1)	48 (66.6)	0.69
Previous myocardial infarction	31 (19.3)	13 (18.1)	0.051
History of heart failure	16 (10)	8 (11.1)	0.81
History of cerebrovascular accident/transient ischemic attack	0	3 (4.2)	0.98
Myocardial infarction			
Q-wave myocardial infarction	128 (80)	58 (80.5)	0.61
Non-Q-wave myocardial infarction	33 (20.3)	15 (20.8)	0.62
Localization of myocardial infarction			
- posterior	105 (65.6)	38 (54.2)	0.61
- posterior with extension to the right			
ventricle	18 (12.3)	10 (13.9)	0.72
- anterior	30 (18.8)	20 (27.8)	0.59
- inferio-posterio-lateral	8 (5)	6 (8.3)	0.79
Acute heart failure (Killip classification)			
I	110 (68,8)	44 (61.1)	0.52
II	31 (19.4)	17 (23.6)	0.64
III	15 (9,4)	10 (13.8)	0.72
IV	3 (1.9)	0	0.95
- Rhythm disturbance	38 (23.8)	20 (27.8)	0.78
Early post-infarction angina	30 (18.8)	16 (22.2)	0.71
Recurrent myocardial infarction	10 (6.3)	3 (4.2)	0.91

Table 1 Baseline clinical characteristics of patients *(Continued)*

Creatine phosphokinase, U/L	339.2 (203.1;699.4)	245 (110.7;523.1)	0.03
Max creatine phosphokinase-MB, U/L	81 (33;179)	66 (35;142)	0.03
Troponin T, ng/ml	1.01 (0.82;3.1)	0.69 (0.17;1.2)	0.01
Left ventricular ejection fraction, %	50 (40;57)	52 (42;53)	0.60
Number of diseased coronary arteries			
Stenosis of a vessels	28 (17.5)	16 (22.2)	0.72
Stenosis of 2 vessels	15 (9.4)	26 (36.1)	0.03
Stenosis of 3 or more vessels	122 (76.3)	14 (43.1)	0.03
Treatment strategy/group of drugs			
Stenting of the infarct-related artery	160 (100)	72 (100)	0,81
Systemic thrombolytic therapy	13 (8.1)	10 (13.8)	0.73
β-blockers	140 (87.5)	72 (100)	0,82
Angiotensin-converting enzyme	145 (90.6)	68 (42.5)	0.59
Calcium channel blocker	120 (78.1)	62 (38.8)	0.97
Diuretics	53 (33.1)	26 (36.1)	0.81
Nitrates	26 (15.6)	15 (20.8)	0.80
Aspirin	160 (100)	71 (98.6)	0.91
Heparin	160 (100)	72 (100)	0.98
Clopidogrel	148 (92.5)	62 (95.8)	0.81
Statins	160 (100.0)	72 (100.0)	0.93

P-value for differences between groups ($P < 0.05$). Data are expressed as number (percentage)
Abbreviations: *HIS* ischemic heart disease; T2DM, type 2 diabetes mellitus

(a 1.6-fold increase) compared to the levels in the control group. Importantly, the concentration of IL-12 was 1.3-fold higher in patients with VO than in those without VO. On day 12, IL-12 levels decreased in both groups, but it did not achieve the control group levels in patients with VO.

More significant changes were observed in IL-6 levels. Patients with VO on day 1 after MI reported a 6.9- and 1.45-fold increase in IL-6 levels compared to the control group and patients without VO. Despite the reduction in the concentration of the cytokine on day 12 in both groups, the values in healthy subjects were not achieved. Importantly, there was a 1.6-fold increase in IL-6 levels in patients with VO compared to patients without VO.

The production of IL-8, a chemokine produced by macrophages and neutrophils, and CRP, an acute phase protein, modulating the immune responses, are activated by proinflammatory cytokines (TNF-α, IL-1β, IL-6 and IL-12). Apparently, this amplifying effect of cytokines has led to the most intense changes in the concentrations

Table 2 Markers of inflammation in patients with myocardial infarction with and without visceral obesity, Me (Q1;Q3)

Variable	Control group, $n = 30$	Patients with visceral obesity, $n = 160$		Patients without visceral obesity, $n = 72$	
		1st day	12st day	1st day	12st day
	1	2	3	4	5
TNF-α, pg/ml	1.2 (0.9;1.4)	1.4 (1.0;1.7) $p_{1-2} = 0.01$	1.9 (1.4;2.0) $p_{1-3} = 0.01$ $p_{2-3} = 0.02$	1.2 (0.7;1.6) $p_{2-4} = 0.002$	1.0 (0.8;2.1) $p_{3-5} = 0.003$
IL -1β, pg/ml	2.2 (2,1;4,3)	5.2 (2.6;6.2) $p_{1-2} = 0,001$	4.9 (2.7;6.6) $p_{1-3} = 0.002$	3.3 (2.0;4.4) $p_{2-4} = 0.003$	2,4 (1.1;5.4) $p_{3-5} = 0.002$
IL −6, pg/ml	2.55 (2,1;3,3)	17.5 (11.7; 25.1) $p_{1-2} = 0.001$	9.5 (3.2; 4.3) $p_{1-3} = 0.01$ $p_{2-3} = 0.02$	12.0 (6.9;18.7) $p_{1-4} = 0.006$ $p_{2-4} = 0.004$	6.1 (2.5;14.1) $p_{1-5} = 0.002$ $p_{3-5} = 0.001$ $p_{4-5} = 0.01$
IL −8, pg/ml	2.4 (2.1;4.1)	58.0 (29.9;69.5) $p_{1-2} = 0.001$	48,3 (40.4;64.4) $p_{1-3} = 0.00$ $p_{2-3} = 0.01$	45.5 (27.4;54.7) $p_{1-4} = 0.005$ $p_{2-4} = 0.004$	43,6 (35,3;52.2) $p_{1-5} = 0.003$ $p_{3-5} = 0.004$
IL −12, pg/ml	60.4 (47.2;88.6)	128.7 (66.4;182.0) $p_{1-2} = 0.001$	98.4 (86.7;261.2) $p_{1-3} = 0.005$ $p_{2-3} = 0.02$	100.1 (48.0;151.7) $p_{1-4} = 0.007$ $p_{2-4} = 0.03$	55.3 (44.0;101.3) $p_{3-5} = 0.02$ $p_{4-5} = 0.01$
CRP, mg/l	1.0 (0.8;1.5)	23.2 (12.1;54.1) $p_{1-2} = 0.008$	11.3 (5.0;21.6) $p_{1-3} = 0.00$ $p_{2-3} = 0.01$	20.2 (12.8;35.0) $p_{1-4} = 0.003$ $p_{2-4} = 0.001$	7.7 (4.7;15.0) $p_{1-5} = 0.005$ $p_{3-5} = 0.004$ $p_{4-5} = 0.01$
IL −10, pg/ml	8.9 (7.4;10.2)	1.9 (0.7;2.5) $p_{1-2} = 0.00$	3.8 (1.1;4.5) $p_{1-3} = 0.00$ $p_{2-3} = 0.01$	5.6 (3.2;6.2) $p_{1-4} = 0.00$ $p_{2-4} = 0.02$	7.8 (6.8;9.7) $p_{1-5} = 0.00$ $p_{3-5} = 0.01$ $p_{4-5} = 0.01$

Data in the table are presented as median (Me) and 25% and 75% quartiles (Q1;Q3)
P-value for differences between groups ($P < 0.05$

of IL-8 and CRP compared to other pro-inflammatory factors. Thus, patients with VO on days 1 and 12 demonstrated a 24.2- and 20.1-fold increase in IL-8 levels compared with healthy subjects. Moreover, this increase was statistically significant compared to patients without VO (Table 2). On day 1 after MI, patients with VO reported a 23.2-fold increase in CRP concentrations compared with the levels in the control group. On day 12, a 2-fold decrease was found in patients with VO, but the levels of the control group were not achieved. The levels of CRP in patients with VO increased 10-fold the levels in the control group. On day 12, patients without VO demonstrated a 7.7-fold increase compared to the levels in the control group.

IL-10 is the central anti-inflammatory cytokines, blocking synthesis of pro-inflammatory cytokines. On day 1 after MI, patients with VO demonstrated a pronounced deficit of IL-10. MI patients with VO reported a 78% reduction in IL-10 levels compared to the control group, whereas patients without VO had a 37% reduction. On day 12, IL-10 increased 2- and 1.4-fold in both groups, respectively. However, a 2-fold decrease in IL-10 levels remained in patients with VO compared with patients without VO.

IL-8/IL-10 ratio was calculated to assess the imbalance of pro- and anti-inflammatory cytokines. On days 1 and 12, the ratio in patients with VO were 30.5 and 12.7, suggesting a 3.8- and 2.3-fold increase compared to the values in patients without VO (8.13 and 5.6, respectively). Increased IL-8/IL-10 ratio was associated with elevated IL-8 levels and decreased IL-10 levels. Thus, the imbalance of pro- and anti-inflammatory cytokines was more pronounced in the presence of visceral obesity.

The logistic regression analysis was performed to identify the most informative variables. The results suggested that among all studied inflammatory markers IL-6 IL-6 (OR 1.9; 95% CI (1.6-2.8) AUC = 0.80, $p = 0.01$) and CRP (OR 1.3; 95% CI (1.1-1.8) AUC = 0.77, p = 0.02) were closely related to visceral obesity.

One year after MI adverse cardiovascular outcome frequently occurred in patients with VO (Fig. 1). There were two cardiac deaths (3.1%), 6 cases (9.3%) of recurrent MI, 19 cases (29.6%) of repeated hospitalizations for unstable angina, whereas only 2 patients without VO (6.6%) were hospitalized for unstable angina. Importantly, there were no cases of cardiac death and recurrent MI in the group of patients without VO.

The results of the logistic regression analysis demonstrated that IL-6 (OR 1.9; 95% CI (1.5-2.1), AUC = 0.84, $p = 0.02$), IL-12 (OR 1.3; 95% CI (1.1-2.0) AUC = 0.75, $p = 0.032$, and IL-10 (OR 0.8; 95% CI (0.5-0.9) AUC = 0.75, $p = 0.04$) had the highest predictive value for occurrence

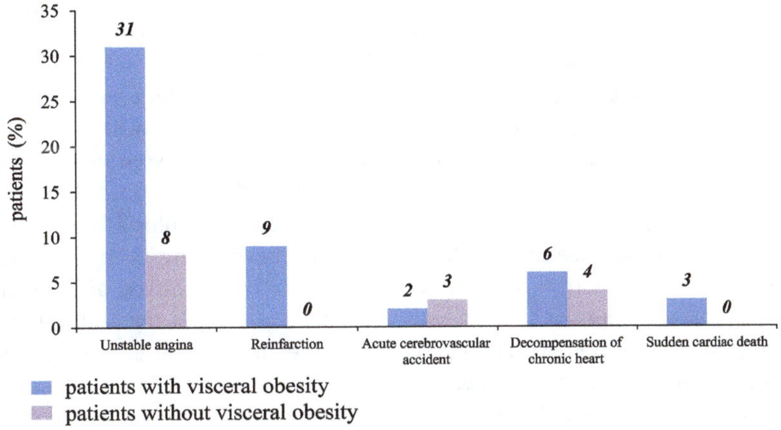

Fig. 1 Basic cardiovascular events within 1 year after myocardial infarction in patients with and without visceral obesity, n (%). The differences between study groups are statistically significant ($P < 0.05$)

of adverse cardiovascular events in patients with VO. Elevated levels of IL-6 and IL-12 were associated with a 1.9- and 1.3-fold increased risk for developing cardiovascular complications, respectively. Moreover, reduced levels of anti-inflammatory cytokine, IL-10, was accompanied by a 20% increased risk, compared to patients without VO.

Discussion

It should be noted that visceral adipose tissue is considered to be one of the most harmful due to its positive association with the development of cardiovascular disease [1]. Excess adiposity is characterized as a chronic state of low-grade inflammation or so-called metabolic inflammation [2]. Adipose tissue-resident immune cells (primarily lymphocytes and macrophages) and hypertrophied adipocytes both contribute to increased circulating levels of proinflammatory cytokines [7]. White adipose tissue (WAT) is the key site mediating systemic inflammation since it is virtually around all organs and tissues, and occupies a large area in obese people [8].

The results of our study suggest that the presence of VO in MI patients is associated with elevated levels of pro-inflammatory factors (TNF-α, IL-1β, IL-6, IL-8, IL-12, CRP), which are mainly produced by macrophages, localized around hypertrophied adipocytes, accumulating in both the subcutaneous and visceral expanding fat depots, even though macrophage infiltration appears to be more prominent in the latter [9].

Along with an increase in the number of adipose tissue macrophages (ATM) for obesity undergo phenotypic changes. In obesity the white oil contains mostly proinflammatory macrophage M1 (40%), while in normal anti-inflammatory predominant population of M2 macrophages. [4]. Activated M1 ATMs are a prominent source of proinflammatory cytokines such as TNF-α and IL-6, IL-8 and may be regarded as effectors of a coordinated inflammatory response. Thus, ATM polarization into M1 to M2, being a more pronounced in visceral obesity, might provide new insights into worsening inflammatory response and reducing anti-inflammatory resistance.

Another important issue that may activate proinflammatory potential in obesity is an increase of expression of Toll-like receptors (TLR2, TLR4) on the membranes of various cell types, such as immune and resident non-immune cells, including adipocytes in VAT [10]. Activation of Toll-like receptors causes the release of transcriptional factors that activate genes responsible for the synthesis of various bioactive molecules, including proinflammatory cytokines (TNF-α, IL-1β, IL-6, IL-8, IL-12) [11].

Ligands can be derived not only from pathogens, but they also can be endogenous, such as heat shock proteins (HSPs) [12], extracellular matrix degradation products (hyaluronan, biglycan, fragments of heparan sulphate) [13], saturated fatty acids (SFAs) of exogenous and endogenous origin are recognized by TLR2 or TLR4 [14].

We have previously reported that elevated levels of circulating FFA in myocardial infarction [15] may contribute to the synthesis of inflammatory mediators through the activation of these receptors in immune, resident non-immune cells as well as in adipose tissue. Moreover, it has been recently suggested that TLR4, TLR2 and their signaling pathways participate in the inflammatory response caused by ischemia reperfusion injury [16].

MI causes the development of aseptic inflammatory acute-phase response, which in severe cases, leads to systemic inflammatory response syndrome [17]. Patients with MI, particularly with VO, demonstrated highly increased CRP levels. Increased CRP levels are observed in any tissue damage and aimed at the reorganization of necrotic myocardial cells and their residues which are highly toxic. Myocardial cells which are dead or damaged under ischemia and reperfusion secrete various endogenous molecules (alarmins) into the extracellular space. Alarmins are ligands of TLRs. Thus, the cells expressing TLRs with further synthesis of proinflammatory cytokines are activated.

In the case of myocardial infarction, obese patients with acute inflammatory responses include adipose tissue, which is already in a state of chronic inflammation and has a significant pro-inflammatory potential due to the macrophage polarization into M1 and a higher expression of TLRs in resident macrophages and adipocytes. However, these changes are more pronounced in VAT. Importantly, the expression of TLRs in circulating blood mononuclear cells is also higher in the presence of obesity. All of these changes ultimately lead to a severe inflammatory response in these patients. This is most obvious, but is not the only mechanism for increasing circulating pro-inflammatory cytokines in blood plasma of obese patients after MI, compared to lean patients.

According to the results of our study, there was insignificant a 1.4- and 1.9-fold increase in TNF-α and IL-1. TNF-α is a proinflammatory cytokine, primarily secreted from myeloid cells via activation of MAPK and NFκB signaling pathways, resulting in the release of other inflammatory cytokines, such as IL-1β and IL-6 [18]. The basic amount of TNF-α is synthesized resident macrophages [19]. Obesity is associated with elevated levels of TNF-α in plasma and adipose tissue, but excess weight loss leads to normalization of this parameter. However, the influence of TNF-α on immune response mostly results from its strengthen effect on the production of other interleukins, such as IL-6 and IL-1 β, rather than from a direct effect [18].

A series of in vitro experiments indicated that adipocytes produce IL-1β in obese people 2 times higher than in lean individuals. Neutralization of IL-1β and TNF-α in the culture medium significantly reduces the synthesis of IL-6 and IL-8 in adipocytes [20, 21]. Further clinical studies confirmed the data of in vitro experiments, indicating that the endogenous release of IL-1β and TNF-α from adipose tissue upregulates the synthesis of IL-6 and IL-8 [22].

According to our data, IL-6 levels increased 6.9-fold in patients with VO. Moreover, a relationship between IL-6 and VO in patients suffered from myocardial infarction may be associated with its synthesis not only by immune cells, but also by adipocytes. Similarly to TNF-α, WAT and plasma IL-6 expression correlate with increased body mass, waist circumference, and free fatty acid levels. IL-6 has been implicated as a marker for VO because VAT releases more IL-6 than SAT [20, 23].

The most significant changes were observed in IL-8 levels, which demonstrated a 24-fold increase. IL-8 belongs to the group of chemokines, providing chemotaxis and adhesion in the area of inflammation of various cell types (neutrophils, monocytes, T-cells, eosinophils and basophils). Monocytes, macrophages, lymphocytes, vascular endothelium, fibroblasts, epithelial cells may also produce IL-8. Its blood levels are elevated in people with obesity, correlating with body weight and TNF-α levels [24]. The main source of IL-8 in adipose tissue may be resident macrophages and adipocytes; thus, its synthesis is higher in visceral adipose tissue than in subcutaneous [24].

Unlike the above-mentioned cytokines, there are no data about possible synthesis of IL-12 in adipose tissue. Its increase is assumed to be associated with the presence of inflammation in the immediate area of myocardial damage. Accumulation of T cells and macrophages in atherosclerotic plaques and the formation of antibodies directed against plaque proteins suggests that adaptive immunity contributes to the development of atherosclerosis [25]. The results of clinical and experimental studies are consistent with this assumption. It has been established that IL-12 is an early inducer and a significant factor in the progression of atherosclerosis. Clinical data suggest using IL-12 blood concentration as a predictor of any adverse events after myocardial infarction within 1 year [26]. According to our data, IL-12 in patients with visceral obesity was also associated with the development of cardiovascular complication in the late post-MI period.

Apparently, intensification of inflammation in MI patients with VO is associated with a pronounced deficit of anti-inflammatory cytokine, IL-10, predominantly expressed by activated T lymphocytes (Th2-type). However, such cells as monocytes, macrophages, dendritic cells and B lymphocytes are involved in its synthesis as well. Lower levels of this cytokine have been found in the peripheral blood of patients with obesity and type 2 diabetes [23]. Suppressing the inflammatory response, IL-10 inhibits the production of IL-1α, IL-1β, TNF-α, IL-6, IL-8 and IL-12, primarily produced by activated monocytes, and reparative processes in myocardium, inhibition of fibrosis, enhancing vascularization. Furthermore, IL-10 may play a significant role in extracellular matrix remodeling by regulating expression of metalloproteinases and their inhibitors [23]. N.G. Frangogiannis et al. suggested that IL-10 may have a role in regulating extracellular matrix metabolism after experimental myocardial ischemia/reperfusion in dogs [26].

According to our data, a decrease in IL-10 levels has obvious adverse effect, particularly pronounced in the presence of VO. Deficiency of IL-10 was accompanied by the development of the imbalance of pro- and anti-inflammatory factors. IL-8/IL-10 ratio in patients with

VO was 3.8 times higher than in lean individuals. In the presence of VO, despite clinical improvement in the post-MI period, adverse cardiovascular events closely related to IL-10 deficiency were registered.

In general, the dynamics of changes in cytokines levels indicates the need to improve the balance of pro- and anti-inflammatory cytokines by introducing new therapeutic approaches (cytokine inhibitors - receptor antibodies, suppression of cytokine synthesis by activated immune cells) regulating the activation process of inflammation. Physicians have much experience with the TNF blockers (infliximab and etanercept) in patients with psoriasis in preventing the development of cardiovascular events.

Conclusion

Cytokine profile in MI patients with VO is characterized by an imbalance caused by elevated pro-inflammatory interleukins and decreased anti-inflammatory interleukins. An increase in the concentration of cytokines was as follows: a 1.3-fold increase in the levels of IL-1 and TNF-α, a 2-fold increase in IL-12 levels, a 6-fold increase in IL-6 levels and a 24-fold increase in IL-8 and CRP levels. Obesity in patients was associated with a marked increase in IL-6 and CRP levels. Dynamics of changes in the concentrations of IL-6, IL-12 and IL-10 is essential for the development of adverse cardiovascular events one year after MI. The obtained results suggest the use of immunomodulators to restore the balance of the pro- and anti-inflammatory cytokines in patients with VO. Drugs affecting the levels of IL-6, −12, −10, namely monoclonal antibody to IL-6 receptor, antibodies to IL-12, IL-10 inducers, seem to be promising in individuals with VO.

Abbreviations

ATM: Adipose tissue macrophages; CAD: Coronary artery disease; CVD: Cardiovascular disease; DM: Diabetes mellitus; MI: Myocardial infarction; SAT: Subcutaneous adipose tissue; TLR: Toll-like receptors; VAT: Visceral adipose tissue; VO: Visceral obesity; WAT: White adipose tissue

Acknowledgements

The authors wish to thank Catherine Anikeeva and Elena Semibratova for assistance in writing this article.

Funding

Not applicable.

Authors' contributions

OG, AK and VM were study design and conception. EU, YA and OA participated in all stages of recruitment of the patients and critically reviewed the manuscript. VK and OB was a principal investigator. All other study investigators conducted the study and collected the data. All authors read and approved the final manuscript.

Competing interests

Not applicable.

Author details

[1]Federal State Budgetary Institution "Research Institute for Complex Issues of Cardiovascular Disease", Kemerovo, Russia. [2]Federal State Budget Educational Institution of Higher Professional Education "Siberian State Medical University" of the Ministry of Healthcare of the Russian Federation, Tomsk, Russia.

References

1. Alexopoulos N, Katritsis D, Raggi P. Visceral adipose tissue as a source of inflammation and promoter of atherosclerosis. Atherosclerosis. 2014;233: 104–12.
2. Shoelson SE, Lee J, Goldfine AB. Inflammation and insulin resistance. J Clinical Investigation. 2006;116:1793–801.
3. Ouchi N, Parker JL, Lugus JJ, Walsh K. Adipokines in inflammation and metabolic disease. Nat Rev Immunol. 2011;11:85–97.
4. Olefsky JM, Glass CK. Macrophages, inflammation, and insulin resistance. Annu Rev Physiol. 2010;72:219–46.
5. D'Ascenzo F, Cerrato E, Appleton D, et al. Prognostic indicators for recurrent thrombotic events in HIV-infected patients with acute coronary syndromes: use of registry data from 12 sites in Europe, South Africa and the United States. Thromb Res. 2014;134(3):558–64. doi:10.1016/j.thromres.2014.05.037.
6. Sjoestrom L. A computed tomography based multicompartment body composition technique and anthropometric predictions of lean body mass, total and subcutaneous adipose tissue. Int J Obes. 1991;15:19–30.
7. Gregor MF, Hotamisligil GS. Inflammatory mechanisms in obesity. Annu Rev Immunol. 2011;29:415–45.
8. Odegaard JI, Chawla A. Pleiotropic actions of insulin resistance and inflammation inmetabolic homeostasis. Science. 2013;339:172–7.
9. Bruun JM, Lihn AS, Pedersen SB, Richelsen B. Monocyte chemoattractant protein-1 release is higher in visceral than subcutaneous human adipose tissue (AT): implication of macrophages resident in the AT. J Clin Endocrinol Metab. 2005;90:2282–9.
10. Ahmad R, Al-Mass A, Atizado V, Al-Hubail A, Al-Ghimlas F, Al-Arouj M, et al. Elevated expression of the toll like receptors 2 and 4 in obese individuals: its significance for obesity-induced inflammation. J Inflamm. 2012;9:48.
11. Takeda K, Akira S. Toll-like receptors. Curr Protoc Immuno. 2007;14:112–21.
12. Asea A. Heat shock proteins and toll-like receptors. Handb Exp Pharmacol. 2008;183:111–27.
13. Piccinini AM, Midwood KS. DAMPening inflammation by modulating TLR signaling. Mediators Inflamm 2010;672395. http://dx.doi.org/10.1155/2010/672395
14. Lee JY, Zhao L, Youn HS, Weatherill AR, Tapping R, Feng L, et al. Saturated fatty acid activates but polyunsaturated fatty acid inhibits Toll-like receptor 2 dimerized with Toll-like receptor 6 or 1. J Biol Chem. 2004;279:16971–9.
15. Gruzdeva O, Uchasova E, Yu D, Belik E, Shurygina E, Barbarash O. Plasminogen activator inhibitor-1, free fatty acids, and insulin resistance in patients with myocardial infarction. Diabetes Metab Syndr Obes. 2013;6:293–301.
16. Satoh M, Shimoda Y, Akatsu T, Ishikawa Y, Minami Y, Nakamura M. Elevated circulating levels of heat shock protein 70 are related to systemic inflammatory reaction through monocyte Toll signal in patients with heart failure after acute myocardial infarction. Eur J Heart Fail. 2006;8:810–5.
17. Kohsaka S, Menon V, Lowe AM, Lange M, Dzavik V, Sleeper LA, et al. Systemic inflammatory response syndrome after acute myocardial infarction complicated by cardiogenic shock. Arch Intern Med. 2005;165:1643–50.
18. Chen G, Goeddel DV. TNF-R1 signaling: a beautiful pathway. Science. 2002;296:1634–5.
19. Weisberg SP, McCann D, Desai M, Rosenbaum M, Leibel RL, Ferrante AW. Obesity is associated with macrophage accumulation in adipose tissue. J Clin Invest. 2003;112:1796–808.
20. Fain JN, Madan AK, Hiler ML, Cheema P, Bahouth SW. Comparison of the release of adipokines by adipose tissue, adipose tissue matrix and adipocytes from visceral and subcutaneous abdominal adipose tissues of obese humans. Endocrinology. 2004;145:2273–82.

21. Moschen AR, Molnar C, Enrich B, Geiger S, Ebenbichler CF, Tilg H. Adipose and liver expression of interleukin (IL)-1 family members in morbid obesity and effects of weight loss. Mol Med. 2011;17:840–5.
22. Fain JN, Bahouth SW, Madan AK. Involvement of multiple signaling pathways in the post bariatric induction of IL-6 and IL-8 mRNA and release in human visceral adipose tissue. Biochem Pharmacol. 2005;69:1315–24.
23. Makki K, Froguel P, Wolowczuk I. Adipose tissue in obesity-Related Inflammation and Insulin Resistance: Cells, Cytokines, and Chemokines. ISRN Inflammation. 2013; 139239. http://dx.doi.org/10.1155/2013/139239
24. Bruun JM, Lihn AS, Madan AK, Pedersen SB, Schiott KM. Fain JN Higher production of IL-8 in visceral vs. subcutaneous adipose tissue. Implication of nonadipose cells in adipose tissue. Am J Physiol Endocrinol Metab. 2004;286:8–13.
25. Hansson GK, Robertson AK, Söderberg-Nauclér C. Inflammation and atherosclerosis. Annu Rev Pathol. 2006;1:297–329.
26. Frangogiannis NG, Mendoza LH, Lindsey ML, Ballantyne CM, Michael LH, Smith CW, et al. The inflammatory response in myocardial infarction. Cardiovasc Res. 2002;53:31–4.

20

The association between periodontal disease and the risk of myocardial infarction

Shuai Xu[1], Mingbao Song[2], Yu Xiong[3], Xi Liu[2], Yongming He[2] and Zhexue Qin[2*]

Abstract

Background: Several meta-analyses have indicated that periodontal disease (PD) are related to cardiovascular diseases (CVDs). However, the association between PD and myocardial infarction (MI) remains controversial. Here we aimed to assess the association between PD and MI by meta-analysis of observational studies.

Methods: PubMed, EMBASE and the Cochrane Library were searched through July, 2016. Observational studies including cohort, cross-sectional and case–control studies reporting odds ratio (OR) or relative risk (RR) with 95% confidence intervals (CIs) were included in the analysis. Either fixed or random-effects model were applied to evaluate the pooled risk estimates. Sensitivity and subgroup analyses were also carried out to identify the sources of heterogeneity. Publication bias was assessed by the Begg's, Egger's test and funnel plot.

Results: We included 22 observational studies with 4 cohort, 6 cross-sectional and 12 case–control studies, including 129,630 participants. Patients with PD have increased risk of MI (OR 2.02; 95% CI 1.59-2.57). Substantial heterogeneity in risk estimates was revealed. Subgroup analyses showed that the higher risk of MI in PD patients exists in both cross-sectional studies (OR 1.71; 95% CI 1.07-2.73) and case–control studies (OR 2.93; 95% CI 1.95-4.39), and marginally in cohort studies (OR 1.18; 95% CI 0.98-1.42). Further, subgroup meta-analyses by location, PD exposure, participant number, and study quality showed that PD was significantly associated with elevated risk of MI.

Conclusion: Our meta-analysis suggested that PD is associated with increased risk of future MI. However, the causative relation between PD and MI remains not established based on the pooled estimates from observational studies and more studies are warranted.

Keywords: Periodontal disease, Myocardial infarction, Observational studies, Meta-analysis

Background

Periodontal disease (PD) is defined as chronic inflammation of the supporting structure of the teeth. PD is estimated to be detectable in 20-50% of the general population and a major cause of tooth loss in adults [1]. The symptoms include bleeding gums (gingivitis), the formation of gingival pockets and bone loss (periodontitis) and finally tooth mobility caused by biofilm and calculus [2]. PD is related to many risk factors, such as inflammation, gender, smoking, genetics and life styles, which were also implicated in cardiovascular diseases (CVD) [3].

A great body of evidence has investigated the association between PD and CVD. Even though a number of meta-analyses indicated the association between PD and CVD, the cause-and-effect relationship between them was still not established with current available evidence according to an American Heart Association scientific statement [4]. Meanwhile, no specified meta-analysis by now has been reported to investigate whether PD was associated with myocardial infarction (MI).

* Correspondence: zhexueqin@126.com; zhexueqin@tmmu.edu.cn
[2]Department of Cardiology, Xinqiao Hospital, Third Military Medical University, 183 Xinqiaozhengjie St., Shapingba District, 400037 Chongqing, China
Full list of author information is available at the end of the article

In 1989, Mattila et al. first reported oral health including PD was related to acute MI [5]. Since then, a variety of literatures explored the nature of the association between PD and MI. Several case–control, cross-section or cohort studies have indicated a significant association between PD and MI [6–17]. However, whether the association is causal is still a matter of debate. Some other studies found no such relationship [18–24]. Given the high prevalence of PD and MI, it is of great value to determine their association.

The purpose of this study was to examine the association between PD and MI in observational studies. By pooling data from individual studies and using meta-analysis, the statistical estimates of the association between PD and incidence of MI were obtained.

Methods

The meta-analysis was performed following the guidelines from Meta-Analysis of Observational Studies in Epidemiology (MOOSE) group [25] and the Preferred Reporting Items for Systematic Reviews and Meta-Analyses (PRISMA) statement [26].

Eligibility criteria

Studies included for the meta-analysis if they referred to observational studies including cross-sectional, case–control, cohort and nested case–control studies. The article should estimate the association between PD and MI and provide the odds ratio (OR) or relative risk (RR) with the corresponding 95% confidence intervals (CIs).

Search strategy

Pubmed, EMBASE and the Cochrane Library Databases were searched to identify relevant studies through July 2016. The medical subject headings (MeSH terms) as well as free text terms were used in the search strategy. The terms applied were as follows: ("periodontal disease" OR "periodontitis" OR "periodontal" OR "periodontal attachment loss" OR "periodontal pocket" OR "alveolar bone loss") AND ("myocardial infarction" OR "acute myocardial infarction" OR "acute coronary syndrome" OR "cardiovascular disease" OR "coronary heart disease" OR "unstable angina") (Additional file 1: Table S1). The search was restricted to studies conducted on human subjects and published in English and Chinese. The bibliographies of the articles found were hand searched for possible additional studies.

Two reviewers (S. Xu and X. Liu) screened the titles and abstracts of the search results and articles were excluded if they did not meet the above-mentioned inclusion criteria.

Quality assessment

Newcastle-Ottawa Quality Assessment Scale was used to assess the quality of the observational studies, including case–control and cohort studies [27] and the Agency for Healthcare Research and Quality (AHRQ) for cross-sectional studies [28]. For case–control and cohort studies, the quality was ranked as followed: low quality = 0-4; moderate quality = 5-7; high quality = 8-9.

To rank the cross-sectional studies, the AHRQ was quantified in the following way. An item would be scored '0', if it was answered 'NO' or 'UNCLEAR'. If it was 'YES', then this item was scored '1'. Article quality was ranked as follows: low quality = 0-3; moderate quality = 4-7; high quality = 8-11 [29].

Data extraction

Two reviewers (S. Xu and X. Liu) extracted the data from all included studies independently. Any discrepancies or uncertainties between the reviewers were resolved by consensus after rechecking the source and discussion with the third reviewer (Z. Qin). A data collection form was used to compile extracted study information and included the following items: first author's surname, publication year, country of origin, sample size, population, study design, enrolled period, age ranges, PD exposure parameter, adjusted OR/RR and their 95% CI, *P* values and adjusting factors.

PD was defined to include self-report diagnosis, or any measure of disease according to clinical, radiographic and microbiological assessment (including pocket probing depth, attachment loss, bleeding on probing, plaque index, gingival index, X-ray and microbiological results). At the very beginning, all related OR/RR based on different PD assessments were extracted. The one selected for final meta-analysis was according to the frequency of each OR/RR in all included studies. The order in this study was clinical attachment loss (CAL), pockets deep and periodontal bone loss.

Data analysis

The OR was used in these studies, while RR and hazard ratio (HR) were considered equivalent. For one study that reported stratified OR/RR in different population, we considered each subgroup analysis as an independent study. Before pooling the data, ORs were transformed into their natural logarithm to stabilize their variance, normalize the distribution and then statistically pooled [30].

The heterogeneity among studies was evaluated by Cochrane Q test and quantified as I^2 metric. For the Q statistic, a *P*-value <0.1 was considered statistically significant heterogeneity. For I^2 statistic, a value of zero was considered no heterogeneity, 25%-49% low, 50%-74% moderate, and above 75% high, respectively. To explore possible reasons for heterogeneity and test the robustness of the association, subgroup analyses were performed based on study design, methodological quality, gender, locations and PD exposure assessment parameters. When obvious heterogeneity across studies exists, the random-effect model was used to calculate the pooled estimates. Otherwise, the fixed-effect model was applied.

Publication bias was assessed by both Begg's rank correlation test and Egger's linear regression test. Funnel plots were also generated to assess the publication bias.

STATA statistical software, version 11.0 (STATA Corporation, College Station, TX, USA) was used for analysis. *P* values were 2-sided and $P < 0.05$ was considered statistically significantly otherwise indicated.

Results

Literature search

Initially, a total of 2558 articles were identified from PubMed (2041 articles), EMBASE (415 articles) and the Cochrane Library Database (102 articles) search. Of these citations, after evaluating the titles and abstracts, 373 studies were chosen for further review by reading the full text. Among them, 353 literatures were excluded because 286 articles were irrelevant, 14 had no OR/RR values, 28 had no clearly MI endpoint, 3 were not treated PD as exposure and 22 had no original data. Finally 22 studies from 20 articles representing 129,630 participants were included in our meta-analysis [6–24, 31]. See Fig. 1 for the flow chart of the study selection process.

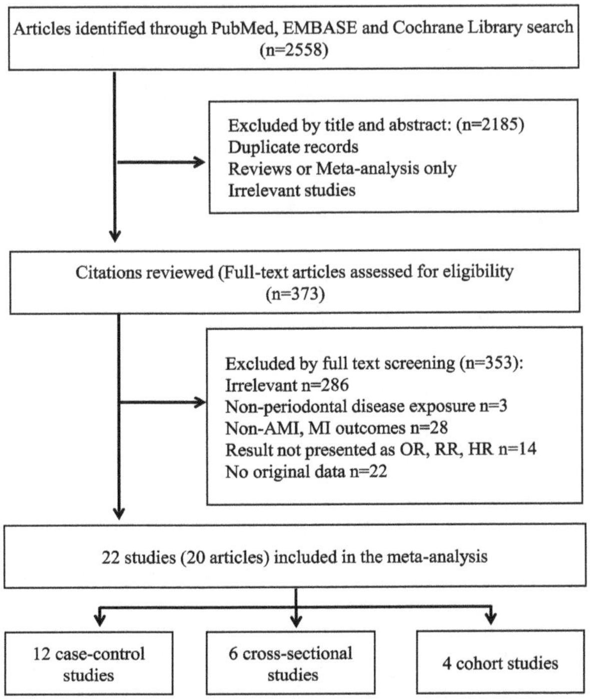

Fig. 1 Flow Chart for study selection

Study characteristics

The characteristics of each study were demonstrated in Table 1, with adjusted covariates of each study presented. Four prospective cohort studies, 6 cross-sectional and 12 case–control studies evaluated the association between PD and MI. Case–control studies included a total of 2912 cases of MI and 3291 controls [6–15, 24]. All studies were published from 1996 to 2016. The reported age ranged from 23 to 83 years. The enrolled years of patients varied from 1982 to 2014. Among 22 studies, 8 were carried out primarily in America [8, 9, 16, 18, 21–23], 5 studies were conducted in Asian countries [12, 13, 20, 31] and 9 studies were from European countries [6, 7, 10, 11, 14, 15, 17, 19, 24]. Sixteen articles reported the OR values between PD and MI, 2 articles gave the HR and 2 articles presented with RR values. In 2 of the studies, OR/RR was less than one [20, 24]. Only two studies did not perform the adjustments for potential confounders [10, 19]. Fourteen studies showed PD was associated with MI [6–17, 31], while 8 studies demonstrated PD was not related to MI [18–24, 31]. PD exposure parameters varied among studies including clinical attachment loss (CAL), probing depth, deep pockets, and periodontal bone loss. The quality of the studies was high overall, without remarkable limitations identified (Additional file 2: Table S2; Additional file 3: Table S3).

Meta-analysis

The OR/RR from 22 studies were pooled and analyzed as presented in Fig. 2. Overall, the PD had statistically significant correlation with MI risk (OR = 2.02, 95% CI 1.59-2.57). A severe statistical heterogeneity among studies was revealed ($Q = 152.77$, $P < 0.001$, $I^2 = 86.3\%$). Sensitivity analysis showed two studies contributed most to the heterogeneity [6, 10]. Although the sensitivity remains marked, the Q value and I^2 decreased to 70.68, and 73.1%, respectively. In the subgroup analysis by type of study (Fig. 3), cohort studies showed marginally increased risk of MI (RR 1.18, 95% CI 0.98-1.42; $I^2 = 64.8\%$, n = 4) [16, 21–23], while PD increased the risk of MI in both cross-sectional studies (OR 1.71, 95% CI 1.07-2.73; $I^2 = 16.7\%$, n = 6) [17–20, 31] and case–control studies (OR 2.93, 95% CI 1.95-4.39; $I^2 = 90.2\%$, n = 12) [6–15, 24].

By removing each study at a time, sensitivity analysis was conducted to determine the influence of each study on the pooled OR. By omitting one study in turn, the pooled OR and 95% CI was not modified significantly (Fig. 4). This sensitivity analysis indicated that the results of this meta-analysis were stable and reliable.

Additionally, publication bias was observed from Egger's Test ($P = 0.013$), Begg's Test ($P = 0.195$), and Funnel plot (Fig. 5). Trim and fill algorithm analysis was

Table 1 The characteristics of the studies included in the analysis

Cohort studies

Author, year	Country	Study design	Sample size (M/F)	Population	Years enrolled (Follow-up)	Age (years)	Exposure	OR/RR (95% CI)	*P* value	Adjusting factors
Joshipura KJ et al., 1996 [21]	USA	Prospective cohort study	44119 male	757 cases	1986-1992 (6)	40-75	PD	1.04 0.86-1.25	NS	Age, BMI, exercise, smoking, alcohol, family history of MI, vitamin E
Howell TH et al., 2001 [22]	USA	Prospective cohort study	2653 male	797 cases	1982-1995 (12.3)	40-84	PD	1.01 0.82-1.24	NS	Age, aspirin, β-carotene treatment, smoking, alcohol, HT, BMI, DM, physical activity, family history of MI
Dorn JM et al., 2010 [23]	USA	Prospective cohort study	884 (668/216)	154 cases	1996-2004 (2.9)	54.5 ± 8.4	CAL	1.48 0.95-2.31	NS	Age, gender, education, DM, EF, HT, physical activity, cholesterol, lipid-lowering medication, BMI, fruit/vegetable intake, CK-MB
Yu YH et al., 2015 [16]	USA	Prospective cohort study	39863 female	642 MI	1992-1995 (15.7)	48.7-60.3	PD	1.39 1.17-1.64	<0.001	Age

Cross-sectional studies

Author, year	Country	Sample size (M/F)	Population	Years enrolled	Age (years)	Exposure	OR/RR (95% CI)	*P* value	Adjusting factors
Bazile A et al., 2002 [18]	USA	80 (48/32)	50 CHD (20 MI)/ 30 control	2002	23-83 (median 54)	CAL	1.23 0.29-5.23	0.775	Age, gender
Buhlin K et al., 2002 [19]	Sweden	1577	1577 (27 MI)	1998	41-84	Deep pockets	1.32 0.51–3.38	0.57	NS
Holmlund A et al., 2006 [17]	Sweden	4254 (1866/2388)	3352 case/902 control	1976-2000	53 ± 14	Periodontal Bone Loss	2.69 1.12-6.46	0.03	Age, gender, smoking
Senba T et al., 2008 [31]	Japan	6,816 M	(MI = 25)	2004	NS	PD	2.34 1.05-5.23	NS	Age
Senba T et al., 2008 [31]	Japan	23,088 F	(MI = 16)	2004	NS	PD	1.76 0.64-4.88	NS	Age
Sujal M. Parkar et al., 2013 [20]	India	60 (42/18)	30 AMI/30 Control	2013	54.3 ± 11.0 (case); 53.1 ± 10.5 (control)	Community periodontal index	0.224 0.03-1.68	0.15	Age, sex, smoking, alcohol, BMI

Case–control studies

Author, year	Country	Sample size (M/F)	Population	Years enrolled	Age (years)	Exposure	OR/RR (95% CI)	P value	Adjusting factors
Persson GR et al., 2003 [6]	Sweden	160 (138/22)	80AMI/80control	2003	63.4 ± 8.9 (case) 61.9 ± 9.1 (control)	CAL	14.1 5.8-34.4	<0.0001	Smoking
Cueto A et al., 2005 [7]	Spain	149 (89/60)	72AMI/77control	2002	62.5 ± 9.9 (case) 58.5 ± 10.2 (control)	CAL	3.31 1.42–7.71	0.005	Sex, age, smoking, HT, DM, exercise, cholesterol
Andriankaja OM et al., 2006 [8]	USA	1337 (765/572)	537MI/ 800control	1997-2001	54.6 ± 8.5 (case) 55.0 ± 0.0 (control)	CAL	2.77 1.95-3.94	<0.001	Age, gender, HT, DM, cholesterol, smoking

Table 1 The characteristics of the studies included in the analysis *(Continued)*

Andriankaja OM et al., 2007 [9]	USA	782 M	415AMI/ 367control	1997-2001	54.5 ± 8.5 (case) 56.5 ± 10.2 (control)	CAL	1.34 1.15–1.57	<0.001	Age, BMI, HT, physical activity, cholesterol, DM, smoking
Andriankaja OM et al., 2007 [9]	USA	593 F	120AMI/ 473Control	1997-2001	55.5 ± 8.7 (case) 54.1 ± 9.8 (control)	CAL	2.08 1.47–2.94	<0.001	Age, BMI, physical activity, HT, cholesterol, DM, smoking
Renvert S et al., 2010 [10]	Sweden	324 (287/ 370)	165ACS/ 159control	2002-2007	31-87	PD	10.3 6.1-17.4	NS	NS
Holmlund A et al., 2011 [11]	Sweden	200 (160/ 40)	100AMI/ 100control	2011	57.1 ± 5.5 (case) 57.9 ± 5.2 (control)	Pockets depth	4.61 1.52-13.94	0.0069	Age, gender, CRP, HT, smoking, IL6, cholesterol, HDL-c, DM, TG, BMI, education,
Khosravi Samani M et al., 2013 [12]	Iran	123	60AMI/63control	2013	54.97 ± 9.68 (case) 55.89 ± 11.9 (control)	CAL	8.79 2.36-32.66	0.001	Age, DM
Li P et al., 2013 [13]	China	155 (113/ 42)	103AMI/ 52control	2013	68 (41-84) (case) 62 (42-78)(control)	CAL	4.89 1.26-18.94	0.02	HT, total cholesterol HDL, BMI, LDL
Willershausen I et al., 2014 [24]	Germany	497 (380/ 117)	248AMI/ 249control	2007-2011	62.3 (51-83)	PD	0.879 0.527-1.466	0.622	Gender, age, smoking
Kodovazenitis G, et al., 2014 [14]	Greece	306 (218/ 88)	204MI/102 control	2007-2009	64.7 ± 12.9 (case) 64.2 ± 10.1 (control)	CAL	2.27 1.22-4.35	0.01	Age, gender, HT, total cholesterol, smoking
Rydén L et al., 2016 [15]	Sweden	1610 (1308/302)	805MI/ 805control	2010-2014	62.5 ± 8	PD	1.28 1.03-1.60	NS	DM, smoking, education, marital status

BMI **body mass index,** ***CAL*** **clinical attachment loss,** ***CI*** **confidence interval,** ***CK-MB*****, creatine phosphokinase-myocardial band,** ***CRP*** **C-response protein,** ***DM*** **diabetes mellitus,** ***EF*** **ejection fraction,** ***HDL-c*** **high-density lipoprotein cholesterol,** ***HT*** **hypertension,** ***MI*** **myocardial infarction,** ***NS*** **not specified,** ***OR*** **odd ratio,** ***PD*** **periodontal disease,** ***RR*** **relative risk,** ***TG*** **triglycerides**
If the studies specified the PD exposure parameters, the detailed PD parameters would be displayed in this table. Otherwise, the PD would be considered as exposure factor

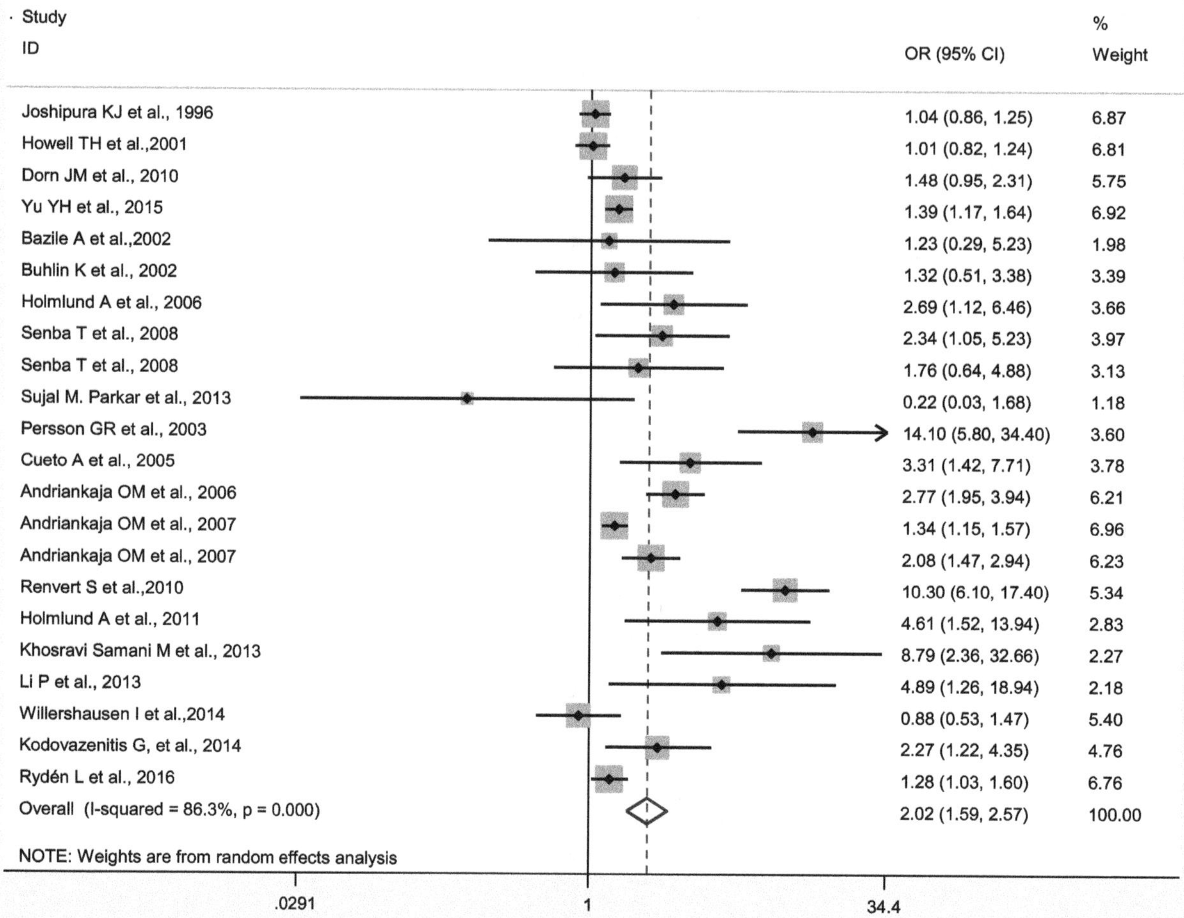

Fig. 2 Meta-analysis of observational studies on periodontal disease and myocardial infarction in a random-effect model. OR, odds ratio; RR, relative ratio; CI, confidence interval

performed and the analysis showed "no trimming performed; data unchanged".

Subgroup analysis

To examine the stability of the studies, subgroup analyses were carried out based on several factors. Patients with PD had increased risk of MI across most subgroups by location, PD exposure parameters and study quality (Table 2). In the gender-specific subgroup, 3 female pooled studies showed an increased risk of MI (OR = 1.64, 95% CI 1.20-2.25) [8, 18, 23], while the pooled results in the 4 male studies were marginally increased (OR = 1.18, 95% CI 0.96-1.44) [9, 21, 22, 31]. Overall, subgroup analyses by various factors demonstrated that patients with PD have a higher risk to develop MI.

Discussion

In this study, we identified a statistical positive correlation between PD and MI. Patients with PD have approximately a 1-fold increase in risk for MI. Given the high prevalence of PD in population [32], this increase might mean a profound public health impact.

Several meta-analyses have reported that subjects with PD have higher odds and higher risks of developing cardiovascular diseases [33–38]. Teeuw et al pooled 25 studies on treatment of periodontitis and demonstrated intervention of PD improved the atherosclerotic profile [39], but the direct evidence of reduction in the risk of cardiovascular events associated with periodontitis treatment remains lacking. Further, a meta-analysis reported that patients with periodontitis compared to controls have increased arterial stiffness [39]. However, the only two interventional studies contradicted with each other

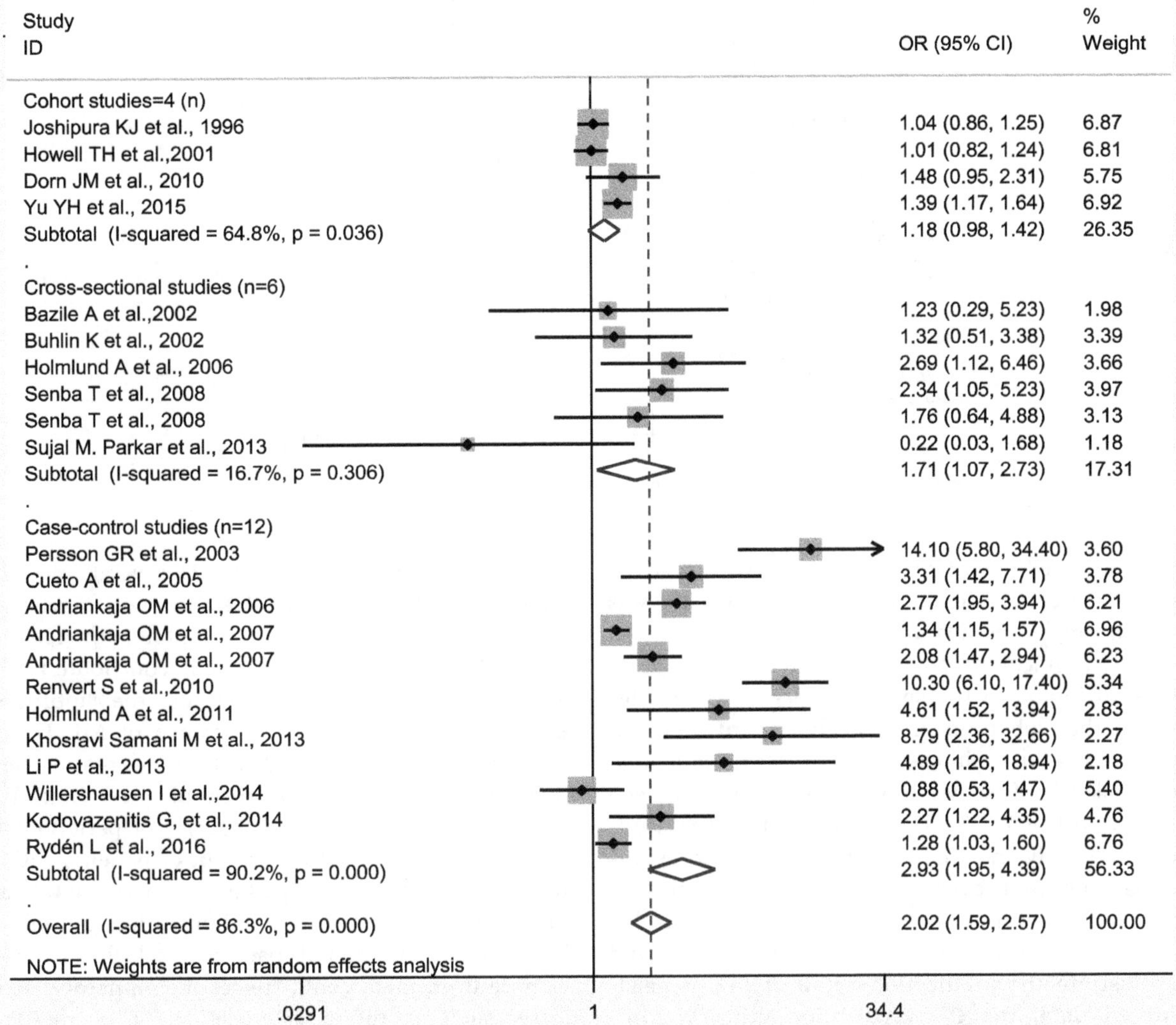

Fig. 3 Association between periodontal disease and myocardial infarction in a random-effect model meta-analyses by study design. OR, odds ratio; RR, relative ratio; CI, confidence interval

on the effects of periodontal treatment on arterial stiffness [40]. Therefore, PD appears to be associated with increased risk of CVD, but the causal relation is still not well established.

Myocardial infarction is one of the most life-threating cardiovascular diseases. Some investigations mentioned the relationship between PD and MI, while dispute exists. In 1996, Joshipural KJ's group followed up a cohort including 44119 males for 6 years and found no overall association between PD and fatal or non-fatal MI in this population [21]. This negative result was further echoed by some other prospective cohort studies [22, 23]. However, a large body of evidence showed there was an association between PD and MI. Very recently a large case–control study indicated that the risk of MI was significantly increased in patients with PD even after adjustment for confounding factors [15]. These disputes required further systemic analyses on the relation between MI and PD. However, to the best of our knowledge, no meta-analyses specified the relation between PD and MI.

In this study, we have showed an overall increased risk for MI in PD patients. The subgroup meta-analyses by study design showed that PD was associated with MI in both cross-sectional and case–control studies, while the relation in the cohort studies was marginal. Likewise, the subgroup analyses by country, PD exposure, participant number and study quality consistently showed an

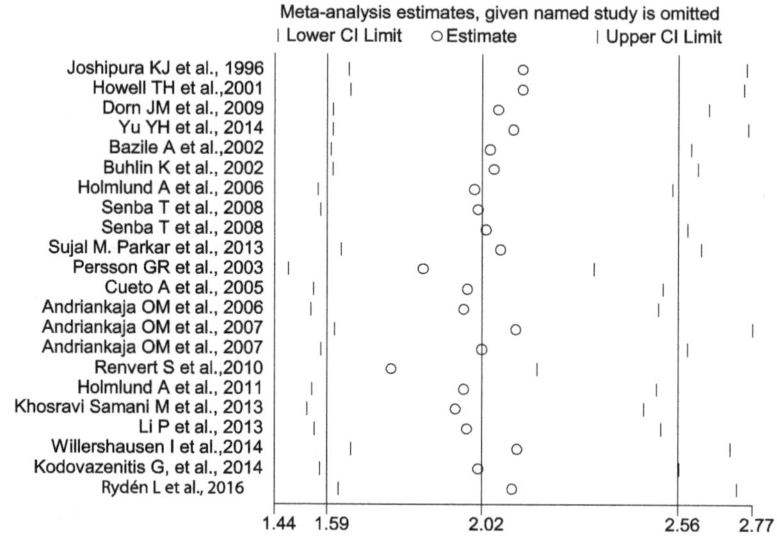

Fig. 4 Sensitivity analysis on meta-analysis between periodontal disease and myocardial infarction

apparent increased risk of MI in PD subjects. Moreover, a marginal but non-significant increase of risk was present in male population. These non-significant findings exist in cohort studies and male participants might be attributed to the small number of studies included in the subgroup meta-analyses. Intriguingly, Rydén L group in their case–control study specified that the risk of a first MI was significantly increased in patients with PD. [15] However, most of the studies did not clarify the MI occurrence which presumably might be first ever MI. Renvert S et al also reported the relation between PD and recurrent MI [10]. First and recurrent MI differentiation would better illustrate the predication value of PD. Regarding limited data, the PD predication efficacy comparison between first and recurrent MI remains unknown.

Although not fully illustrated, several mechanisms were speculated to be involved in such a relation between PD and MI. The periodontal pathogen burden and its by-products might not only contribute to the development of atherosclerosis but also the rupture of atherosclerotic plaques and occurrence of MI. Dozens of literature has demonstrated that periodontal bacteria are detected in from atherosclerotic plaques. Ohki T et al. further suggested that three species of periodontal bacteria were present in the thrombi of patients with acute MI [41]. This finding suggested that periodontal bacteria might play a role in plaque inflammation and instability. Meanwhile, periodontal bacteria and the lipopolysaccharide from them could trigger inflammatory factor release, such as tumor necrosis factor α, interleukins, whose roles are well established in atherogenesis and rupture of developed lesions [42]. Further, C-reactive

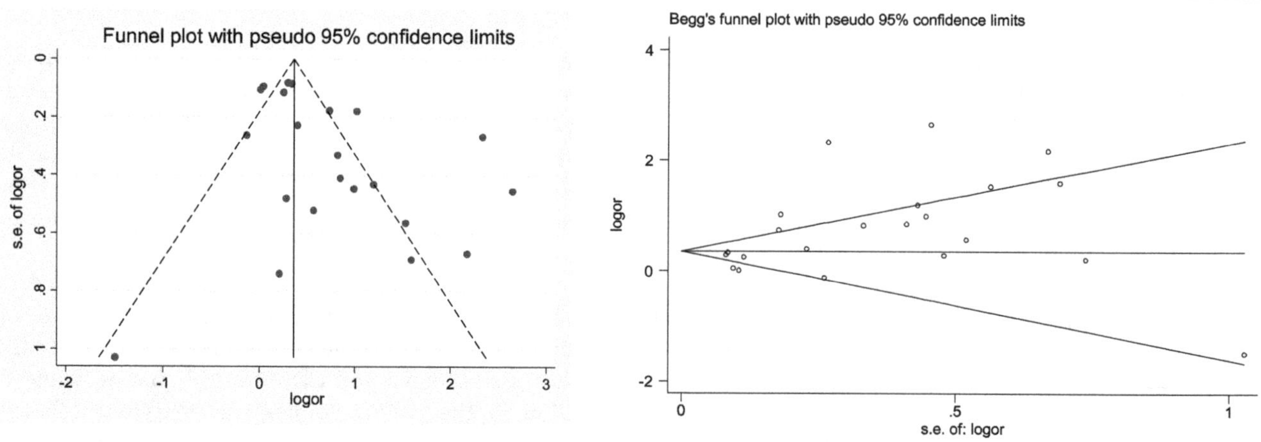

Fig. 5 Funnel plot of the included studies for publication bias

Table 2 Subgroup analysis

Group	Number of studies	Pooled RR	95% CI	*P* (heterogeneity)	I^2 (%)
All studies	22	2.02	1.59-2.57	0.000	86.3%
Location					
America	8	1.44	1.16-1.78	0.000	81.1%
Asia	9	2.93	1.52-5.65	0.000	90.7%
Europe	5	2.44	1.01-5.86	0.0033	61.8%
Gender					
Female	3	1.64	1.20-2.25	0.117	53.4%
Male	4	1.18	0.96-1.44	0.026	67.6%
Exposure					
CAL	10	2.66	1.80-3.94	0.000	82.5%
Others	12	1.65	1.20-2.27	0.000	87.3%
Study quality					
High	12	2.29	1.61-3.25	0.000	91.0%
Low and moderate	10	1.66	1.20-2.29	0.001	66.5%
Number of participants					
> 1000	9	1.46	1.16-1.83	0.000	76.8%
< 1000	13	2.69	1.68-4.30	0.000	88.3%

protein (CRP), a non-specific acute-phase factor participating in the systemic response to inflammation, helps to improve the risk prediction of cardiovascular events. Patients with PD also have increased serum levels of CRP relative to unaffected subjects [43]. The level of infection with periodontal pathogens is positively correlated with CRP level [44]. These evidence suggests that CRP might underlie the relation between PD and MI. In addition, platelet aggregation and thrombo-embolic events could be activated by periodontal pathogens themselves and many other cytokines [38].

Heterogeneity among studies was revealed in this analysis, although the relation between PD and MI has similar tendency in the overall and subgroup analysis. The significant heterogeneity was also reported in meta-analysis on PD and cardiovascular diseases [45, 46]. By nature, the diagnosis of PD was quite variable and included a series of parameters, such as attachment loss, bone loss pocket, probing depth, bleeding on probing, plaque index, gingival index, X-ray and microbiological results, teeth loss and the Russell periodontal index. Different PD assessment resulted in discrepancy when analyzing the relation between PD and MI. Renvert S' group compared 5 PD parameters and their combination, founding that comprehensive PD data should be used in studies of associations between periodontitis and heart diseases [47]. Many other risk factors including age, smoking, and diabetes are common in both PD and MI. These factors could be taken into consideration as confounding factor. Different confounding factors were adjusted as demonstrated in Table1. This different adjustment could also affect the adjusted OR/RR when investigating the relation between PD and MI. Moreover, study design, study quality, number of participants and location were examined to find the sources of heterogeneity. The subgroup analysis showed these factors did not appreciably change the heterogeneity among studies. Further, sensitivity analyses showed no alterations to the pooled OR by omitting each study. Together, the significant heterogeneity should be considered when interpreting the results in this study, although the strong relation between PD and MI are observed.

Most of the studies that exclude for the meta-analysis in this study also supported a positive association between PD and MI. A population-based study showed periodontitis was associated with an increased risk of major adverse cardiac events including MI occurrence [48]. Other studies also indicated that PD may be associated with MI in Turkish and Iran population [49, 50]. Vice versa, there was higher prevalence of edentulousness and advanced PD in the hospitalized MI group than that in the non-MI group [51]. A case–control study also showed MI patients exhibited an unfavorable dental chronic infection compared with healthy patients. These data from the other angle suggests an association between PD and MI.

Several limitation of this meta-analysis should be noted. First, limited by the nature of observational studies, the causality between PD and MI cannot be inferred from our findings. Second, as aforementioned, definitions for PD in each study included in the analysis were not identical. Although we set rules when extracting data, this discrepancy in the assessments for PD seemed not to be eliminated nor even decreased obviously. Additionally, the differences in the study design, population and criteria to measure the exposure may weaken the evidence and lead to considerable heterogeneity. Although further analysis were performed, the sources of the heterogeneity remained not clear. The meta-regression analysis might further explain the source of heterogeneity. For the paucity of the data, these analyses were not conducted. Finally, the concrete mechanisms to explain the PD and MI relation still need further investigation, though possible mechanisms were discussed above. Further prospective studies are warranted to establish the association between PD and MI, while it might also be helpful to confirm the relation with randomized, controlled interventional trials including medication to control the pain and inflammation and surgery to remove the inflamed tissue and reduce the bone damage.

Conclusion

In conclusion, our meta-analysis yielded a statistically significant association between PD and MI. Subgroup analyses also confirmed the elevated risk for MI in PD subjects, although heterogeneity should be noted. More studies including large-scale prospective cohort studies and randomized controlled trials are warranted.

Abbreviations

AHRQ: Agency for healthcare research and quality; CAL: Clinical attachment loss; CIs: Confidence intervals; CRP: C-reactive protein; CVDs: Cardiovascular diseases; HR: Hazard ratio; MI: Myocardial infarction; MOOSE: Meta-analysis of observational studies in epidemiology; OR: Odds ratio; PD: Periodontal disease; PRISMA: Preferred reporting items for systematic reviews and meta-analyses; RR: Relative risk

Acknowledgements

None.

Funding

Study design, data collection, analysis and interpretation of data and writing the manuscript has been conducted by staff of the Third Military Medical University, Chongqing, China.

Authors' contributions

S. Xu and Z. Qin designed this study. S. Xu and X. Liu searched the databases and selected the studies according to the criteria and exclusion criteria. M. Song and Y Xiong helped develop search strategies. S. Xu, Y. He and M. Song extracted data and conducted the statistics. Z. Qin wrote the draft of the paper. All authors participated in the process of discussion, review, and revision of the paper.

Competing interests

None.

Author details

[1]Department of Stomatology, Xinqiao Hospital, Third Military Medical University, 400037 Chongqing, China. [2]Department of Cardiology, Xinqiao Hospital, Third Military Medical University, 183 Xinqiaozhengjie St., Shapingba District, 400037 Chongqing, China. [3]Department of Stomatology, Southwest Hospital, Third Military Medical University, 400038 Chongqing, China.

References

1. Albandar JM, Brunelle JA, Kingman A. Destructive periodontal disease in adults 30 years of age and older in the United States, 1988-1994. J Periodontol. 1999;70(1):13–29.
2. Pihlstrom BL, Michalowicz BS, Johnson NW. Periodontal diseases. Lancet. 2005;366(9499):1809–20.
3. You Z, Cushman M, Jenny NS, Howard G. Regards. Tooth loss, systemic inflammation, and prevalent stroke among participants in the reasons for geographic and racial difference in stroke (REGARDS) study. Atherosclerosis. 2009;203(2):615–9.
4. Lockhart PB, Bolger AF, Papapanou PN, Osinbowale O, Trevisan M, Levison ME, et al. Periodontal disease and atherosclerotic vascular disease: does the evidence support an independent association?: a scientific statement from the American Heart Association. Circulation. 2012;125(20):2520–44.
5. Mattila KJ, Nieminen MS, Valtonen W, Rasi VP, Kesaniemi YA, Syrjala SL, et al. Association between dental health and acute myocardial infarction. BMJ. 1989;298(6676):779–81.
6. Rutger Persson G, Ohlsson O, Pettersson T, Renvert S. Chronic periodontitis, a significant relationship with acute myocardial infarction. Eur Heart J. 2003; 24(23):2108–15.
7. Cueto A, Mesa F, Bravo M, Ocana-Riola R. Periodontitis as risk factor for acute myocardial infarction. A case control study of Spanish adults. J Periodontal Res. 2005;40(1):36–42.
8. Andriankaja OM, Genco RJ, Dorn J, Dmochowski J, Hovey K, Falkner KL, et al. The use of different measurements and definitions of periodontal disease in the study of the association between periodontal disease and risk of myocardial infarction. J Periodontol. 2006;77(6):1067–73.
9. Andriankaja OM, Genco RJ, Dorn J, Dmochowski J, Hovey K, Falkner KL, et al. Periodontal disease and risk of myocardial infarction: the role of gender and smoking. Eur J Epidemiol. 2007;22(10):699–705.
10. Renvert S, Ohlsson O, Pettersson T, Persson GR. Periodontitis: a future risk of acute coronary syndrome? A follow-up study over 3 years. J Periodontol. 2010;81(7):992–1000.
11. Holmlund A, Hedin M, Pussinen PJ, Lerner UH, Lind L. Porphyromonas gingivalis (Pg) a possible link between impaired oral health and acute myocardial infarction. Int J Cardiol. 2011;148(2):148–53.
12. Samani MK, Jalali F, Ahadi SMS, Hoseini SR, Sattari FD. The relationship between acute myocardial infarction and periodontitis. Caspian J Intern Med. 2013;4(2):667–71.
13. Li P, He L, Sha YQ, Luan QX. Periodontal status of patients with post-acute myocardial infarction. Beijing da xue xue bao. 2013;45(1):22–6.
14. Kodovazenitis G, Pitsavos C, Papadimitriou L, Vrotsos IA, Stefanadis C, Madianos PN. Association between periodontitis and acute myocardial infarction: a case-control study of a nondiabetic population. J Periodontal Res. 2014;49(2):246–52.
15. Ryden L, Buhlin K, Ekstrand E, de Faire U, Gustafsson A, Holmer J, et al. Periodontitis Increases the Risk of a First Myocardial Infarction: A Report From the PAROKRANK Study. Circulation. 2016;133(6):576–83.
16. Yu YH, Chasman DI, Buring JE, Rose L, Ridker PM. Cardiovascular risks associated with incident and prevalent periodontal disease. J Clin Periodontol. 2015;42(1):21–8.
17. Holmlund A, Holm G, Lind L. Severity of periodontal disease and number of remaining teeth are related to the prevalence of myocardial infarction and hypertension in a study based on 4,254 subjects. J Periodontol. 2006;77(7):1173–8.
18. Bazile A, Bissada NF, Nair R, Siegel BP. Periodontal assessment of patients undergoing angioplasty for treatment of coronary artery disease. J Periodontol. 2002;73(6):631–6.
19. Buhlin K, Gustafsson A, Håkansson J, Klinge B. Oral health and cardiovascular disease in Sweden. J Clin Periodontol. 2002;29(3):254–9.
20. Parkar SM, Modi GN, Jani J. Periodontitis as risk factor for acute myocardial infarction: A case control study. Heart Views. 2013;14(1):5–11.

21. Joshipura KJ, Rimm EB, Douglass CW, Trichopoulos D, Ascherio A, Willett WC. Poor oral health and coronary heart disease. J Dent Res. 1996;75(9):1631–6.
22. Howell TH, Ridker PM, Ajani UA, Hennekens CH, Christen WG. Periodontal disease and risk of subsequent cardiovascular disease in U.S. male physicians. J Am Coll Cardiol. 2001;37(2):445–50.
23. Dorn JM, Genco RJ, Grossi SG, Falkner KL, Hovey KM, Iacoviello L, et al. Periodontal disease and recurrent cardiovascular events in survivors of myocardial infarction (MI): the Western New York Acute MI Study. J Periodontol. 2010;81(4):502–11.
24. Willershausen I, Weyer V, Peter M, Weichert C, Kasaj A, Munzel T, et al. Association between chronic periodontal and apical inflammation and acute myocardial infarction. Odontology. 2014;102(2):297–302.
25. Stroup DF, Berlin JA, Morton SC, Olkin I, Williamson GD, Rennie D, et al. Meta-analysis of observational studies in epidemiology: a proposal for reporting. Meta-analysis Of Observational Studies in Epidemiology (MOOSE) group. JAMA. 2000;283(15):2008–12.
26. Liberati A, Altman DG, Tetzlaff J, Mulrow C, Gotzsche PC, Ioannidis JP, et al. The PRISMA statement for reporting systematic reviews and meta-analyses of studies that evaluate healthcare interventions: explanation and elaboration. BMJ. 2009;339:b2700.
27. Stang A. Critical evaluation of the Newcastle-Ottawa scale for the assessment of the quality of nonrandomized studies in meta-analyses. Eur J Epidemiol. 2010;25(9):603–5.
28. Owens DK, Lohr KN, Atkins D, Treadwell JR, Reston JT, Bass EB, et al. AHRQ series paper 5: grading the strength of a body of evidence when comparing medical interventions–agency for healthcare research and quality and the effective health-care program. J Clin Epidemiol. 2010;63(5):513–23.
29. Hu J, Dong Y, Chen X, Liu Y, Ma D, Liu X, et al. Prevalence of suicide attempts among Chinese adolescents: A meta-analysis of cross-sectional studies. Compr Psychiatry. 2015;61:78–89.
30. Walter SD, Cook RJ. A comparison of several point estimators of the odds ratio in a single 2 x 2 contingency table. Biometrics. 1991;47(3):795–811.
31. Senba T, Kobayashi Y, Inoue K, Kaneto C, Indue M, Toyokawa S, et al. The association between self-reported periodontitis and coronary heart disease - From my health up study. J Occup Health. 2008;50(3):283–7.
32. Brown LJ, Brunelle JA, Kingman A. Periodontal status in the United States, 1988-1991: prevalence, extent, and demographic variation. J Dent Res. 1996; 75 Spec No:672-683.
33. Leng WD, Zeng XT, Kwong JS, Hua XP. Periodontal disease and risk of coronary heart disease: An updated meta-analysis of prospective cohort studies. Int J Cardiol. 2015;201:469–72.
34. Khader YS, Albashaireh ZS, Alomari MA. Periodontal diseases and the risk of coronary heart and cerebrovascular diseases: a meta-analysis. J Periodontol. 2004;75(8):1046–53.
35. Janket SJ, Baird AE, Chuang SK, Jones JA. Meta-analysis of periodontal disease and risk of coronary heart disease and stroke. Oral Surg Oral Med Oral Pathol Oral Radiol Endod. 2003;95(5):559–69.
36. Humphrey LL, Fu R, Buckley DI, Freeman M, Helfand M. Periodontal disease and coronary heart disease incidence: a systematic review and meta-analysis. J Gen Intern Med. 2008;23(12):2079–86.
37. Beck JD, Offenbacher S. The association between periodontal diseases and cardiovascular diseases: a state-of-the-science review. Ann Periodontol. 2001;6(1):9–15.
38. Bahekar AA, Singh S, Saha S, Molnar J, Arora R. The prevalence and incidence of coronary heart disease is significantly increased in periodontitis: a meta-analysis. Am Heart J. 2007;154(5):830–7.
39. Teeuw WJ, Slot DE, Susanto H, Gerdes VE, Abbas F, D'Aiuto F, et al. Treatment of periodontitis improves the atherosclerotic profile: a systematic review and meta-analysis. J Clin Periodontol. 2014;41(1):70–9.
40. Vidal F, Cordovil I, Figueredo CM, Fischer RG. Non-surgical periodontal treatment reduces cardiovascular risk in refractory hypertensive patients: a pilot study. J Clin Periodontol. 2013;40(7):681–7.
41. Ohki T, Itabashi Y, Kohno T, Yoshizawa A, Nishikubo S, Watanabe S, et al. Detection of periodontal bacteria in thrombi of patients with acute myocardial infarction by polymerase chain reaction. Am Heart J. 2012;163(2):164–7.
42. Libby P. Inflammation in atherosclerosis. Arterioscler Thromb Vasc Biol. 2012; 32(9):2045–51.
43. Slade GD, Ghezzi EM, Heiss G, Beck JD, Riche E, Offenbacher S. Relationship between periodontal disease and C-reactive protein among adults in the Atherosclerosis Risk in Communities study. Arch Intern Med. 2003;163(10):1172–9.
44. Dye BA, Choudhary K, Shea S, Papapanou PN. Serum antibodies to periodontal pathogens and markers of systemic inflammation. J Clin Periodontol. 2005;32(12):1189–99.
45. Blaizot A, Vergnes JN, Nuwwareh S, Amar J, Sixou M. Periodontal diseases and cardiovascular events: meta-analysis of observational studies. Int Dent J. 2009;59(4):197–209.
46. Martin-Cabezas Rodrigo SN. Petit Catherine, Agossa K′evimy, Gaertner S′ ebastien, Tenenbaum Henri, Davideau Jean-Luc, et al. Association between periodontitis and arterial hypertension: A systematic review and meta-analysis. Am Heart J. 2016;180:98–112.
47. Renvert S, Ohlsson O, Persson S, Lang NP, Persson GR. Analysis of periodontal risk profiles in adults with or without a history of myocardial infarction. J Clin Periodontol. 2004;31(1):19–24.
48. Chou SH, Tung YC, Lin YS, Wu LS, Lin CP, Liou EJ, et al. Major Adverse Cardiovascular Events in Treated Periodontitis: A Population-Based Follow-Up Study from Taiwan. PLoS One. 2015;10(6):e0130807.
49. Emingil G, Buduneli E, Aliyev A, Akilli A, Atilla G. Association between periodontal disease and acute myocardial infarction. J Periodontol. 2000; 71(12):1882–6.
50. Amoian B, Maboudi A, Abbasi V. A periodontal health assessment of hospitalized patients with myocardial infarction. Caspian J Intern Med. 2011;2(2):234–9.
51. Wozakowska-Kaplon B, Wlosowicz M, Gorczyca-Michta I, Gorska R. Oral health status and the occurrence and clinical course of myocardial infarction in hospital phase: a case-control study. Cardiol J. 2013;20(4):370–7.

21

Myocardial infarction during anaphylaxis in a young healthy male with normal coronary arteries- is epinephrine the culprit?

W. D. Jayamali*, H. M. M. T. B. Herath and Aruna Kulathunga

Abstract

Background: Anaphylaxis is an acute, potentially fatal medical emergency. Myocardial injury or infarction in the setting of an anaphylaxis can be due the anaphylaxis itself, when it is known as Kounis syndrome or it can also be due to the effect of epinephrine treatment. Epinephrine is considered as the cornerstone in management of anaphylaxis. Myocardial infarction secondary to therapeutic doses of adrenaline is a rare occurrence and only a few cases have been reported in literature. The mechanism of myocardial injury was considered to be due to coronary vasospasm secondary to epinephrine as the coronary angiograms were normal on these occasions.

Case presentation: A 21-year- old previously healthy male got admitted to the local hospital with an urticarial rash and difficulty in breathing, one hour after ingestion of prawns for which he was known to be allergic. He was treated with 0.5 ml of intramuscular adrenaline (1:1000) which was administered to the lateral side of the thigh, following which he developed palpitations and tightening type central chest pain. Electrocardiogram showed ST segment depressions in leads III, aVF and V1 to V5 and he was transferred to a tertiary care hospital. The second electrocardiogram, done 2 h later, showed resolution of ST segment depressions but new T inversions in leads I and aVL. Troponin I was elevated with a titer of 2.15 ng/ml. He was treated with sublingual GTN in the emergency treatment unit and the symptoms resolved. Transthoracic 2D echocardiogram and stress testing with treadmill was normal and CT coronary angiogram revealed normal coronary arteries.

Conclusion: Here we present a case of a young healthy adult with no significant risk factors for coronary artery disease who developed myocardial infarction following intramuscular administration of therapeutic dose of adrenalin for an anaphylactic reaction. The postulated mechanism is most likely an alpha receptor mediated coronary vascular spasm. However the use of adrenaline in the setting of life threatening anaphylaxis is life saving and the benefits far outweigh the risks of adverse effects. Therefore the purpose of reporting this case is not to discourage the use of adrenaline in anaphylaxis but to make aware of this potential adverse effect which can occur in the acute setting.

Keywords: Anaphylaxis, Epinephrine, Myocardial infarction

* Correspondence: dhanushka.withanage1987@gmail.com
National Hospital, Colombo, Sri Lanka

Background

Myocardial infarction occurring in the context of an anaphylactic reaction can occur due two possible reasons. One being the anaphylaxis itself causing allergic myocardial infarction, known as Kounis syndrome and the other being the use of epinephrine resulting in myocardial injury. Epinephrine is considered as the cornerstone in the management of anaphylaxis. Intramuscular injection of 1:1000 adrenaline to a maximum dose of 0.5 mg is recommended in the management of anaphylaxis [1, 2]. Intravenous use is less often used in anaphylaxis. There have been a few cases of myocardial infarction occurring as a result of therapeutic doses adrenaline for anaphylaxis, reported in the previous case reports [3–7].The mechanism of myocardial injury was considered to be due to coronary vasospasm secondary to epinephrine as the coronary angiograms were normal in these occasions.

Here we report a case of a young healthy male who developed myocardial infarction following administration of therapeutic dose of intramuscular adrenaline for an anaphylaxis.

Case presentation

A 21-year-old Sri Lankan male developed urticaria and difficulty in breathing one hour after ingestion of prawns, for which he was known to be allergic. He got admitted to the local hospital 2 h after the onset of symptoms. On admission to the local hospital he was dyspnoeic with a respiratory rate of 28/min and widespread rhonchi. His pulse rate was 94 beats per minute and the blood pressure was 100/70 mmHg. He was treated with intravenous hydrocortisone 200 mg, intravenous chlorpheniramine 10 mg and 0.5 ml of adrenaline (1:1000 solution) intramuscularly to the upper lateral side of the thigh (vastus lateralis). Ten minutes after the administration of adrenalin, he developed palpitations and tightening type central chest pain with autonomic symptoms. The pain lasted for about 30 min and resolved spontaneously. The first electrocardiogram (ECG), which was taken at the local hospital showed a sinus tachycardia and ST segment depressions in leads III, aVF and V1 to V5(Fig. 1). He was not given any treatment for the chest pain in the local hospital and was transferred to our hospital about 2 h from the onset of the pain.

On admission to our hospital, he was not dyspnoeic and his pulse rate was 100 beats per minute and the blood pressure was 100/60 mmHg. His respiratory rate was 18/min and had a few rhonchi on auscultation. Rest of the examination was normal. The second ECG which was done in our hospital, 2 h after the 1st one, showed resolution of ST segment depressions but new T inversions in leads I and aVL (Fig. 1). These T in versions persisted in subsequent ECGs (Fig. 1). Troponin I done 6 h after the event was positive with a titer 2.15 ng/ml (<0.5). The test was repeated on the second day and it was still positive with a tire of 0.69 ng/ml. He was given sublingual glyceryl trinitrate 0.4 mg single dose after admission to our hospital. However antiplatelets and statins were not given and anticoagulation was not started as the most likely cause was assumed to be coronary vasospasm rather than plaque rupture.

He was previously healthy and did not have any risk factors for premature coronary vascular disease such as smoking. He has had a history urticaria to prawns but there was no previous history of anaphylaxis. He did not have asthma. There was no family history of diabetes, ischemic heart disease or premature deaths due to cardiovascular diseases. He worked as a computer operator trainee and was unmarried.

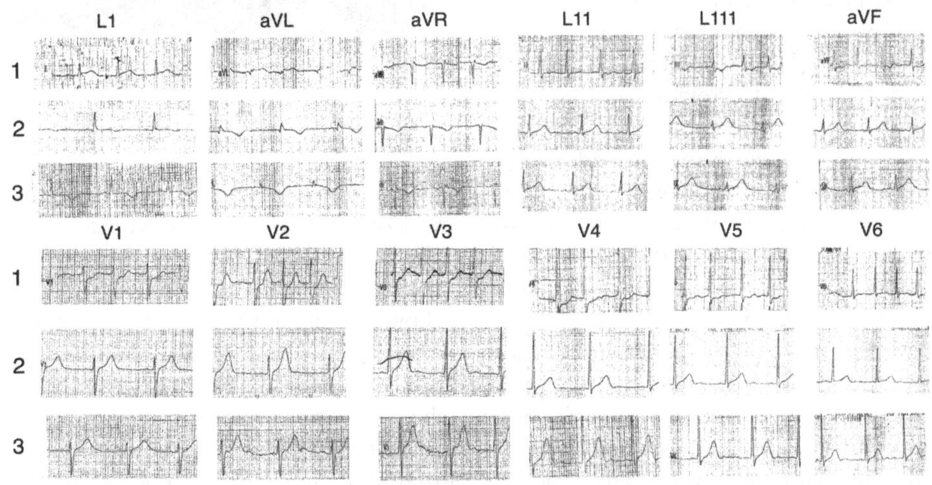

Fig. 1 Electrocardiograms taken after adrenaline administration. 1 = The first ECG which taken at the local hospital (15 min after the chest pain / 25 min after the adrenalin) showing a sinus tachycardia of 109/min and ST segment depression in leads III, aVF and V1 to V5. 2 = The Second ECG taken 2 h after the 1st one showing resolution of ST segment depressions and new T inversions in leads I and aVL. 3 = T inversions persisted in subsequent ECGs

Further investigations which were done at our unit included transthoracic 2D echocardiogram which revealed an ejection fraction of 60% with no wall motion abnormalities. We did not proceed with a coronary angiogram as the patient was a young healthy adult and the cardiology team concluded that coronary artery vasospasm to be the likely cause for the myocardial ischaemia rather than atherosclerotic coronary artery disease. Subsequent stress ECG with treadmill was normal and CT coronary angiogram revealed normal coronary arteries (Fig. 2). Complete blood count and renal functions were normal. Chest x ray was also normal. Fasting blood sugar was 98 mg/dl and the lipid profile was normal.

Patient was asymptomatic during the hospital stay and was discharged after 2 days. At subsequent reviews he remained asymptomatic.

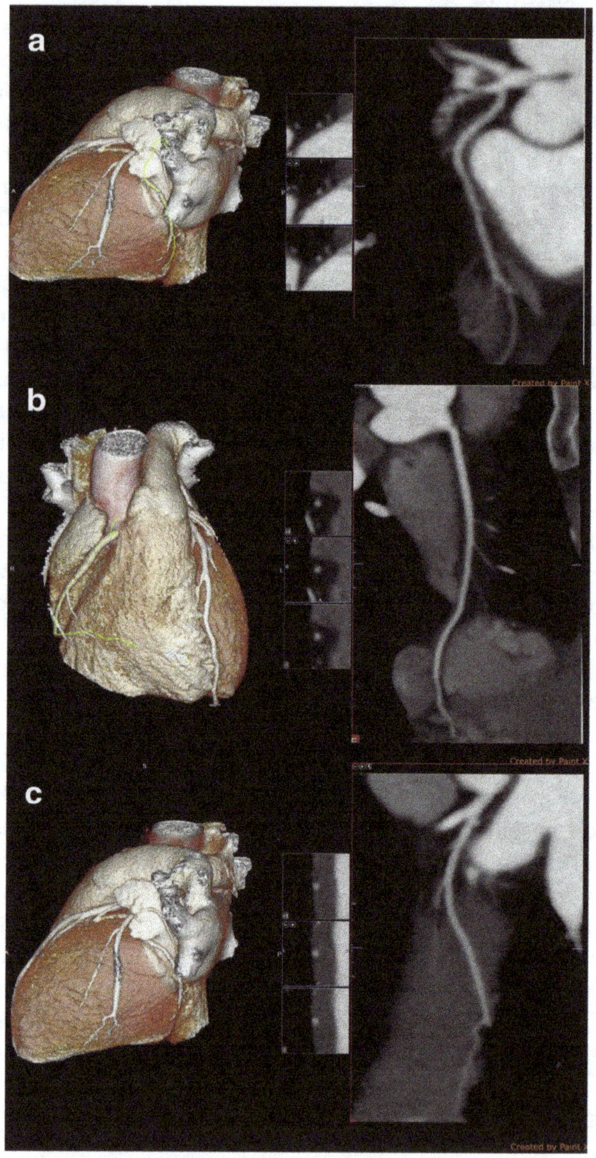

Fig. 2 Normal CT coronary angiogram. **a** = Normal left circumflex artery. **b** = Normal Right coronary artery and posterior descending artery. **c** = Normal Ramus intermedius artery

Discussion and conclusion

The patient presented in this case fulfilled the criteria for an acute myocardial infarction according to the universal definition of myocardial infarction as the patient had elevated cardiac troponins above 99th centile of the upper limit with a falling pattern with clinical evidence of ischemic type chest pain and significant new ST and T wave changes [8]. It is most likely type 2 myocardial infarction according to the third universal classification of myocardial infarction because the most likely underlying mechanism is coronary vasospasm [8].

Myocardial injury or infarction in the setting of an anaphylaxis can be due the anaphylaxis itself, when it is known as Kounis syndrome or can also due to the effect of epinephrine treatment. Kounis syndrome or allergic angina is an acute coronary syndrome occurring in association with conditions that involves mast cell activation such as hypersensitivity reaction,anaphylactic or anaphylactoid conditions [9–11].The chemical mediators that are involved are neutral proteases including tryptase and chymase, arachidonic acid products, histamine, platelet activating factor and a variety of cytokines and chemokines. It is believed that these mediators induce coronary vasospasm resulting in myocardial ischemia and infarction. Kounis syndrome consists of 3 variants. Type I is where patients with normal coronary arteries without predisposing factors for coronary artery disease develop coronary artery spasm with normal cardiac biomarkers or infarction with elevated biomarkers. This is most likely due to endothelial dysfunction or microvascular angina. The type II variant includes patients with inactive but quiescent preexisting atheromatous plaques, in whom the allergic insult leads to plaque erosion or rupture, leading to acute coronary event. The type III variant includes coronary artery stent thrombosis secondary to allergic reaction [9, 10]. There were several reported cases of patients where they have developed acute coronary syndrome following allergic reaction,-most of which have occurred prior to receiving epinephrine and only one occasion where it occurred after the use of epinephrine [12, 13].

Epinephrine induced myocardial infarction in the setting of management of anaphylaxis has been reported only on a few occasions. There have been five reported cases where therapeutic doses of epinephrine had caused myocardial infarction [3–7]. Out of these reports one was after intravenous injection, another after intramuscular use of epinephrine and two cases following subcutaneous injection and one other where a subcutaneous epi pen auto injector use. The cases by Shaver and colleagues,

Ferry and colleagues, Rubio and colleagues and Saff and colleagues were similar to our patient as the patients were previously healthy individuals and have developed myocardial infarction after use of epinephrine and normal coronary arteries were demonstrated later. However in the case reported by Cunnigton and colleagues, the patient described had been on propranolol before the incident and they have identified it as a potential predisposing factory for epinephrine induced vasospasm.

Our patient was a 21 year old young healthy male who did not have any modifiable or non-modifiable risk factors for coronary artery disease. He had minimal cardiovascular symptoms up to two hours from the onset of allergy, but developed chest pain and palpitations 10 min following administration of epinephrine with associated ECG changes and elevated cardiac biomarkers. This temporal relationship is in more favor of epinephrine as the cause of myocardial infarction rather than the Kounis syndrome, but still it cannot be excluded. A likely mechanism postulated for the myocardial infarction by epinephrine was coronary vasospasm induced by it as the subsequent CT coronary angiogram demonstrated normal coronary vasculature.

Epinephrine has a high affinity for beta1, beta 2, alpha 1 and alpha 2 receptors in cardiac and smooth muscles of the vascular walls [14]. Stimulation of Beta 1 and Beta 2 leads to increased cardiac contractility and rate and dilates coronary arteries whereas alpha 1 and 2 receptors mediate vasoconstriction including that of the coronary vasculature. At low doses, beta-adrenergic effects are predominant whereas at higher doses, alpha effects are more pronounced. [14]. Yasue and his colleagues did an experimental study on four patients with prinzmetal's variant form of angina and demonstrated severe coronary artery spasm induced by administration of epinephrine and propranolol together [15].

Even though our patient developed myocardial infarction following intramuscular administration of epinephrine it was considered to be a relatively safe route of epinephrine administration [16]. From the limited data available regarding the safest route of administration of epinephrine in anaphylaxis it is demonstrated that intravenous route is associated with more cardiovascular events than the intramuscular route. This was shown in an observational study done by Campbell and his colleagues on 573 patients who presented with anaphylaxis and managed with epinephrine administered by various routes [17]. Risk of overdose of epinephrine in this group was higher with the intravenous route as well. Intravenous overdose of epinephrine was a known cause of coronary vasospasm [18]. However even local infiltration of therapeutic doses of epinephrine with the purpose of reducing bleeding is known to cause coronary vasospasm [19]. Patients who are at risk of developing coronary artery spasms following administration of epinephrine is an area that needs to be explored. Old age, preexisting coronary artery disease and being on a beta blocker were some of the risk factors for epinephrine induced myocardial ischemia based on available evidence [11, 20, 21].

However even though there are no randomized controlled trials available on the use of adrenaline in anaphylaxis it is clearly evident from the available literature that early use of adrenaline is life saving and associated with a better outcome than delayed use [22, 23]. Therefore even though myocardial ischemia could occur on rare occasions even with therapeutic doses of adrenalin, this should not prevent the early use of adrenaline as a lifesaving medication. There are no absolute contraindications for the use of adrenaline in the setting of life threatening anaphylaxis as the risk of anaphylaxis is far greater than the risk of adverse effects [24].The attending physician should be aware and be vigilant of the possible adverse effects of adrenaline and take necessary remediable steps if they occur.

Most occasions of myocardial injury secondary of adrenaline were treated with nitrates with intravenous infusions or sublingual administration and calcium channel blockers [3, 6]. Our patient was treated with sublingual nitrates in the emergency unit and was not started on further treatment as he remained asymptomatic.

Here we presented a case of a young healthy adult with no significant risk factors for coronary vascular disease who developed myocardial infarction following a therapeutic dose of intramuscular administration of adrenalin for an anaphylactic reaction. Even though intra muscular administration of adrenalin is considered a safe route, this case illustrates that on rare occasions myocardial ischemia could result. The postulated mechanism is most likely an alpha 1 receptor mediated coronary vascular spasm. However the use of adrenaline in the setting anaphylaxis is life saving and the benefits far outweighs the risks of adverse effects. Therefore the purpose of reporting this case is not to discourage the use of adrenaline in anaphylaxis but to make aware of this potential adverse effect which can occur in the acute setting.

Abbreviations

ECG: Electrocardiogram

Acknowledgements

This case report was supported by doctors working in ward 55, national hospital of Sri Lanka, in acquisition, analysis and interpretation of data. The CARE guidelines were followed for this case presentation.

Funding

No source of funding.

Authors' contributions

Dr. WDJ collected data, followed up the patient and did the literature review and drafted the manuscript. Dr. HMMTBH helped with the literature review and did the preliminary corrections of the manuscript. A.K corrected the manuscript. All authors read and approved the final manuscript.

Competing interests

The authors declare that they have no competing interests

References

1. World allergy organization guidelines for the assessment and management of anaphylaxis. World Allergy Organization Journal. 2011;4(2):13.
2. Working group of the resuscitation council(UK); Emergency treatment of anaphylactic reactions,Guidelines for health care providers: 2008;77(2):157-69.
3. Shaver KJ, Adams C, Weiss SJ. Acute myocardial infarction after administration of low dose intravenous epinephrine for anaphylaxis. CJEM. 2006 Jul;8(4):289–94.
4. Cunnington C, McDonald JE, Singh RK;Epinphrine induced myocardial infarction in severe anaphylaxis:is non-selective beta blockade a contributory factor?: Am J Emerg Med 2013 Apr;31(4):759,e1-2. Epub 2013 Feb 4.
5. Ferry BR, Henry RL, Kern MJ. Epinephrine induced myocardial infarction in a patient with angiographycally normal coronary arteries. Am Heart J. 1986;111:1193–5.
6. Rubio CJA, Oteo DJF, Maicas BC, et al. An adrenaline induced vasospasm as the form of presentation of vairent angina. Rev Esp Cardiol. 1999;52(4):273–6.
7. Saff R, Naggas A, Flink JN. Myocardial infarction induced by coronary vasosoasm after self-administration of epinephrine. Annals of allergy. 1993 May;70(5):396–8.
8. Thygesen K, Alpert JS, Jaffe AS, Simoons M. L et al. Third universal definition of myocardial infarction European Heart Journal. 2012;33:2551–67. doi: 10. 1093/eurheartj/ehs184.
9. Kounis NG. Kounis syndrome (allergic angina and allergic myocardial infarction): a natural paradigm? Int J Cardiol. 2006;110:7–14.
10. Kounis NG. Coronary hypersensitivity disorder: the Kounis syndrome. Clin Ther. 2013;35(5):563–71.
11. Lieberman P, Simons FE.Clin Exp Allergy. 2015 Aug;45(8):1288–95. doi: 10. 1111/cea.12520. Review. Erratum in: Clin Exp Allergy. 2015 Dec;45(12):1914. PMID: 25711241.
12. Gangadharan V, Bhatheja S, Balbissi KA; Kounis syndrome - an atopic monster for the heart. Cardiovascular Diagnosis and Therapy. 2013;3(1):47.
13. Gikas A, Lazaros G, Kontou-Fili K. Acute ST-segment elevation myocardial infarction after amoxycillin-induced anaphylactic shock in a young adult with normal coronary arteries: a case report. BMC Cardiovasc Disord. 2005;5: 6. Published online 2005 Feb 25. doi: 10.1186/1471-2261-5-6.
14. Overgaard CB. Dzaik.Inotroohs and vasopressors:review of physiology and clinical use in cardiovasculardisease. Circulation. 2008;2008(118):1047–56.
15. Yasue H, Touyama M, Kat o H, et al. Prinzmetal's variant form of angina as a manifestation of alpha adrenergic receptor mediated coronary artery spasms: documentation by coronary arteriography. Am Heart J. 1976;91:148–55.
16. Wood JP, Traub SJ, Lipinski C. Saftey of epinephrine for anaphylaxis in emergency setting. World J Emerg Med. 2013;4(4):245–51.
17. Campbell RL,Bellolio MF, Hess EP; Epinephrine in anaphylaxis:higher risk of cardiovascular complication and overdose after administration of intravenous bolus epinephrine compared with intramuscular epinephrine;J Allergy Clin Immunol Pract ; 2015,vol.3 (1)76-80,doi10.
18. Karch SB. Coronary artery spasm induced by intravenous epinephrine overdose. Am J Emerg Med. 1989;7:485–8.
19. Lee JY, Hong SJ, Chon JY, Kwon SY. Cardiac arrest induced by submucosal injection of epinephrine in a patient with variant angina. Rhinology. 2010; 48(2):251–3.
20. McLean-Tooke APC, Bethune CA, Spickett GP. Adrenaline in the treatment of anaphylaxis:what is the evidence? BMJ. 2003 Dec 6;327(7427):1332–5.
21. Lang DM. Anaphylactoid and anaphylactic reactions. Hazards of beta blockers. Drug Saftey. 1995;12(5):299–304.
22. Sampson HA, Mendelson L, Rosen JP. Fatal and near fatal anaphylactic reactions to food in children and adolescents. NEJM. 1992;327:380–4.
23. Soreide E, Buxrud T, Harboe S. Severe anaphylactic reactions outside hospital:aetiology,symptoms and treatment. Acta Anaesthesiol Scand. 1988;32:339–42.

22

Do heart failure status and psychosocial variables moderate the relationship between leisure time physical activity and mortality risk among patients with a history of myocardial infarction?

Rony Oosterom-Calo[1,2*], Saskia J. te Velde[2], Wim Stut[1], Yaacov Drory[3], Johannes Brug[4,5] and Yariv Gerber[4]

Abstract

Background: Leisure time physical activity (LTPA) is inversely related to mortality risk among patients with a history of myocardial infarction (MI). The aims were to explore if heart failure (HF) status and psychosocial variables moderate the association.

Methods: Participants ($n = 1169$) were from a multi-center prospective cohort study. Information on LTPA (none, irregular,1–150, 151–300 and >300 weekly minutes), depression, social support and other prognostic indicators were collected 10–13 years after index MI. Cox regressions were conducted, adjusting for potential confounders. In case of significant moderation by HF-status or psychosocial variables, stratified analyses were performed.

Results: During follow-up (M = 8.4 years), 25.6 % of the sample had died. LTPA was inversely associated with mortality (p for trend < 0.01 in all models). HF did not, but psychosocial variables did, moderate the association. In the LTPA category 1–150 weekly minutes, patients with a high level of depression had a lower mortality risk in comparison to those with a low level (hazard ratios (95 % confidence intervals) were 0.43 (0.25, 0.75) versus 0.69 (0.36, 1.32)), and patients with a low level of social support had a lower mortality risk in comparison to those with a high level (0.40 (0.21, 0.77) versus 0.71 (0.39, 1.27)). In the category >300 min, patients with a high level of social support had a lower mortality risk than those with a low level (0.38 (0.19, 0.79) versus 0.51 (0.30, 0.87)).

Conclusions: LTPA was inversely related to mortality risk of post-MI patients. HF did not moderate the relationship; depression and social support partially did.

Keywords: Leisure time physical activity, Post-MI, Heart failure, Mortality, Exercise, Psychosocial variables, Depression, Social support

Background

Physical activity (PA) is recommended to patients that have survived a myocardial infarction (MI) [1]. Physical activity is defined as any bodily movement produced by contraction of skeletal muscles resulting in energy expenditure above the basal level [1]. It may be promoted in a counseling intervention [1, 2] and as part of a cardiac rehabilitation program, including exercise-based training and lifestyle counseling components [3]. Such interventions have shown that performance of PA or exercise can reduce the risk of mortality by follow-up [3, 4]. The association between *leisure time physical activity* (LTPA), including leisurely walking and other recreational and sports activities, on clinical outcomes, also deserves attention. Previous work [5] has demonstrated a strong association between LTPA and mortality among post- MI patients, when comparing performance of no LTPA to

* Correspondence: rony.calo@philips.com
[1]Philips Research, Eindhoven, The Netherlands
[2]EMGO Institute for Health and Care Research and the Department of Epidemiology and Biostatistics, VU University Medical Center, Amsterdam, The Netherlands
Full list of author information is available at the end of the article

performance of weekly regular LTPA and irregular LTPA. Building on the previous work, in the current work we explore differences in mortality risk also based on the number of regular weekly LTPA minutes by refining the category of regular weekly LTPA to include more categories, in order to understand if patients who performed more regular LTPA had a lower mortality risk than those who performed less regular LTPA.

To further explore the benefits of LTPA in post-MI patients, it is worthwhile to uncover which groups of patients may benefit the most from LTPA. Patients at a higher risk of mortality may have a greater need for preventive measures, including performance of LTPA, to reduce the risk. Heart failure (HF) may be an important modifier of the relationship between performance of LTPA and mortality risk, because although on the one had post-MI HF patients have worse prognosis [6] compared to patients who did not develop HF [7], PA performance may be a protective factor among HF patients by reducing the risk of cardiovascular events and mortality [8]. Since post-MI patients who developed HF are at risk of mortality not only due to having had an MI in the past, but also due to their HF, LTPA, as a protective factor may demonstrate a larger effect in terms of reduction of mortality risk. The first aim of the current work is thus to assess whether HF is a modifying factor in the relationship between LTPA and mortality risk.

Also psychosocial factors may have an effect on prognosis [9]. A systematic review and meta-analysis reveals that two years after initial assessment of coronary heart disease (CHD), depressed patients are more than twice as likely to die as non-depressed patients [10] and that socially unsupported post-MI patients have a 2–3-fold higher risk of mortality [11]. Since depressed and socially unsupported patients have a higher risk of mortality than non-depressed and socially supported patients, and therefore more room for improvement in terms of reduction of mortality risk, they may benefit relatively more from LTPA. Specifically, in their case, LTPA may be a protective factor due to having had an MI in the past, as well as due to their psychosocial status, and may therefore demonstrate a larger effect on mortality risk. The second aim is therefore to assess if depression and/or social support moderate the relationship between LTPA and mortality risk among patients with a history of MI.

Finally, a secondary question remains as to whether these high-risk patients actually participate in LTPA. Patients with HF have a reduced exercise tolerance [12], making it difficult for them to exercise. They may therefore be less likely to perform activity than post-MI patients who are HF-free. This could mean that the patients who may benefit the most from LTPA may also be less likely to engage in it, and therefore do not gain the potential benefits. The third aim is therefore to assess the relationship between HF status and LTPA.

In summary, we hypothesize that (1) more LTPA is inversely related to mortality risk (Fig. 1), (2) HF status moderates this relationship, such that HF patients benefit relatively more from higher levels of LTPA, (3) depression and (4) social support moderate the relationship between LTPA and mortality risk, such that more depressed and less social supported patients benefit relatively more from higher levels of LTPA, and (5) patients with HF perform less LTPA.

Method

Study design and sample

Data were drawn from the Israel Study of First Acute Myocardial Infarction, a longitudinal prospective

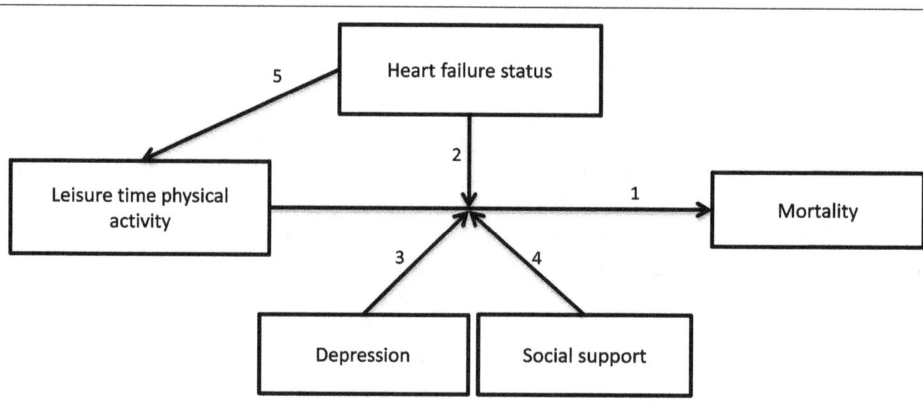

Fig. 1 Conceptual model depicting the hypothesized associations between the variables[1]. [1]Hypothesis 1: Leisure time physical activity will be related to reduced mortality rates; Hypothesis 2: Heart failure status will moderate the relationship between leisure time physical activity and mortality, such that heart failure patients will benefit more than HF-free patients; Hypothesis 3: Depression will moderate the relationship between leisure time physical activity and mortality, such that patients with high scores will benefit more than patients with low depression scores; Hypothesis 4: Social support will moderate the relationship between leisure time physical activity and mortality, such that patients with low scores will benefit more than patients with high social support scores; Hypothesis 5: Patients with HF, high depression scores and/or low social support scores will perform less leisure time physical activity

cohort study investigating the effects of various socio-demographic, medical and psychosocial variables on long-term clinical outcomes and quality of life in patients hospitalized for index MI [13, 14]. The total sample included patients aged 30–65 years, who were admitted to one of eight medical centers in central Israel between February 1992 and February 1993. The parent study was approved by the Ethics Committees of all medical centers involved (Wolfson, Holon; Sheba, Tel Hashomer; Tel Aviv Sourasky, Tel Aviv; Meir, Kfar Sava; Assaf Harofeh, Zerifin; Beilinson, Petach Tikvah; Hasharon, Petach Tikvah; and Laniado, Netanya) and ratified by the Institutional Ethics Committee of Tel Aviv University, and participants gave written informed consent.

Data collection

Within the Israel Study of First Acute Myocardial Infarction, demographic, socioeconomic and clinical data were collected from medical records and structured interviews one week, 3-6 months, 1–2 years, 5 years and 10–13 years following index MI hospitalization. We used data collected at the latter measurement point, because extensive data on clinical and psychosocial factors were measured in all survivors, in contrast to other measurement points, which targeted a sub-sample, and because it is the most recent measurement point, in which HF is more common (patients are older). Data were obtained through structured interviews, questionnaires, and review of medical records. The data on the following variables was used for the current analysis: Age, sex, educational level, occupational status, HF status, comorbidity status, smoking status, obesity, participation in cardiac rehabilitation, relevant medication prescriptions, depression and social support.

Variable measures

Outcome variable

Follow-up mortality data were obtained through 2011. Death was determined through data from the Israeli Population Registry.

Leisure time physical activity To assess LTPA, patients were asked to rate their LTPA (walking and other activities including gym, exercise at home such as on an exercise bicycle or treadmill, swimming, tennis, soccer/basketball/volleyball, or other) as regular (weekly), irregular (not weekly), or none. Patients that rated their LTPA as regular were asked to report the average frequency and duration of each session [5]. Regular LTPA was divided into three categories: 1–150, 150–300, or >300 weekly minutes. There were therefore five LTPA categories, including no LTPA, irregular LTPA and the three regular LTPA categories.

Heart failure status HF was defined according to clinical history (previous HF-related hospitalization) and a New York Heart Association (NYHA) classification of III-IV.

Psychosocial variables

Depression was assessed using the depression subscale of the Mental Health Inventory (MHI). The MHI includes 38 items, rated on a 7-point likert scale, ranging from 1 (very strongly disagree) to 7 (very strongly agree). The psychonomic properties of the MHI were assessed on a Israeli sample [15]; the depression subscale had an internal consistency (α) of 0.88. Social support was assessed using the Multidimensional Scale of Perceived Social Support (MSPSS) [16], which has an internal consistency (α) of .92 to .95 for its three subscales [17]. This scale is used to measure the perceived availability of support and includes twelve items, which assess three sources of support: Family, friends, and a significant other. Items are rated on a 7-point likert scale, ranging from 1 (very strongly disagree) to 7 (very strongly agree). The MSPSS has been used in previous research on this dataset [18].

Confounders

Socio-demographic data

Educational level was assessed by asking patients to indicate the number of years of formal education they have received. Occupational status was assessed by asking patients to indicate if they are working, retired, never worked, or stopped working for another reason than retirement.

Clinical variables

The clinical variables included conditions other than HF and smoking status. Although there was data available for many conditions within the Israel Study of First Acute Myocardial Infarction, conditions other than HF regarding which information was available (including diabetes, peripheral vascular disease, cerebrovascular disease, cancer, ulcer disease, chronic renal disease, chronic obtrusive pulmonary disease) were selected for inclusion in the current study based on their appearance in the Charlson Comorbidity Index [19]. Conditions were classified dichotomously (having versus not having a condition other than HF). Smoking status, obtained by information from structured interviews [13, 20] was classified as never smoked, previously smoked, or currently smoking. Information on weight and height was used to calculate body mass index (BMI) by dividing the weight by the height squared. Obesity was categorized in three categories, based on the World Health Organization's (WHO) categorization [21], including below normal until normal weight (BMI < 25, pre-obese (25 < =BMI <

30), and obese (30 < =BMI). Below normal weight and normal weight were grouped in one category due to the small number of below normal weight participants in the sample ($N = 4$).

Treatment-related variables

Medication prescriptions were extracted from personal interviews and questionnaires. Patients were asked to indicate if they have ever participated in cardiac rehabilitation.

Statistical analyses

Baseline data are presented as percentage or mean (standard deviation). Baseline characteristics across LTPA categories were compared using the using the Mantel–Haenszel chi-square test for trend for categorical variables and generalized linear models for continuous variables. To test the first hypothesis, cox proportional hazards models were constructed to evaluate covariate-adjusted hazards ratios (HR's) and 95 % confidence intervals (CI's) associated with LTPA categories. The reference category was defined at no LTPA. Five models, taking into account risk factors for poor post-MI prognosis, were constructed. These models adjusted for: sex and age (basic model, i.e., Model 1); sex, age, educational level and occupational status (demographic model, i.e., Model 2); sex, age, HF status, having a comorbidity, smoking status and obesity (clinical model, i.e., Model 3); sex, age, having received cardiac rehabilitation, being prescribed ACE inhibitors, beta blockers, aspirin, and statins (treatment-related model, i.e., Model 4); and finally, sex, age, depression and social support (psychosocial model, i.e., Model 5). In addition, in order to test the association linearly, the models were tested with LTPA as a continuous variable. The proportional hazards assumption was tested by plotting partial residuals against survival time (i.e. survival, in days, at follow up), with no violations detected.

To test whether the estimated HR's for the HF and HF-free patients were statistically different from each other, interaction terms between HF-status and each of the LTPA categories were added to the basic model described above. The basic model was selected since it was the most parsimonious of the constructed models and since LTPA was associated with less mortality in all models, including the basic one. A p cutoff value of 0.10 was used as the significance level for the interaction terms, due to difficulties in detecting moderation effects [22], and based on strategies for detecting moderator variables reported elsewhere [23]. In case of significant interaction terms (i.e. $p < 0.10$), HR's for each group were presented separately. In case of non-significant interaction terms, stratified analyses were only performed to check whether estimated HR's for each group were indeed similar, or were different but with wide and overlapping confidence intervals.

To test the third and fourth hypotheses, regarding moderation effects of depression and social support, it was tested whether the estimated HR's for high depression/high social support and low depression/low social support were statistically different from each other by adding interaction terms between depression/social support and each of the LTPA categories to the basic model described above. To explore whether associations between LTPA categories and mortality differed between patients with high and low depression scores, and between socially supported and unsupported patients, stratified analyses were conducted, when significant interaction terms (i.e. $p < 0.10$) were observed, by comparing high to low depression/social groups. Groups were defined using the median scores as a cutoff. Again, in case of non-significant interaction terms, stratified analyses were only performed to check whether estimated hazard ratios for each group were indeed similar, or were different but with wide and overlapping confidence intervals.

To test the fifth hypothesis, the relationship of LTPA with HF status was evaluated using a one-way analysis of variance. Bonferroni post-hoc analyses were performed to test for differences in HF status among LTPA categories. A $p < 0.05$ was regarded as statistically significant. For interaction terms $p < 0.10$ was regarded significant, due to a lower power to detect significant interactions.

Results

The sample included 1169 patients, who completed the measurement at the fifth interview 10–13 years after index MI (see Additional file 1: Table S1 for sample characteristics). At this time point, 237 (20 %) had developed HF (see Additional file 2: Table S2 for the characteristics of the HF subsample). During a median of 8.4 years follow-up after the fifth interview, 303 deaths occurred (26 % of the sample), of which 122 were in HF cases (i.e., 51 % of the HF cases) and 179 in HF-free cases (i.e., 19 % of the HF-free cases). Of the 303 deaths, 51 % performed no LTPA, 19 % performed irregular LTPA, 13 % performed 1–150 and 8 % performed 151–300 and 8 % performed > 300 weekly minutes of LTPA.

Of the post-MI patients, 37.7 % reported being inactive, 19.1 % reported being irregularly active, 14.5 % reported performing less than 150 weekly minutes of LTPA, 14.5 % reported performing 151–300 weekly minutes of LTPA, and 13.8 % reported performing more than 300 weekly minutes of LTPA. Men performed more LTPA than women (p for trend < 0.01). Educational level and having participated in the past in cardiac rehabilitation were positively related to LTPA (p for trend < 0.01). Having HF, having at least one other comorbidity than HF and depression were negatively related to LTPA (p for trend < 0.01). Out of the inactive participants, 35 % had died by follow-up, followed by 26 % of the irregularly active participants, 17 % of the regularly active participants who had performed 1–150, 14.7 % who performed 151–300, and 22.6 % who performed >300 weekly minutes.

Is more LTPA related to a reduced mortality risk?

Patients who performed irregular, 1–150, 151–300, or >300 weekly minutes of LTPA all had a lower mortality risk than patients who performed no LTPA ($p < 0.01$ for all; Table 1). In addition to the significant categorical relationships, also linear relationships were found; significant linear trends of LTPA were found in all models (p for trend <0.01 for all).

Does heart failure status moderate the relationship between leisure time physical activity and reduced mortality risk?

No interaction of HF by LTPA was found (all interaction terms were $p > 0.30$; see Additional file 3: Table S3). Further exploration by means of analyses stratified by HF status confirmed that the observed estimates for the two groups were very similar.

Does depression moderate the relationship between leisure time physical activity and survival?

Patients with a high level of depression, who performed 1–150 min of weekly LTPA, had a lower mortality risk than patients with a high level of depression who performed no LTPA ($p = 0.08$; Table 2). Patients with a low level of depression did not have a reduction in mortality risk associated with performance 1–150 min of weekly LTPA. There was no difference in terms of mortality risk between depressed and non-depressed patients who performed irregular, 151–300 or >300 weekly minutes of LTPA (all interaction terms had a $p > 0.10$).

Does social support moderate the relationship between leisure time physical activity and mortality risk?

The interaction between social support and LTPA was significant for the category 1–150 min ($p = 0.09$; Table 2). Patients with a low level of social support who performed 1–150 min of weekly LTPA had a lower mortality risk compared to patients with a low level of social support who performed no LTPA. Patients who had a high level of social support did not have a reduction in mortality risk associated with performance of 1–150 weekly minutes of LTPA. The interaction was borderline significant for the category >300 min ($p = 0.10$). Patients with high social support who performed >300 min had a lower mortality risk than patients with a high social support who performed no LTPA. A similar relationship was not observed in patients who had a low level of social support. All other interaction terms of LTPA categories by social support were found non-significant ($p > 0.10$).

Is heart failure status related to performance of leisure time physical activity?

Heart failure status was significantly related to LTPA (p for trend <0.01). Bonferroni post-hoc analyses demonstrated that patients who performed no LTPA were more likely to have HF than those in all other LTPA categories ($p < 0.01$). Patients who performed irregular LTPA were more likely to have HF in comparison to those that performed 151–300 weekly minutes of LTPA ($p = 0.04$). Differences between all other LTPA categories were non-significant.

Discussion

A persistent, inverse association between LTPA and mortality risk was demonstrated in the current study in a sample of post-MI patients, irrespective of HF status and when adjusting for basic, demographic, clinical, treatment-related and psychosocial covariates. These

Table 1 Hazard ratios (95 % CI's) for the relationships between leisure time physical activity categories and survival in the post-MI

	Model 1	Model 2	Model 3	Model 4	Model 5
	HR (95 % CI)	HR (95 % CI)	HR (95 % CI)	HR (95 % CI)	HR (95 % CI)
No LTPA (reference)	1	1	1	1	1
Irregular LTPA	0.66 (0.49, 0.90)	0.66 (0.49, 0.90)	0. 76 (0.55, 1.03)	0.69 (0.51, 0.93)	0.79 (0.55, 1.13)
1–150 min	0.49 (0.34, 0.71)	0.49 (0.34, 0.71)	0.64 (0.44, 0.93)	0.52 (0.36, 0.75)	0.53 (0.34, 0.82)
151–300 min	0.30 (0.19, 0.47)	0.33 (0.21, 0.52)	0.40 (0.25, 0.66)	0.33 (0.21, 0.52)	0.39 (0.24, 0.65)
>300 min	0.39 (0.26, 0.58)	0.39 (0.26, 0.58)	0.50 (0.33, 0.76)	0.41 (0.28, 0.61)	0.49 (0.31, 0.76)
p for trend [a]	<0.01	<0.01	<0.01	<0.01	<0.01

HR hazard ratio, *95%CI* 95 % confidence interval, *LTPA* Leisure time physical activity
Model 1: Basic model, adjusted for age and sex; Model 2: demographic model = Model 1 + adjustments for educational level and occupational status; Model 3: clinical model = Model 1 + adjustments for HF status, having a comorbidity, smoking status and obesity; Model 4: treatment-related model = Model 1 + adjustments for having received cardiac rehabilitation, being prescribed ACE inhibitors, beta blockers, aspirin, and statins; Model 5 : psychosocial model = Model 1 + adjustments for depression and social support
[a]Based on Cox regression analyses with LTPA as a continuous variable

Table 2 Hazard ratios (95 % confidence Intervals) in the stratified analysis comparing mortality risk related to leisure time physical activity of patients with high versus low depression and high versus low social support

	High depression[a] HR [b] (95 % CI)	Low depression[a] HR [b] (95 % CI)	p-value interaction term	High social support[a] HR [b] (95 % CI)	Low social support[a] HR [2] (95 % CI)	*p*-value interaction term
No LTPA: Reference category	1	1		1	1	
Irregular LTPA	0.80 (0.52, 1.24)	0.63 (3.4, 1.15)	0.63	0.82 (0.47, 1.43)	0.69 (0.44, 1.09)	0.56
1–150 min	0.43 (0.25, 0.75)	0.69 (0.36, 1.32)	0.08	0.71 (0.39, 1.27)	0.40 (0.21, 0.77)	0.09
151–300 min	0.28 (0.13, 0.58)	0.45 (0.23, 0.88)	0.41	0.40 (0.20, 0.80)	0.30 (0.14, 0.62)	0.45
>300 min	0.48 (0.29, 0.81)	0.42 (0.20, 0.86)	0.82	0.38 (0.19, 0.79)	0.51 (0.30, 0.87)	0.10
p for trend	>0.01	>0.01	0.39	>0.01	>0.01	0.56

HR hazard ratio, *CI* confidence interval, *LTPA* leisure time physical activity
[a]Based on a cutoff value of median depression = 7 and median social support = 5.6
[b]HR adjusting for age and sex

results replicate previous work demonstrating the survival benefits related to being active for post-MI patients [5]. The current work adds to previous investigations through the refinement of the regular weekly LTPA variable into three categories based on minutes of LTPA per week, and by exploring potential moderators for the association, thereby allowing making practical recommendations for LTPA promotion. Moreover, previous studies with HF patients have focused on exercise training [24, 25] and on PA following a counseling intervention [4]. This is the first study to focus specifically on PA conducted at leisure time among HF patients.

Our hypothesis regarding the moderating effects of HF status on the inverse relationship between LTPA and mortality risk was not met. This indicates that HF patients were just as likely to benefit from LTPA as HF-free patients with a history of MI. Therefore, interventions to promote LTPA may be beneficial for inactive patients with and without HF. It may be necessary, however, to target interventions separately at the two groups because HF and HF free post-MI patients differ from each other on a number of characteristics, including age [7].

Depression and social support partially moderated the relationship between LTPA and mortality risk. It was found that patients with high depression scores, as well as those with low social support scores, appear to benefit from *any* amount of regular, weekly, LTPA, i.e. that low levels of LTPA are already beneficial for these groups. It was also found that performing more than 300 min of LTPA was more strongly related to survival in the high social support group than in the low social support group, although both groups benefitted from conducting more than 300 min of LTPA.

Finally, it was found that patients with HF were less likely to perform LTPA in comparison to those without HF. This indicates that in particular HF patients may have a need for LTPA promotion interventions, especially in light of the fact that they benefit from LTPA just as much as the HF-free patients. There is evidence that preventive interventions targeting specifically the HF patient population, can be effective [4]. More research is necessary to clarify the direction of causality, however, as there is also evidence that patients who are less active are more likely to develop HF [26].

There are a number of strengths in the current work. The results make an important contribution to current knowledge about the relationship among LTPA and mortality risk among post-MI patients. It replicates results regarding the survival benefits of PA performed at leisure among patients with a history of MI, but using a more refined LTPA variable, thereby contributing to more specific recommendations regarding LTPA promotion. It is the first study exploring the moderating effects of HF status on this relationship. Since prognosis is low among HF patients [6] this association is of particular importance. The inverse association between LTPA performance and mortality risk was evaluated in models that adjusted for a range of relevant variables, thereby increasing the confidence in the observed effects.

There are also a number of limitations. Based on the results, it is unclear if certain characteristics of active patients, for example a better health status, can account for the observed associations between LTPA and survival. Known mortality risk factors were adjusted for in the statistical models, but it is still possible that factors beyond the scope of the current work account for the findings. A limiting factor of the current work is that the baseline mortality risk of participants was not taken into account. However, with survival analyses it is not possible to estimate the baseline risk. Performing another type of analysis, such as logistic regression, would not have been preferable in this case, because it would have not been possible to take time into account in the model. Selection bias may have also been a limitation. The selection of HF patients was based on hospitalization history and a NYHA III-IV class, rather than the Framingham criteria for HF diagnosis [27]. Furthermore, patients who died before index MI, as well as patients who died during index hospitalization, were not included. Finally, LTPA measurement was not optimal, because it was self-reported, rather than assessed with objective measurement techniques such as accelerometers [28]. It is often difficult for economic and pragmatic reasons to assess LTPA with accelerometers in prospective cohort studies, but some studies have done this [29–31], although notably with smaller sample sizes. Furthermore, the self-report measure of LTPA provided information regarding duration of LTPA but not on exercise intensity or about more specific modes of physical activity, and effects of LTPA may be dependent on intensity and may be different for specific activities.

Conclusions

In conclusion, in a sample of post-MI Israeli patients, LTPA positively predicted reductions in mortality risk, irrespective of HF status, although HF patients were less likely to be physically active than HF-free patients. There was some evidence that depression and social support moderate the inverse relationship between LTPA and mortality risk, indicating that more depressed patients and patients with less social support may already benefit from relatively fewer weekly minutes of LTPA. These findings have implications for LTPA promotion among patients with a history of MI.

Additional files

Additional file 1: Table S1. Baseline characteristics of the post-MI patient sample. Baseline characteristics of the post-MI sample categorized according to amount of LTPA performed. (DOC 61 kb)

Additional file 2: Table S2. Baseline characteristics of the HF subsample. Baseline characteristics of the subsample of post-MI patients who developed HF categorized according to amount of LTPA performed. (DOC 58 kb)

Additional file 3: Table S3. Hazard ratio's (CI's) in the stratified analysis comparing HF to HF-free cases' mortality risk related to LTPA categories. Results of the stratified analysis comparing the mortality risk in relation to LTPA of post-MI patients who did and did not develop HF. (DOC 41 kb)

Abbreviations

BMI: Body mass index; CI: Confidence interval; HF: Heart failure; HR: Hazards ratio; LTPA: Leisure time physical activity; MI: Myocardial infarction; WHO: World health organization;

Acknowledgements

One of the authors of this study, and founder of the Israel Study of First Acute Myocardial Infarction, Professor Yaacov Drory, passed away at the time of writing this article. Professor Drory was a dedicated cardiologist and researcher, who published numerous papers and books and made a great and unique contribution to the field of preventive cardiology and cardiac rehabilitation.

The following investigators and institutions took part in the Israel Study Group on First Acute Myocardial Infarction: Yaacov Drory, MD, Principal Investigator, Department of Rehabilitation, Sackler Medical School, Tel Aviv University, Tel Aviv; Yeheskiel Kishon, MD, Michael Kriwisky, MD, and Yoseph Rosenman, MD, Wolfson Medical Center, Holon; Uri Goldbourt, PhD, Hanoch Hod, MD, Eliezer Kaplinsky, MD, and Michael Eldar, MD, Sheba Medical Center, Tel Hashomer; Itzhak Shapira, MD, Amos Pines, MD, Margalit Drory, MSW, Arie Roth, MD, Shlomo Laniado, MD, and Gad Keren, MD, Tel-Aviv Sourasky Medical Center, Tel-Aviv; Daniel David, MD, Morton Leibowitz, MD, and Hana Pausner, MD, Meir Medical Center, Kfar Sava; Zvi Schlesinger, MD, and Zvi Vered, MD, Assaf Harofeh Medical Center, Zerifin; Alexander Battler, MD, Alejandro Solodky, MD, and Samuel Sclarovsky, MD, Beilinson Medical Center, Petach Tikvah; Izhar Zehavi, MD, and Rachel Marom-Klibansky, MD, Hasharon Medical Center, Petah Tikvah; and Ron Leor, MD, Laniado Medical Center, Netanya.

We would like to thank Professor Jos Twisk for his statistical advice.

Funding

No financial support was received.

Authors' contributions

ROC conceived of the study, conducted the analysis and wrote the manuscript. SJtV assisted with the analysis, provided statistical consultation and extensive comments on the manuscript. WS provided consultation on the research topic and extensive comments on the manuscript. YD conceived of the parent study, founded the Israel Study on First Acute Myocardial Infarction and led the collection of data analyzed in the current study. JB provided consultation on the research topic and on the analysis as well as extensive comments on the manuscript. YG guided and supported the analysis, provided consultation in relation to the parent study and the data as well as extensive comments on the manuscript. All authors read and approved the final manuscript.

Competing interests

The authors declare that they have no competing interests.

Author details

[1]Philips Research, Eindhoven, The Netherlands. [2]EMGO Institute for Health and Care Research and the Department of Epidemiology and Biostatistics, VU University Medical Center, Amsterdam, The Netherlands. [3]Department of Rehabilitation, Sackler School of Medicine, Tel Aviv University, Tel Aviv, Israel. [4]Department of Epidemiology and Preventive Medicine, School of Public Health, Sackler Faculty ofMedicine, Tel Aviv University, Tel Aviv, Israel. [5]AmsterdamSchool for Communication Research, University of Amsterdam, Amsterdam, The Netherlands.

References

1. Corra U, Piepoli MF, Carre F, Heuschmann P, Hoffmann U, et al. Secondary prevention through cardiac rehabilitation: physical activity counselling and exercise training: key components of the position paper from the Cardiac Rehabilitation Section of the European Association of Cardiovascular Prevention and Rehabilitation. Eur Heart J. 2010;31:1967–74.
2. Piepoli MF, Guazzi M, Boriani G, Cicoira M, Corra U, et al. Exercise intolerance in chronic heart failure: mechanisms and therapies. Part I. Eur J Cardiovasc Prev Rehabil. 2010;17:637–42.
3. Giannuzzi P, Temporelli PL, Marchioli R, Maggioni AP, Balestroni G, et al. Global secondary prevention strategies to limit event recurrence after myocardial infarction: results of the GOSPEL study, a multicenter, randomized controlled trial from the Italian Cardiac Rehabilitation Network. Arch Intern Med. 2008;168:2194–204.
4. Wal M, Veldhuisen D, Veeger N, Rutten F, Jaarsma T. Compliance with non-pharmacological recommendations and outcome in heart failure patients. Eur Heart J. 2010;31:1486–93. doi:10.1093/eurheartj/ehq1091. Epub2010Apr1430.
5. Gerber Y, Myers V, Goldbourt U, Benyamini Y, Scheinowitz M, et al. Long-term trajectory of leisure time physical activity and survival after first myocardial infarction: a population-based cohort study. Eur J Epidemiol. 2011;26:109–16.
6. Mosterd A, Cost B, Hoes AW, de Bruijne MC, Deckers JW, et al. The prognosis of heart failure in the general population: The Rotterdam Study. Eur Heart J. 2001;22:1318–27.

7. Emanuelsson H, Karlson BW, Herlitz J. Characteristics and prognosis of patients with acute myocardial infarction in relation to occurrence of congestive heart failure. Eur Heart J. 1994;15:761–8.
8. Miura Y, Fukumoto Y, Miura T, Shimada K, Asakura M, et al. Impact of physical activity on cardiovascular events in patients with chronic heart failure. A multicenter prospective cohort study. Circ J. 2012;77:2963–72.
9. Hemingway H, Marmot M. Evidence based cardiology: psychosocial factors in the aetiology and prognosis of coronary heart disease. Systematic review of prospective cohort studies. BMJ. 1999;318:1460–7.
10. Barth J, Schumacher M, Herrmann-Lingen C. Depression as a risk factor for mortality in patients with coronary heart disease: a meta-analysis. Psychosom Med. 2004;66:802–13.
11. Mookadam F, Arthur HM. Social support and its relationship to morbidity and mortality after acute myocardial infarction: systematic overview. Arch Intern Med. 2004;164:1514–8.
12. McMurray J, Adamopoulos S, Anker S, Auricchio A, Bohm M, et al. ESC guidelines for the diagnosis and treatment of acute and chronic heart failure 2012: The Task Force for the Diagnosis and Treatment of Acute and Chronic Heart Failure 2012 of the European Society of Cardiology. Developed in collaboration with the Heart Failure Association (HFA) of the ESC. Eur J Heart Fail. 2012;14:803–69. doi:10.1093/eurjhf/hfs1105.
13. Gerber Y, Rosen LJ, Goldbourt U, Benyamini Y, Drory Y. Smoking status and long-term survival after first acute myocardial infarction a population-based cohort study. J Am Coll Cardiol. 2009;54:2382–7.
14. Gerber Y, Benyamini Y, Goldbourt U, Drory Y. Neighborhood socioeconomic context and long-term survival after myocardial infarction. Circulation. 2010; 121:375–83.
15. Florian V, Drory Y. The mental health inventory: psychometric properties and normative data in the Israeli population. Psychologia. 1990;2:26–35.
16. Zimet GD, Powell SS, Farley GK, Werkman S, Berkoff KA. Psychometric characteristics of the multidimensional scale of perceived social support. J Pers Assess. 1990;55:610–7.
17. Zimet GD, Dahlem NW, Zimet SG, Farley GK. The multidimensional scale of perceived social support. J Pers Assess. 1988;52:30–41.
18. Drory Y, Kravetz S, Hirschberger G. Long-term mental health of men after a first acute myocardial infarction. Arch Phys Med Rehabil. 2002;83:352–9.
19. Charlson ME, Pompei P, Ales KL, MacKenzie CR. A new method of classifying prognostic comorbidity in longitudinal studies: development and validation. J Chronic Dis. 1987;40:373–83.
20. Gerber Y, Koren-Morag N, Myers V, Benyamini Y, Goldbourt U, et al. Long-term predictors of smoking cessation in a cohort of myocardial infarction survivors: a longitudinal study. Eur J Cardiovasc Prev Rehabil. 2011;18:533–41.
21. Organization WH. Preventing and managing the global epidemic [report of a WHO Consultation on Obesity]. Geneva: World Health Organization; 1997.
22. McClelland GH, Judd CM. Statistical difficulties of detecting interactions and moderator effects. Psychol Bull. 1993;114:376.
23. Stone-Romero EF, Liakhovitski D. Strategies for detecting moderator variables: a review of conceptual and empirical issues. Research in personnel and human resources management. 2002;21:333–72.
24. Belardinelli R, Georgiou D, Cianci G, Purcaro A. Randomized, controlled trial of long-term moderate exercise training in chronic heart failure: effects on functional capacity, quality of life, and clinical outcome. Circulation. 1999;99:1173–82.
25. O'Connor CM, Whellan DJ, Lee KL, Keteyian SJ, Cooper LS, et al. Efficacy and safety of exercise training in patients with chronic heart failure: HF-ACTION randomized controlled trial. JAMA. 2009;301:1439–50.
26. He J, Ogden LG, Bazzano LA, Vupputuri S, Loria C, et al. Risk factors for congestive heart failure in US men and women: NHANES I epidemiologic follow-up study. Arch Intern Med. 2001;161:996–1002.
27. McKee PA, Castelli WP, McNamara PM, Kannel WB. The natural history of congestive heart failure: the Framingham study. N Engl J Med. 1971;285:1441–6.
28. Prince S, Adamo K, Hamel M, Hardt J, Gorber S, et al. A comparison of direct versus self-report measures for assessing physical activity in adults: a systematic review. Int J Behav Nutr Phys Act. 2008;5:56.
29. Tucker JM, Tucker LA, Lecheminant J, Bailey B. Obesity increases risk of declining physical activity over time in women: A prospective cohort study. Obesity (Silver Spring). 2013;21(12):E715–20.
30. Hamer M, Kivimaki M, Steptoe A. Longitudinal patterns in physical activity and sedentary behaviour from mid-life to early old age: a substudy of the Whitehall II cohort. J Epidemiol Community Health. 2012;66:1110–5.

23

Effects of the concomitant administration of xanthine oxidase inhibitors with zofenopril or other ACE-inhibitors in post-myocardial infarction patients

Claudio Borghi[1,4*], Stefano Omboni[2], Giorgio Reggiardo[3], Stefano Bacchelli[1], Daniela Degli Esposti[1], Ettore Ambrosioni[1] and on behalf of the SMILE Working Project

Abstract

Background: Oxidative stress is increased in hyperuricemic patients with acute myocardial infarction (AMI). Use of *sulfhydryl* ACE-inhibitors (ACEIs), such as zofenopril or captopril, plus xanthine oxidase inhibitors (XOIs), may potentially result in enhanced antioxidant effects and improved survival.

Objective: We verified the benefit of such combination in a randomly stratified sample of 525 of the 3630 post-AMI patients of the four randomized prospective SMILE (Survival of Myocardial Infarction Long-term Evaluation) studies.

Methods: One hundred sixty-five (31.4%) patients were treated with XOIs (79 under zofenopril, 86 placebo, lisinopril or ramipril), whereas 360 were not (192 zofenopril, 168 placebo or other ACEIs). In these four groups, we separately estimated the 1-year combined risk of major cardiovascular events (MACE, death or hospitalization for cardiovascular causes).

Results: MACE occurred in 10.1% of patients receiving zofenopril + XOIs, in 18.6% receiving placebo or other ACEIs + XOIs, in 13.5% receiving zofenopril without XOIs and in 22.0% receiving placebo or other ACEIs, but no XOIs ($p = 0.034$ across groups). Rate of survival free from MACE was significantly larger under treatment with zofenopril + XOIs than with other ACEIs with no XOIs [hazard ratio: 2.29 (1.06–4.91), $p = 0.034$]. A non-significant trend for superiority of zofenopril + XOIs combination was observed vs. zofenopril alone [1.19 (0.54–2.64), $p = 0.669$] or vs. placebo or other ACEIs + XOIs [1.82 (0.78–4.26), $p = 0.169$].

Conclusions: Our retrospective analysis suggests an improved survival free from MACE in post-AMI patients treated with a combination of an urate lowering drug with antioxidant activity and an ACEI, with best effects observed with zofenopril.

Keywords: Acute myocardial infarction, Hyperuricemia, Angiotensin-converting enzyme inhibitors, Xanthine oxidase inhibitors

* Correspondence: claudio.borghi@unibo.it
[1]Unit of Internal Medicine, Policlinico S. Orsola, University of Bologna, Bologna, Italy
[4]Divisione di Medicina Interna, Policlinico S.Orsola, Via Massarenti 9, 40138 Bologna, Italy
Full list of author information is available at the end of the article

Background

Reduced myocardial antioxidant activity and increased oxidant damage have been described in animal models of coronary artery disease and heart failure (HF), and markers of oxidative stress are elevated in the same patients [1]. Among potential stimuli that contribute to myocardial failure progression, the over-activation of xanthine oxidase (XO) plays a central role. XO is an enzyme involved in the last two steps of purine catabolism that ultimately results in uric acid production [2]. The degree of activation of XO is directly related to the the circulating levels of uric acid that can be considered as an indirect marker of oxidative stress in several clinical conditions [2]. Serum uric acid is a potent antioxidant, but it can also promote oxidative stress at high concentrations and in surroundings with low pH or low levels of other antioxidants [3]. In vitro, uric acid may affect vascular smooth muscle and mononuclear cells that are important in pathophysiology of cardiovascular (CV) diseases [4]. Indeed, significantly increased serum uric acid levels have been identified in 25% of patients with heart failure and reduced ejection fraction and have been associated with worsening symptoms and increased mortality [5, 6]. Vascular activity of XO may also increase the oxidative stress that underlies endothelial dysfunction. XO inhibition with allopurinol 300 mg once daily for one month was compared with placebo to investigate its potential in endothelial function improvement after HF. Allopurinol significantly ameliorated endothelium-dependent vasodilation and reduced markers of oxidative stress [7]. In patients with HF allopurinol administration improved left ventricular ejection fraction [8], diastolic function, and coronary flow reserve [9] on the short-term, but showed no definitive benefits on the long-term [10]. In a placebo controlled cross-over study involving patients with chronic stable angina, treatment with allopurinol (600 mg per day) for 6 weeks showed anti-ischemic properties [11]. Thus, current evidence suggest that XOIs may have important cardioprotective activities [12].

Zofenopril is a potent sulfhydryl angiotensin-converting enzyme (ACE) inhibitor, characterized by high lipophilicity, selective cardiac ACE-inhibition, and antioxidant and tissue protective activities [13]. The effects of zofenopril treatment in terms of circulating adhesion molecules, oxidative stress parameters and endothelium-dependent vasodilation were analyzed in essential mildly hypertensive patients. Zofenopril has demonstrated a sustained antioxidant activity and reduced endothelial activation compared to carboxylic ACE-inhibitor ramipril and the beta-adrenoceptor blocker atenolol [14]. The analysis of the overall population of more than 3600 patients with coronary heart disease (CHD) and enrolled in the Survival of Myocardial Infarction Long-Term Evaluation (SMILE) project, showed that the treatment with zofenopril was associated with a lower risk of mortality and morbidity as compared to placebo or other ACE-inhibitors. The beneficial effect of zofenopril was associated with some degree of anti-ischemic effects and confirmed in patients with preserved or impaired left ventricular function [15–18].

Considering the importance of the over-activation of XO in presence of hyperuricemia, we investigated the effects of the concomitant andministration of XO inhibitors and ACE-inhibitors in post-acute myocardial infarction (AMI) patients. We also postulated that the antioxidant activity of zofenopril may be more beneficial in comparison to other ACE-inhibitors in patients with AMI treated with XO inhibitor (XOI). Therefore, in this meta-analysis we assessed subgroups of patients involved in the SMILE studies who were concomitantly treated with XOIs to verify the potential enhanced antioxidant effect and survival improvement after zofenopril treatment.

Methods

Study design

The present meta-analysis aimed to evaluate the 1-year combined occurrence of death or hospitalization for CV causes in patients involved in the SMILE studies who were treated with XOIs. Briefly, the SMILE studies were double-blind, randomized, parallel-group studies that compared the efficacy and safety of zofenopril with placebo plus standard therapy for AMI excluding ACE-inhibitors (SMILE-1 and 3) [15, 18], lisinopril (SMILE-2) [17] or ramipril (SMILE-4) [16]. The inclusion criteria for the SMILE studies were as follows: i) early AMI (< 24 h), not eligible for thrombolytic therapy because of late admission to the intensive care unit or with contra-indication to systemic fibrinolysis (SMILE-1) [15], ii) confirmed diagnosis of AMI and a prior thrombolytic treatment within 12 h of the onset of clinical symptoms of AMI (SMILE-2) [17]; iii) recent AMI (within 6 ± 1 weeks) with preserved left ventricular ejection fraction (> 40%), treated with a thrombolytic treatment and with ACE-inhibitors (SMILE-3) [18]; and iv) early AMI (< 24 h) , treated or not with thrombolysis, with primary percutaneous transluminal angioplasty or coronary artery by-pass graft, and with clinical and/or echocardiographic evidence of left ventricular dysfunction (SMILE-4) [16]. The main exclusion criteria were: i) the presence of cardiogenic shock (Killip class IV); ii) severe hypotension (SBP < 90–100 mmHg), iii) severe hypertension (DBP > 115 mmHg and/or SBP > 200 mmHg) iv) a serum creatinine concentration > 2.5 mg/dL or renal failure; v) bilateral renal artery stenosis; vi) hemodynamically significant valvular disease; vii) current treatment with ACE-inhibitors or angiotensin II-receptor blockers (or acetylsalicylic acid for the SMILE-4), and hypersensitivity to these drugs; viii) inability or unwillingness to give informed consent.

Patients were studied between January 1991 (SMILE-1 study) and July 2009 (SMILE-4 study) and randomized double-blind to receive zofenopril, placebo, lisinopril or ramipril, in addition to standard recommended therapy for AMI. Duration of treatment and follow-up were depending on the study and ranged 6 to 48 weeks.

Patients who at the randomization visit were treated with preparation inhibiting uric acid production, namely allopurinol, tisopurine, febuxostat and other anti-gout medications (collectively defined in this paper as XOIs) were allowed to continue this therapy during the studies.

All studies were conducted according with the Guidelines for Good Clinical Practice and the Declaration of Helsinki and were approved by the Ethics Committee of each participating center. Written informed consent was obtained from each patient before enrollment.

Statistical analysis

The primary study endpoint was the 1-year combined occurrence of death or hospitalization for CV causes (major CV events or MACE) and it was calculated after weighing for the number of subjects contributing from each study. All patients treated with at least one dose of study medication and providing at least once the measure of the primary efficacy assessment were included in the analysis. The efficacy endpoint was compared across four different treatment groups: patients taking zofenopril with concomitant XOIs, zofenopril without XOIs, placebo or any other ACE-inhibitor (lisinopril or ramipril) plus XOIs, placebo or other ACEI-inhibitors without XOIs. Since in the pooled dataset of the SMILE Studies the number of subjects treated with XOIs was small (165, of which 79 treated with zofenopril and 86 with placebo, lisinopril or ramipril) compared to those not treated with XOIs (3465, of which 1729 under zofenopril and 1736 under placebo or other ACE-inhibitors), the control group was re-sampled with a 2:1 ratio, using a stratified random sampling method, in order to allow a balanced comparison across the four study groups.

Hazard ratios (HRs) and 95% confidence intervals (CIs) were calculated by a Cox proportional-hazard regression model in which treatment group, gender (males vs. females), age and concomitant cardiovascular risk factors (previous angina, congestive heart failure, arterial hypertension, diabetes mellitus, hypercholesterolemia, peripheral arterial occlusive disease, coronary revascularization) were included as a covariate. In order to account for different duration of follow up among the four studies, the relative risk of CV morbidity and mortality was assessed using a time-dependent Cox regression model and corresponding survival curves were drawn. In addition, a confirmatory Kaplan-Meier survival analysis with Log Rank (Mantel-Cox) test was run by considering events at the time of their occurrence, without applying any missing handling procedure.

Furthermore, we ran a confirmatory analysis by using the propensity score approach to balance non-equivalent study groups on observed potential confounding variables, in order to get more accurate estimates of the effect of treatment with XOIs. The propensity score was estimated by applying a logistic regression analysis, where the outcome was the treatment variable and predictor variables were the covariates [19, 20]. Accordingly, we estimated propensity scores with the observed covariates as predictors, and treatment assignment (dummy coded 0 = no treatment with XOIs, 1 = treatment with XOIs) as dependent variable. The selected model included as predictors: age, gender, body mass index, blood pressure, cardiovascular medical history, diagnosis of diabetes, diagnosis of hypertension, fasting plasma glucose, total and HDL cholesterol. After fitting the model according to a stepwise approach, the patients in the two treatment groups were stratified according to the aforementioned predictors and ranked in five equal-sized strata or quintiles (Q). The Q I represented patients with the best and the Q V included those with the worst risk profile; thus, patients inside each Q had a similar overall risk. The choice of five strata was based on the Cochran method [21], which showed that five strata are able to remove approximately 90% of the bias due to a single continuous covariate [22]. To validate the propensity score model we tested each of the covariates (predictors) in a two way (2 conditions × 5 strata) analysis of variance (continuous variables) or using a logistic regression (dichotomous categorical variables).

Homogeneity of patients' baseline characteristics were compared by a Chi-square test (discrete variables) or a Student t-test (continuous variables). The minimum level of statistical significance was $p < 0.05$. Data were represented as mean ± SD or 95% confidence interval or as absolute (n) and relative (%) frequencies.

Results

Patient population

The pooled data set included in this analysis consisted of 525 patients of whom 271 (51.6%) were treated with zofenopril, 147 (28.0%) with placebo and 107 (20.4%) with ramipril or lisinopril. One-hundred-sixty-five (31.4%) of the 525 patients were treated with XOIs (79 under zofenopril and 86 under placebo or other ACE-inhibitors), whereas the remaining 360 (68.6%) were not (192 zofenopril and 168 placebo or other ACE-inhibitors) (Fig. 1).

Demographic and clinical baseline characteristics were comparable among the four groups except for the prevalence of diabetes and differences in body mass index and diastolic blood pressure (Table 1). Regarding the drugs used during the study no statistically significant difference was observed in the use of cardiovascular therapy across the four study groups (Table 2).

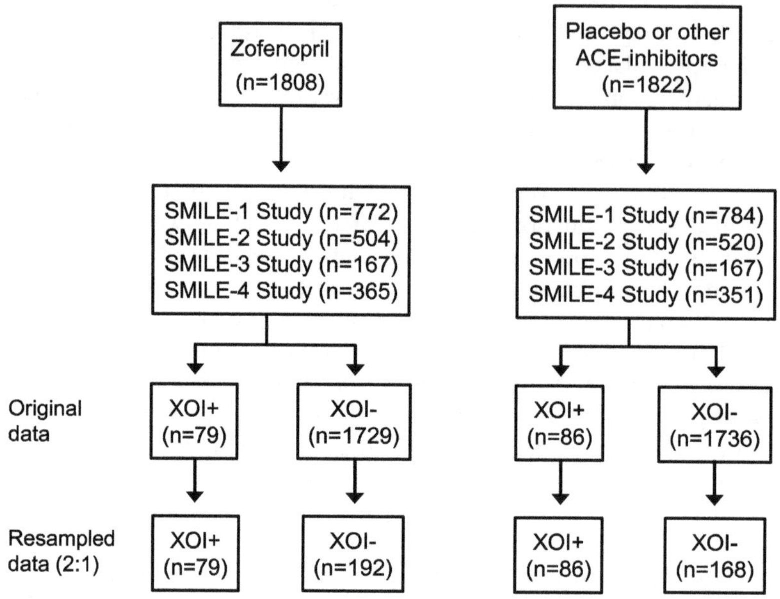

Fig. 1 Flow-chart of the patients in the study. ACE: Angiotensin Converting Enzyme; XOI+: patients treated with xanthine oxidase inhibitors; XOI-: patients not treated with xanthine oxidase inhibitors

Table 1 Demographic and clinical characteristics of the study population summarized by type of treatment (with, + or without, – concomitant xanthine oxidase inhibitors)

	Zofenopril+ ($n = 79$)	Zofenopril-($n = 192$)	Placebo or other ACE-inhibitors+ ($n = 86$)	Placebo or other ACE-inhibitors- ($n = 168$)	*p*-value
Age (years)	62.0 ± 10.3	60.2 ± 10.2	62.0 ± 10.3	62.9 ± 11.0	0.112
Gender					
Male	*57 (72.2)*	*151 (78.6)*	*71 (82.6)*	*119 (70.8)*	*0.121*
Female	*22 (27.8)*	*41 (21.4)*	*15 (17.4)*	*49 (29.2)*	
BMI (kg/m^2)	26.8 ± 3.3	28.2 ± 4.2	27.4 ± 3.9	26.3 ± 3.8	< 0.001
Systolic BP (mmHg)	139.8 ± 22.4	134.0 ± 20.0	135.5 ± 21.0	136.4 ± 22.8	0.251
Diastolic BP (mmHg)	85.2 ± 13.8	80.8 ± 12.3	83.1 ± 12.3	83.3 ± 11.9	0.046
Heart Rate (bpm)	78.9 ± 14.5	77.7 ± 16.1	77.6 ± 16.1	76.1 ± 15.1	0.503
LVEF (%)	46.6 ± 8.4	44.9 ± 10.0	45.1 ± 5.9	45.1 ± 13.2	0.946
Killip Class					
I	38 (48.1)	80 (41.7)	44 (51.2)	75 (44.6)	0.477
II	35 (44.3)	101 (52.6)	39 (45.3)	85 (50.6)	0.519
III-IV	4 (5.1)	11 (5.7)	3 (3.5)	8 (4.8)	0.884
CV risk factors	68 (86.1)	154 (80.2)	70 (81.4)	137 (81.5)	0.728
Diabetes	21 (26.6)	44 (22.9)	27 (31.4)	70 (41.7)	0.001
Hypercholesterolemia	19 (24.1)	47 (24.5)	17 (19.8)	38 (22.6)	0.848
Hypertension	47 (59.5)	97 (50.5)	46 (53.5)	87 (51.8)	0.592

Data are shown as absolute (n) and relative (%) frequencies for categorical variables and as means (±SD) for continuous variables. *P*-values refer to the statistical significance of the difference across the four treatment groups. BMI: Body Mass Index; *SD* Standard Deviation, *BP* Blood Pressure, *LVEF* Left Ventricular Ejection Fraction, *CV* Cardiovascular

Table 2 Concomitant cardiovascular drug treatments during the follow-up period by type of treatment (with, + or without, – concomitant xanthine oxidase inhibitors

	Zofenopril+ ($n = 79$)	Zofenopril-($n = 192$)	Placebo or other ACE-inhibitors+ ($n = 86$)	Placebo or other ACE-inhibitors- ($n = 168$)	p-value
ACE-inhibitors	2 (2.5)	6 (3.1)	2 (2.3)	3 (1.8)	0.879
Angiotensin II receptor blockers	–	2 (1.0)	–	–	0.323
Beta-blockers	37 (46.8)	95 (49.5)	39 (45.4)	85 (50.6)	0.837
Calcium channel blockers	6 (7.6)	19 (9.9)	6 (7.0)	13 (7.7)	0.814
Diuretics	13 (16.5)	40 (20.8)	20 (23.3)	38 (22.6)	0.682
Nitrates	31 (39.2)	96 (50.0)	50 (58.1)	92 (54.8)	0.067
Antiarrhythmic drugs	6 (7.6)	16 (8.3)	5 (5.8)	13 (7.7)	0.910
Antithrombotic agents (including ASA)	70 (88.6)	151 (78.6)	69 (80.2)	141 (83.9)	0.219
Lipid lowering drugs (including statins)	32 (40.5)	61 (31.8)	28 (32.6)	52 (31.0)	0.480
Other cardiovascular drugs	11 (13.9)	31 (16.2)	12 (13.9)	22 (13.1)	0.866

Data are shown as absolute (n) and relative (%) frequencies. *P*-values refer to the statistical significance of the difference across the four treatment groups. *ACE* Angiotensin Converting Enzyme, *ASA* Acetyl Salicylic Acid

Cardiovascular outcomes according to treatment group

MACE occurred in 24 of 165 patients (14.5%) treated with concomitant XOIs and in 63 of 360 patients (17.5%) not treated with XOIs, with a 20% non-statistically significant ($p = 0.398$) lower risk of achieving the end-point under XOIs [hazard ratio: 0.80 (0.48, 1.34)]. Eight (10.1%) patients receiving zofenopril with XOIs, 16 (18.6%) receiving placebo or other ACE-inhibitors with XOIs, 26 (13.5%) receiving zofenopril without XOIs and 37 (22.0%) receiving placebo or other ACE-Inhibitors without XOIs reported a MACE during the study ($p = 0.034$ across groups) (Fig. 2a).

Survival MACE free rate was significantly larger in patients receiving zofenopril with XOIs than in those who were treated with placebo or other ACE-inhibitors without XOIs [hazard ratio: 2.29 (1.06, 4.91), Cox regression analysis $p = 0.034$] (Fig. 2d). A non-significant trend for superiority was observed for zofenopril with XOIs compared to zofenopril alone [1.19 (0.54, 2.64), $p = 0.669$] (Fig. 2b) or to placebo or other ACE-inhibitors with XOIs [1.82 (0.78, 4.26), $p = 0.169$] (Fig. 2c).

In the Kaplan-Meier analysis, survival time without any events was significantly longer in patients treated with zofenopril and XOIs [10.9 (10.2, 11.7) months] than in those treated with placebo or other ACE-inhibitors without XOIs [9.5 (8.7, 10.2) months; Log rank test $p = 0.033$) (Fig. 3c). Average survival time free from cardiovascular events was only marginally lower in patients treated with zofenopril without XOIs [10.7 (10.2, 11.2) months; $p = 0.709$ vs. zofenopril plus XOIs) and in those treated with placebo or ACE-Inhibitors with XOIs [9.9 (8.9, 10.8) months; $p = 0.170$ vs. zofenopril with XOIs] (Fig. 3a and b).

Propensity analysis

A statistically significant difference was observed across the five groups for the predictors included in the propensity analysis, except for body mass index (QI: 27.3 ± 3.6 kg/m^2; QII: 27.8 ± 3.8 kg/m^2; QIII: 27.0 ± 3.6 kg/m^2; QIV: 27.3 ± 4.4 kg/m^2; QV: 26.7 ± 4.3 kg/m^2; $p = 0.329$) and the prevalence of diabetes (QI:28.6%; QII: 34.3%; QIII: 37.1%; QIV: 33.3%; QV: 21.0%; $p = 0.095$) and hypercholesterolemia (QI:15.2%; QII: 24.8%; QIII: 25.7%; QIV: 27.6%; QV: 21.9%; $p = 0.238$) (Table 3). After adjusting for the propensity score, the rate of MACE was still non-significantly ($p = 0.456$) lower in XOI-treated patients [hazard ratio: 0.84 (0.34, 2.10)].

The rate of MACE significantly ($p = 0.043$) increased at increasing Q. Differences in the effect of the various study drugs were observed within each Q of the propensity score. A superior effect of concomitant treatment with XOIs (and in particular of zofenopril with XOIs) vs. treatment without XOIs (in particular placebo or ACE-inhibitors without XOIs) was observed in Q I (MACE under zofenopril plus XOIs: 0% vs. 20.8% under placebo or other ACE-inhibitors without XOIs) and Q II (4.5% vs. 17.2%) low risk category and in the Q IV (16.7% vs. 28.1%) and Q V (20.0% vs. 25.5%) high risk category.

Figure 4a, shows cumulative survival without events during 1-year of follow-up in the whole study population and after stratification for propensity score in all the treated patients: the trend for a superior effect of treatment including a XOI was observed for all Qs except for Q III. When patients treated with placebo were excluded from the analysis (thus including only patients treated with zofenopril or other ACE-inhibitors), the analysis confirmed a trend to a higher chance of survival in case of concomitant treatment with XOIs in the lowest and highest Qs, whereas for intermediate risk (QIII) a benefit of XOI treatment was not observed (Fig. 4b).

Discussion

This retrospective analysis on SMILE pooled patients demonstrated that the combination of an ACE-inhibitor

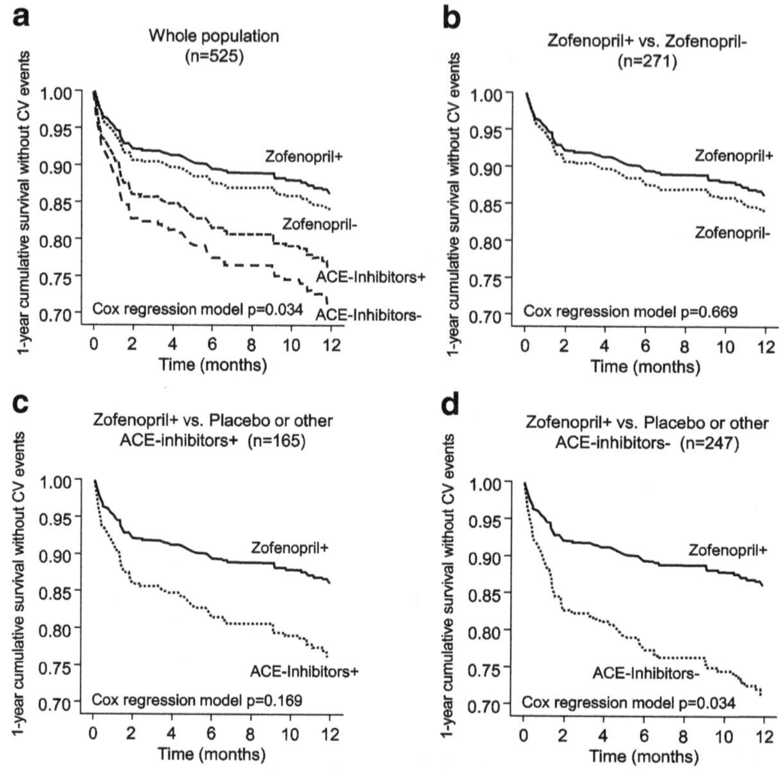

Fig. 2 Cumulative survival without events during 1-year of follow-up (based on Cox regression analysis), in (**a**) the whole population of patients treated (+) or not treated (-) with Xantine-oxidase inhibitors, (**b**) patients receiving zofenopril with xanthine oxidase inhibitors (+) as respect to those treated with zofenopril alone (-), (**c**) those treated with zofenopril (zofenopril+) vs. placebo or other angiotensin converting enzyme (ACE)-inhibitors both in combination with and xanthine-oxidase inhibitors (ACE-inhibitors+) and (**d**) those treated with zofenopril and xanthine-oxidase inhibitors (zofenopril+) vs. placebo or other ACE-inhibitors without XOIs (ACE-inhibitors-). *P*-values for the between-group comparison are reported in each panel

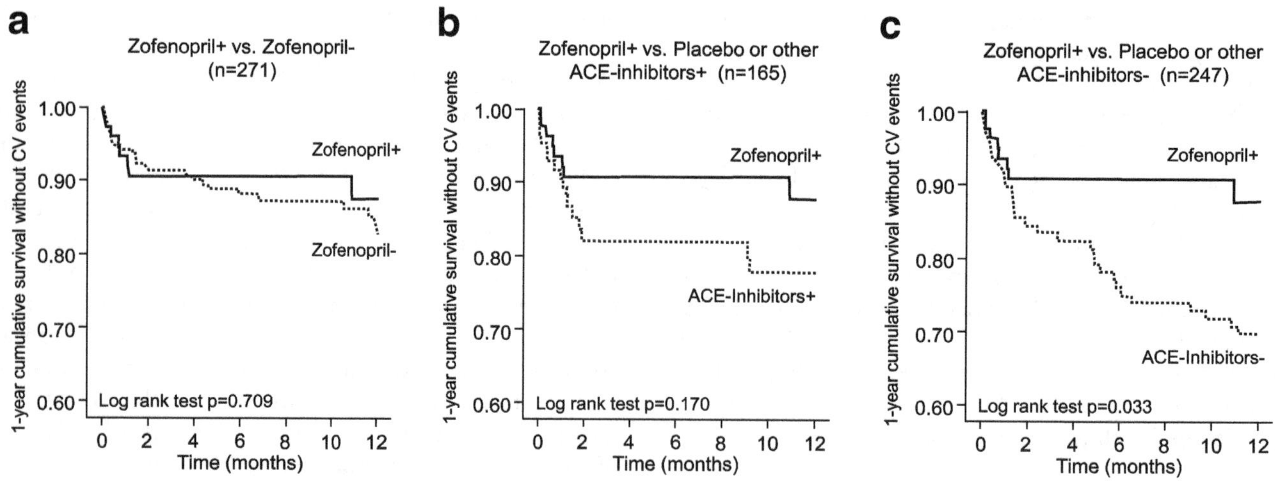

Fig. 3 Kaplan-Meier curves for survival without events during 1-year of follow-up, in patients receiving zofenopril with xanthine oxidase inhibitors or XOIs (+) as respect to those treated with zofenopril without (–) XOIs, those treated with placebo or other angiotensin converting enzyme (ACE)-inhibitors plus XOIs, those treated with placebo or other ACE-inhibitors without concomitant XOIs. *P*-values for the between-group comparison based on Log Rank Test are reported in each panel

Table 3 Baseline demographic characteristics of the study population stratified by propensity subgroups (quintiles, Q)

Characteristics	Propensity group					*p*-value for propensity score analysis
	Q I (*n* = 105)	Q II (*n* = 105)	Q III (*n* = 105)	Q IV (*n* = 105)	Q V (*n* = 105)	
	≤0.0095	0.0096–0.0205	0.0206–0.0412	0.0413–0.0849	≥0.0850	
Age (years, mean ± SD)	51.6 ± 8.8	58.1 ± 10.2	61.9 ± 8.2	65.0 ± 7.1	71.4 ± 6.6	< 0.001
Gender (n, %)						
Male	*98 (93.3)*	*88 (83.8)*	*87 (82.9)*	*73 (69.5)*	*52 (49.5)*	< 0.001
Female	*7 (6.7)*	*17 (16.2)*	*18 (17.1)*	*32 (30.5)*	*53 (50.5)*	
BMI (kg/m^2, means ± SD)	27.3 ± 3.6	27.8 ± 3.8	27.0 ± 3.6	27.3 ± 4.4	26.7 ± 4.3	0.329
Systolic BP (mmHg, means±SD)	127.4 ± 18.9	129.8 ± 19.0	139.1 ± 20.1	138.5 ± 23.0	144.4 ± 22.2	< 0.001
Diastolic BP (mmHg, means±SD)	77.1 ± 11.7	79.8 ± 11.4	83.3 ± 11.1	84.7 ± 12.6	88.5 ± 12.4	< 0.001
Heart rate (bpm, means ± SD)	73.1 ± 13.1	74.5 ± 13.0	74.1 ± 12.6	81.0 ± 14.8	83.9 ± 15.4	< 0.001
LVEF (%, means ± SD)	48.8 ± 10.2	45.9 ± 10.1	45.7 ± 9.1	42.7 ± 9.4	41.1 ± 10.3	0.002
CV Risk Factors (n, %)	48 (45.7)	80 (76.2)	93 (88.6)	103 (98.1)	105 (100.0)	< 0.001
Diabetes (n, %)	30 (28.6)	36 (34.3)	39 (37.1)	35 (33.3)	22 (21.0)	0.095
Hypercholesterolemia (n, %)	16 (15.2)	26 (24.8)	27 (25.7)	29 (27.6)	23 (21.9)	0.238
Hypertension (n, %)	29 (27.6)	50 (47.6)	61 (58.1)	66 (62.9)	71 (67.6)	< 0.001

Data are shown as absolute (n) and relative frequencies (%) for categorical variables and as means (±SD) for continuous variables. *P*-values refer to the statistical significance of the difference across the five Qs. *SD* Standard Deviation, *BMI* Body Mass Index, *LVEF* Left Ventricular Ejection Fraction, *SBP* Systolic Blood Pressure, *DBP* Diastolic Blood Pressure, *HR* Heart Rate

and XOIs may be protective against MACE after AMI compared to treatment with an ACE-inhibitor without XOIs. A combination treatment of zofenopril and XOI seems to promote a statistically significant longer survival time without any events than treatment with other ACEIs not combined with XOIs, whereas a non-statistically significant trend to a large benefit of the XOI + zofenopril combination is observed vs. the combination of another ACE-inhibitor and XOI or vs. zofenopril alone. Possible explanations for our findings, as well as limitations of the present retrospective analysis, will be discussed in the next paragraphs.

In our population, the prevalence of patients who needed preparation inhibiting uric acid production was slightly higher than gout prevalence reported from 2000 to 2005 in European countries (4.5% vs 1.4%) [23]. This may be explained with the observation that there is an independent relationship between hyperuricemia and AMI [24] and patients with gout have an increased risk of AMI [25].

The analysis of pooled data confirmed the results of individual SMILE studies. In each SMILE study, treatment of AMI patients with zofenopril effectively reduced the risk of mortality and hospitalization for cardiovascular causes compared to placebo and other ACE-inhibitors, such as lisinopril and ramipril [26]. The results of pooled SMILE studies supported the notion that there are differences in terms of efficacy between different ACE-inhibitors, and that, in contrast to previous observations, a class effect is unlikely [27]. As a matter of fact, Hansen et al. investigated the risk of mortality and re-infarction after a first episode of AMI and demonstrated that there was none difference in terms of clinical efficacy between ACE inhibitors. However, in this study zofenopril was not included and the only sulfhydryl ACE inhibitor was captopril [27]. Zofenopril demonstrated higher anti-atherosclerotic and antioxidant effects than captopril in the arterial wall of hypercholesterolemic apoE(−/−) mice [28]. In rat models of experimental cardiac ischemia/reperfusion (IR) injury, zofenopril prevented the changes that usually occurred during IR injury and reduced lipid peroxidation, protein oxidation, and nitric oxide levels as well as XO and myeloperoxidase activities and increased the catalase and superoxide dismutase activities [29]. In untreated normocholesterolemic patients with moderate essential hypertension without clinically evident target organ damage, a 12-weeks treatment with zofenopril significantly reduced malondialdehyde levels, plasma NOx and asymmetrical dimethyl-L-arginine concentrations, compared to enalapril that was ineffective [30]. Consistently, the long term treatment with zofenopril in mildly hypertensive patients resulted in a favorable nitric oxide/oxidative stress profile and showed a slower progression of intima- media thickening of the carotid artery beyond lowering arterial pressure [31].

The present retrospective analysis is based on the observation that clinical benefits of early zofenopril treatment in post-AMI phase are related also to its antioxidant properties and, therefore, the combination with XOIs may have an enhanced effect. Previous studies have investigated the opportunity of a therapy with

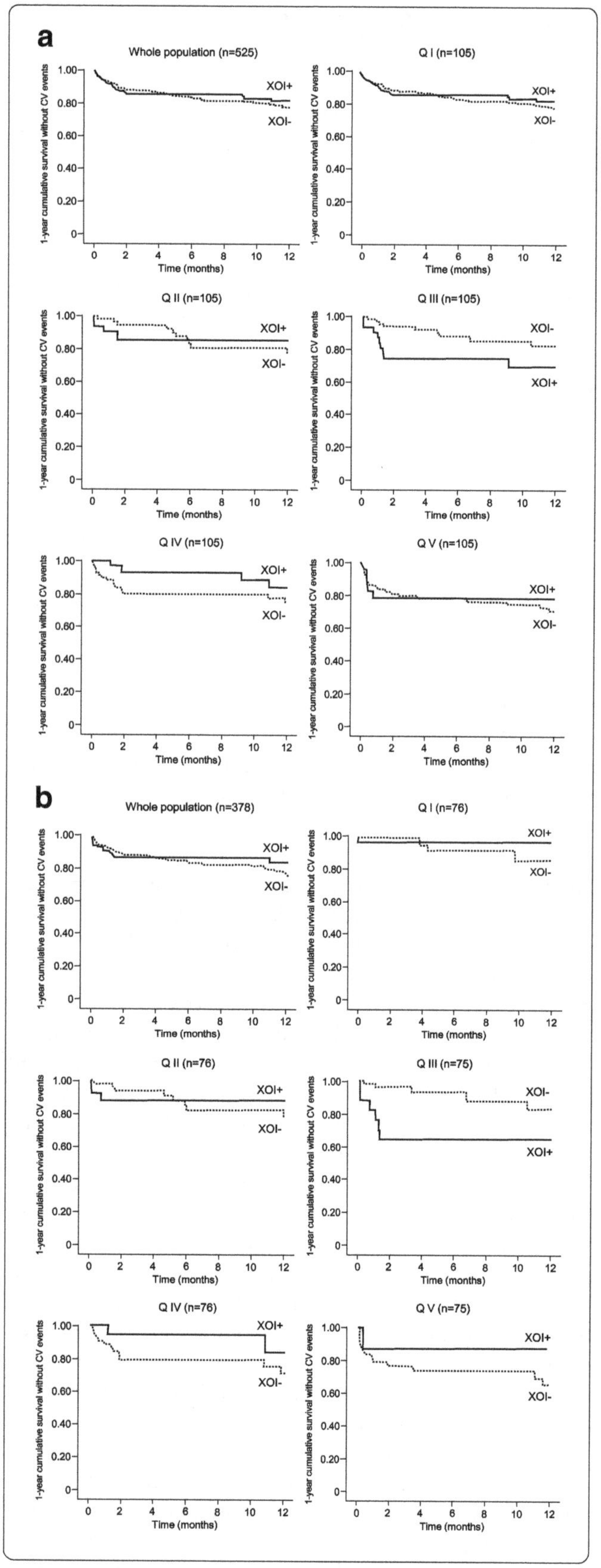

Fig. 4 Cumulative survival without events during 1-year of follow-up in the whole study population and after stratification for propensity score (quintiles, Q), according to presence (+) or absence (–) of concomitant treatment with xanthine oxidase inhibitors XOIs. Data are shown for all treated patients (**a**) and after excluding patients treated with placebo (**b**)

oxypurinol 600 mg daily in addition to an ACE-inhibitors or angiotensin receptor blocker and a beta-blocker in patients with moderate-to-severe HF. Oxypurinol significantly reduced serum uric acid by approximately 2 mg/dL, but did not improve the clinical status in unselected patients and when patients were stratified according to uric acid levels patients with elevated uric acid levels ($\geq$ 9.5 mg/dL, $n = 108$) responded favorably to oxypurinol, whereas patients with UA < 9.5 mg/dL exhibited a trend towards worsening [32]. In our study, patients were clustered according to XOI treatment and not to uric acid levels. Therefore, we selected patients who already needed a preparation inhibiting uric acid production and had a therapy. These patients had major benefits in post-AMI phase when they were treated with zofenopril than lisinopril or ramipril. Further larger studies should be recommended to identify which population of hyperuremic patients may achieve major clinical benefits with zofenopril treatment post-AMI.

This study has some main limitations. First of all, it was a retrospective analysis and the number of patients concomitantly treated with ACE inhibitors and XOI in post-AMI phase was limited. This may explain why some comparisons (e.g. those between zofenopril and other ACE-inhibitors) did not achieve statistical significance. We tried to overcome this limitation in two ways: we down-sampled the control population of patients not treated with XOI, thus balancing the comparisons (yet, however, limited to a small sample), and we applied a propensity score analysis [19]. The latter confirmed the superiority of concomitant treatment with XO in terms of prevention of MACE and supported a better efficacy of a combination including zofenopril. However, we acknowledge that, given the retrospective nature of our study, the sample size could have been underpowered to demonstrate the study goal. Second, despite a very similar design of the four SMILE studies, there were some differences in the inclusion criteria, treatment duration, and follow-up. Our analysis included both thrombolyzed and non-thrombolyzed patients and those with and without left ventricular dysfunction; in addition, clinical effect was observed at different time-points. Thus, the patients considered in this study may be representative of those who could be encountered in post-AMI phase in clinical practice. However, in assessments of differences between treatments, variations in baseline characteristics may decrease the sensitivity of such analyses to show interaction.

Finally, we have no information about the exact type of XOI used by patients and the duration of treatment in the patients of these groups and thus we cannot know whether differences in outcomes may be related to differences in the type or duration of treatment. We also do not have information on serum levels of uric acid at baseline and during the follow-up period and thus we do not know the actual effectiveness of XOI treatment.

Conclusions

Our retrospective analysis on patients involved in the four SMILE studies suggests that concomitant use of zofenopril and urate lowering drugs with antioxidant activity (XOIs) may further improve survival free from MACE in post-AMI patients. Further prospective studies should be recommended to compare the activity of different ACE-inhibitors in hyperuremic patients and establish a treatment schedule to gain major clinical benefits.

Abbreviations

ACE: Angiotensin-Converting Enzyme; AMI: Acute Myocardial Infarction; CHD: Coronary Heart Disease; CI: Confidence Interval; CV: Cardiovascular; HDL: High Density Lipoprotein; HF: Heart Failure; HR: Hazard Ratio; IR: Ischemia / Reperfusion; MACE: Major Cardiovascular Events; NOx: Nitric Oxide; Q: Quintile; SD: Standard Deviation; SMILE: Survival of Myocardial Infarction Long-Term Evaluation; XO: Xanthine Oxidase; XOI: Xanthine Oxidase Inhibitors

Funding

This work was financially supported by Menarini International Operations Luxembourg S.A. through an unconditional and unrestricted grant. The funding source did not influence or commented on planned methods, protocol, data analysis and the draft report.

Authors' contributions

CB conceived the study analyses. GR performed the analyses. SO wrote the paper and critically revised the results of the analyses. SB, SSE and EA critically revised the final manuscript. All authors read and approved the final manuscript.

Competing interests

Competing interest of Prof Claudio Borghi: consultancy for Boheringer Ingelheim, Menarini International, Sanofi, Amgen, Takeda, Novartis, Ely Lilly and Servier. None of the other authors has any conflict of interest to disclose.

Author details

[1]Unit of Internal Medicine, Policlinico S. Orsola, University of Bologna, Bologna, Italy. [2]Clinical Research Unit, Italian Institute of Telemedicine, Varese, Italy. [3]Mediservice S.r.l., Agrate Brianza, Italy. [4]Divisione di Medicina Interna, Policlinico S.Orsola, Via Massarenti 9, 40138 Bologna, Italy.

References

1. Mallat Z, Philip I, Lebret M, Chatel D, Maclouf J, Tedgui A. Elevated levels of 8-iso-prostaglandin F2alpha in pericardial fluid of patients with heart failure: a potential role for in vivo oxidant stress in ventricular dilatation and progression to heart failure. Circulation. 1998;97(16):1536 9.
2. Trkulja V, Car S. On-admission serum uric acid predicts outcomes after acute myocardial infarction: systematic review and meta-analysis of prognostic studies. Croat Med J. 2012;53(2):162–72.
3. Feig DI, Kang DH, Johnson RJ. Uric acid and cardiovascular risk. N Engl J Med. 2008;359(17):1811–21.
4. Duan X, Ling F. Is uric acid itself a player or a bystander in the pathophysiology of chronic heart failure? Med Hypotheses. 2008;70(3):578–81.
5. Anker SD, Doehner W, Rauchhaus M, Sharma R, Francis D, Knosalla C, Davos CH, Cicoira M, Shamim W, Kemp M, Segal R, Osterziel KJ, Leyva F, Hetzer R, Ponikowski P, Coats AJ. Uric acid and survival in chronic heart failure: validation and application in metabolic, functional, and hemodynamic staging. Circulation. 2003;107(15):1991–7.
6. Kittleson MM, St John ME, Bead V, Champion HC, Kasper EK, Russell SD, Wittstein IS, Hare JM. Increased levels of uric acid predict haemodynamic compromise in patients with heart failure independently of B-type natriuretic peptide levels. Heart. 2007;93(3):365–7.
7. Farquharson CA, Butler R, Hill A, Belch JJ, Struthers AD. Allopurinol improves endothelial dysfunction in chronic heart failure. Circulation. 2002;106(2):221–6.
8. Cingolani HE, Plastino JA, Escudero EM, Mangal B, Brown J, Perez NG. The effect of xanthine oxidase inhibition upon ejection fraction in heart failure patients: La Plata study. J Card Fail. 2006;12(7):491–8.
9. Erdogan D, Tayyar S, Uysal BA, Icli A, Karabacak M, Ozaydin M, Dogan A. Effects of allopurinol on coronary microvascular and left ventricular function in patients with idiopathic dilated cardiomyopathy. Can J Cardiol. 2012; 28(6):721–7.
10. Givertz MM, Anstrom KJ, Redfield MM, Deswal A, Haddad H, Butler J, Tang WH, Dunlap ME, LeWinter MM, Mann DL, Felker GM, O'Connor CM, Goldsmith SR, Ofili EO, Saltzberg MT, Margulies KB, Cappola TP, Konstam MA, Semigran MJ, McNulty SE, Lee KL, Shah MR, Hernandez AF, Network NHFCR. Effects of xanthine oxidase inhibition in Hyperuricemic heart failure patients: the xanthine oxidase inhibition for Hyperuricemic heart failure patients (EXACT-HF) study. Circulation. 2015;131(20):1763–71.
11. Noman A, Ang DS, Ogston S, Lang CC, Struthers AD. Effect of high-dose allopurinol on exercise in patients with chronic stable angina: a randomised, placebo controlled crossover trial. Lancet. 2010;375:2161–7.
12. Opie LH. Allopurinol for heart failure: novel mechanisms. J Am Coll Cardiol. 2012;59:809–12.
13. Evangelista S, Manzini S. Antioxidant and cardioprotective properties of the sulphydryl angiotensin-converting enzyme inhibitor zofenopril. J Int Med Res. 2005;33(1):42–54.
14. Pasini AF, Garbin U, Nava MC, Stranieri C, Pellegrini M, Boccioletti V, Luchetta ML, Fabrizzi P, Lo Cascio V, Cominacini L. Effect of sulfhydryl and non-sulfhydryl angiotensin-converting enzyme inhibitors on endothelial function in essential hypertensive patients. Am J Hypertens. 2007;20(4):443–50.
15. Ambrosioni E, Borghi C, Magnani B. The effect of the angiotensin-converting-enzyme inhibitor zofenopril on mortality and morbidity after anterior myocardial infarction. The survival of myocardial infarction long-term evaluation (SMILE) study investigators. N Engl J Med. 1995;332(2):80–5.
16. Borghi C, Ambrosioni E, Novo S, Vinereanu D, Ambrosio G, Party S-W. Comparison between zofenopril and ramipril in combination with acetylsalicylic acid in patients with left ventricular systolic dysfunction after acute myocardial infarction: results of a randomized, double-blind, parallel-group, multicenter, European study (SMILE-4). Clin Cardiol. 2012;35(7):416–23.
17. Borghi C, Ambrosioni E. Survival of myocardial infarction long-term Evaluation-2 working P. Double-blind comparison between zofenopril and lisinopril in patients with acute myocardial infarction: results of the survival of myocardial infarction long-term Evaluation-2 (SMILE-2) study. Am Heart J. 2003;145(1):80–7.
18. Borghi C, Ambrosioni E, Survival of Myocardial Infarction Long-term Evaluation Study G. Effects of zofenopril on myocardial ischemia in post-myocardial infarction patients with preserved left ventricular function: the Survival of Myocardial Infarction Long-term Evaluation (SMILE)-ISCHEMIA study. Am Heart J. 2007;153(3):445. e7–14
19. D'Agostino RB. Propensity scores in cardiovascular research. Circulation. 2007;115:2340–3.
20. Williamson EJ, Forbes A, White IR. Variance reduction in randomized trials by inverse probability weighting using the propensity score. Statist Med. 2013;33:721–37.
21. Cochran WG. The effectiveness of adjustment by sub-classification in removing bias in observational studies. Biometrics. 1968;24:295–313.
22. Rosembaum PR, Rubin DB. Reducing bias in observational studies using subclassification on the propensity score. J Am Stat Assoc. 1984;79:516–24.

23. Annemans L, Spaepen E, Gaskin M, Bonnemaire M, Malier V, Gilbert T, Nuki G. Gout in the UK and Germany: prevalence, comorbidities and management in general practice 2000-2005. Ann Rheum Dis. 2008;67(7):960–6.
24. Krishnan E, Baker JF, Furst DE, Schumacher HR. Gout and the risk of acute myocardial infarction. Arthritis Rheum. 2006;54(8):2688–96.
25. Liu SC, Xia L, Zhang J, Lu XH, Hu DK, Zhang HT, Li HJ. Gout and risk of myocardial infarction: a systematic review and meta-analysis of cohort studies. PLoS One. 2015;10(7):e0134088.
26. Borghi C, Omboni S, Reggiardo G, Bacchelli S, Degli Esposti D, Ambrosioni E. Cardioprotective role of zofenopril in patients with acute myocardial infarction: a pooled individual data analysis of four randomised, double-blind, controlled, prospective studies. Open Heart. 2015;2(1):e000220.
27. Hansen ML, Gislason GH, Kober L, Schramm TK, Folke F, Buch P, Abildstrom SZ, Madsen M, Rasmussen S, Torp-Pedersen C. Different angiotensin-converting enzyme inhibitors have similar clinical efficacy after myocardial infarction. Br J Clin Pharmacol. 2008;65(2):217–23.
28. de Nigris F, D'Armiento FP, Somma P, Casini A, Andreini I, Sarlo F, Mansueto G, De Rosa G, Bonaduce D, Condorelli M, Napoli C. Chronic treatment with sulfhydryl angiotensin-converting enzyme inhibitors reduce susceptibility of plasma LDL to in vitro oxidation, formation of oxidation-specific epitopes in the arterial wall, and atherogenesis in apolipoprotein E knockout mice. Int J Cardiol. 2001;81(2–3):107–115; discusssion 15–6.
29. Altunoluk B, Soylemez H, Oguz F, Turkmen E, Fadillioglu E. An angiotensin-converting enzyme inhibitor, zofenopril, prevents renal ischemia/reperfusion injury in rats. Ann Clin Lab Sci. 2006;36(3):326–32.
30. Napoli C, Sica V, de Nigris F, Pignalosa O, Condorelli M, Ignarro LJ, Liguori A. Sulfhydryl angiotensin-converting enzyme inhibition induces sustained reduction of systemic oxidative stress and improves the nitric oxide pathway in patients with essential hypertension. Am Heart J 2004;148(1):e5.
31. Napoli C, Bruzzese G, Ignarro LJ, Crimi E, de Nigris F, Williams-Ignarro S, Libardi S, Sommese L, Fiorito C, Mancini FP, Cacciatore F, Liguori A. Long-term treatment with sulfhydryl angiotensin-converting enzyme inhibition reduces carotid intima-media thickening and improves the nitric oxide/ oxidative stress pathways in newly diagnosed patients with mild to moderate primary hypertension. Am Heart J. 2008;156(6):1154. e1–8
32. Hare JM, Mangal B, Brown J, Fisher C Jr, Freudenberger R, Colucci WS, Mann DL, Liu P, Givertz MM, Schwarz RP, Investigators O-C. Impact of oxypurinol in patients with symptomatic heart failure. Results of the OPT-CHF study. J Am Coll Cardiol. 2008;51(24):2301–9.

24

Allopurinol use and the risk of acute cardiovascular events in patients with gout and diabetes

Jasvinder A. Singh[1,2,3,4*], Rekha Ramachandaran[2], Shaohua Yu[2] and Jeffrey R. Curtis[2,3]

Abstract

Background: Few studies, if any, have examined cardiovascular outcomes in patients with diabetes and gout. Both diabetes and gout are risk factors for cardiovascular disease. The objective of this study was to examine the effect of allopurinol on the risk of incident acute cardiovascular events in patients with gout and diabetes.

Methods: We used the 2007–2010 Multi-Payer Claims Database (MPCD) that linked health plan data from national commercial and governmental insurances, representing beneficiaries with United Healthcare, Medicare, or Medicaid coverage. In patients with gout and diabetes, we assessed the current allopurinol use, defined as a new filled prescription for allopurinol, as the main predictor of interest. Our outcome of interest was the occurrence of the first Incident hospitalized myocardial infarction (MI) or stroke (composite acute cardiovascular event), after which observations were censored. We employed multivariable-adjusted Cox proportional hazards models that simultaneously adjusted for patient demographics, cardiovascular risk factors and other medical comorbidities. We calculated hazard ratios [HR] (95% confidence intervals [CI]) for incident composite (MI or stroke) acute cardiovascular events. We performed sensitivity analyses that additionally adjusted for the presence of immune diseases and colchicine use, as potential confounders.

Results: There were 2,053,185 person days (5621.3 person years) of current allopurinol use and 1,671,583 person days (4576.5 person years) of prior allopurinol use. There were 158 incident MIs or strokes in current and 151 in prior allopurinol users, respectively. Compared to previous allopurinol users, current allopurinol users had significantly lower adjusted hazard of incident acute cardiovascular events (incident stroke or MI), with an HR of 0.67 (95% CI, 0. 53, 0.84). Sensitivity analyses, additionally adjusted for immune diseases or colchicine use, confirmed this association.

Conclusions: Current allopurinol use protected against the occurrence of acute cardiovascular events in patients with gout and diabetes. The underlying mechanisms for this potential cardio-protective effect of allopurinol need further exploration.

Keywords: Allopurinol, Acute cardiovascular events, Gout, Diabetes, Myocardial infarction, Stroke, Predictors

* Correspondence: Jasvinder.md@gmail.com
[1]Medicine Service, VA Medical Center, 700 19th St S, Birmingham, AL 35233, USA
[2]Department of Medicine at School of Medicine, University of Alabama at Birmingham, 510, 20th street South, Faculty office tower (FOT), Birmingham, AL 35294, USA
Full list of author information is available at the end of the article

Background

Chronic inflammatory conditions, such as rheumatoid arthritis and gout, are associated with significant increase in cardiovascular morbidity and mortality. Several studies have reported a higher risk of cardiovascular disease in patients with gout [1–3]. The evidence supporting the association of hyperuricemia with increased cardiovascular risk [1, 4–7] indicates that this may be at least one potential mechanism for this increased cardiovascular risk in patients with gout.

Allopurinol, a purine analog, acts as a competitive substrate for xanthine oxidase, an enzyme that converts hypoxanthine to xanthine and xanthine into uric acid. Thus, it reduces the level of serum urate and acts as a urate-lowering therapy (ULT). Xanthine oxidase generates superoxide anions and other oxidative free radicals that are associated with oxidative stress [8]. Allopurinol reduces uric acid production and oxidative stress, processes that have been hypothesized to be associated with endothelial dysfunction, inflammation and progression of atherosclerosis [9]. Thus, allopurinol might have beneficial effects on cardiac physiology [10, 11].

Recent studies have debated whether allopurinol has a true cardio-protective effect, i.e., does it reduce the risk of outcomes such as myocardial infarction (MI)? A case-control study with a prevalent user design using the French pharmacoepidemiology database found that allopurinol use did not significantly reduce the risk of non-fatal MI, odds ratio (OR) was 0.80 (95% CI, 0.59, 1.09) [12]. In contrast, in a nested case-control study using Spanish primary care database, current allopurinol use and not past use, was associated with reduction in non-fatal MI with odds ratios of 0.52 (95% CI, 0.33 to 0.83) and 0.99 (95% CI, 0.61, 1.61), respectively [13]. Yet another study of gout patients using Scottish database reported that compared to non-use, allopurinol use was associated with higher (not lower) adjusted hazards of cardiovascular hospitalization (including coronary artery disease (CAD), hypertensive heart disease, heart failure, stroke, other cardiovascular diseases) of 1.25 (95% CI, 1.10, 1.41) [14]. These three studies differed in the main outcome assessed (MI vs. non-fatal MI vs. cardiovascular hospitalization including heart failure) and the country setting (France vs. Spain vs. Scotland), which could have explain the differences in the results between these three studies.

Key limitations of the previous studies included the use of a prevalent- user design [12, 14], the potential lack of adequate statistical power [12, 13], a short follow-up [13], potential survival bias since non-fatal MI cases were included [12–14], and the non-exclusion of patients with previous MI [14]. A prevalent-user design (used in 2 of the 3 studies) is likely more biased than a new-user design, due to the potential inclusion of factors on the causal pathway and the lack of an ability to capture early events (especially harmful effects) after starting a medication. Incident user design, in which medication exposure time begins with a new start of a medication, allows for more valid treatment comparisons compared to mixing ongoing users with new users in the same analysis [15]. Thus, based on the current knowledge, it is unclear whether allopurinol treatment is independently associated with better cardiac outcomes.

Gout is commonly associated with several comorbidities, such as hypertension, diabetes etc. One-third of gout patients have diabetes [16]. Diabetes, as a major cardiovascular disease risk factor, affects 26 million Americans, is among the top 10 causes of death in the U.S., and cost $245 billion in direct and indirect costs in 2012 [17]. Despite the common occurence of both conditions and associated morbidity, studies of cardiovascular outcomes in patients with gout and diabetes are lacking.

We were interested in investigating cardiovascular (CV) events in patients with gout and concomitant diabetes, since this group of patients is at high risk of CV events, given that diabetes is an established CV risk factor and hyperuricemia (the key underlying abnormality in gout) has been implicated as a CV risk factor [1, 4–7]. Therefore our study objectives were to assess whether in patients with gout with diabetes, allopurinol therapy was associated with cardiovascular benefit as demonstrated by a lower incidence of acute cardiovascular events (myocardial infarction [MI] or stroke).

Methods

Study methods and results are reported as recommended by the Strengthening of Reporting in Observational studies in Epidemiology (STROBE) statement [18].

Study cohort and participants

The Institutional Review Board at the University of Alabama at Birmingham (UAB) approved the study. We conducted a retrospective cohort study using the Multi-Payer Claims Database (MPCD) that linked health plan data from national commercial and governmental insurances, representing beneficiaries with United Healthcare, Medicare, or Medicaid coverage during 2007–2010. MPCD data contain patients' demographic and insurance coverage information from enrollment files, claims for inpatient and outpatient services, and prescription medications.

For this analysis, we examined patients who had a diagnosis of both gout and diabetes. Gout was defined as the occurrence of an inpatient admission or 2 outpatient visits with a physician encounter at least 7 days apart and the presence of International Classification of Diseases, ninth revision, clinical modification [ICD-9-CM] codes 274.xx for gout, shown to have a positive predictive value >90% [19]. Diabetes was ascertained by the presence of two ICD-9-CM codes of 250.xx associated with physician encounter visits at least 7 days apart but ≤365 days and the use of a diabetes-specific medication [20], also a validated definition with high positive predictive value >90% [21–23]. The person was diabetes-eligible and gout-eligible "completely" the day he/she satisfied both diseases' eligibility criteria. The index date (follow up start) of the study cohort was defined as the day when the criteria for both disease eligibility and the 365 days of continuous coverage were satisfied. The baseline period was defined as 365 days before the start of follow up for each eligible participant episode. An individual was allowed to have more than 1 episode satisfying the 365 days of continuous coverage and at least 1 day for follow up, a standard methodology to maximize use of all data in the incident user design.

Study outcome

The study outcome of interest was incident acute cardiovascular event, a composite of incident hospitalized MI or incident hospitalized stroke, in patients with gout and diabetes. We excluded patients with MI, stroke or coronary artery disease (CAD) in the baseline 365-day period for these analyses, using diagnoses for incident or prevalent cardiovascular disease (410, 412, 430–438, 428, 429.2x) (Additional file 1), in order to analyze the first incident MI and the first incident stroke.

Incident MI and incident stroke were defined as inpatient hospitalization with respective ICD-9-CM codes for MI or stroke with at least 1-day hospital stay, unless death occurred (Additional file 1). This approach is accurate for case identification with high positive predictive value >90% for these diagnoses and other cardiovascular risk factors [23–25].

We censored observation if there was an outpatient diagnosis of 410.x1 or an inpatient or outpatient diagnosis of 410 other than 410.x1 and 412 in the MI analyses but allowed for a 2-day "grace period" in which MI hospitalizations were sought. For example, someone with an outpatient diagnosis of MI who was hospitalized for it within 24 h with hospital length of stay >1-day would have met the MI definition. For stroke analyses, we censored patients with grace period of 2-days after the occurrence of an outpatient diagnosis of stroke (430.xx, 431.xx, 433.x1, 436.xx, 434.xx except 434.x0) or an inpatient or outpatient diagnosis of 430–438 other than that of stroke ICD-9-codes (listed above). This approach was used due to uncertainties about the clinical relevance of an outpatient diagnosis of MI or stroke and to exclude prevalent cases of MI or stroke.

Exposure of interest

The study exposure of interest was the new use of allopurinol, defined based on a filled prescription for allopurinol, with no prior filled prescription of allopurinol for previous 183 days. We considered exposure days of medications from 2007 to 2010 allowing up to 30 days of stock to be carried over (if the medication was refilled slightly early). We allowed the days of supply of allopurinol to be a maximum of 120 days only. A new medication episode started if a patient had complete coverage but no filled prescription of allopurinol in previous 183 days. For the main analysis that used a new user design, we defined various time-varying allopurinol use categories for each person-day of follow-up as either current use (present day covered by allopurinol) or prior use (present day not covered by allopurinol, but prior period with allopurinol exposure) based on medication episodes. Each patient could contribute person-time to each of these groups, as per standard methodology in an incident user design, to allow maximal use of data.

Covariates and confounders

Study covariates measured in the baseline period were age, gender and race/ethnicity. We categorized age in 5-year age group categories and race/ethnicity into Asian, Hispanic, Black, White, other and missing. Cardiovascular risk factors other than diabetes (hypertension, hyperlipidemia), and other medical comorbidities, including chronic obstructive pulmonary disease (COPD) and renal failure were assessed based on the presence of respective ICD-9-CM codes during the study period prior to occurrence of outcome, as time-varying variables (Additional file 1). Comorbidities were categorized as present or absent.

Statistical analyses

We calculated summary statistics as proportion or mean (standard deviation). Unadjusted comparisons were performed using chi-square or t-tests, as appropriate. Crude incidence rates for MI and stroke were calculated for current and prior allopurinol users. We used the new user design as our main analysis to assess the association of allopurinol use with outcomes of interest [15].

We performed unadjusted and age-adjusted Cox regression analyses to obtain hazards of the composite acute cardiovascular event (incident MI or incident stroke) with allopurinol use. Multivariable-adjusted Cox regression analyses were performed next to account for demographics, cardiovascular risk factors (hypertension, hyperlipidemia), and comorbidities (COPD, renal failure). Hazard ratios for incident acute cardiovascular event were calculated, based on allopurinol use, current, vs. prior (referent). We performed statistical analyses using SAS version 9.2. A p-value <0.05 was considered significant.

We performed several sensitivity analyses to test the robustness of findings by: (1) additionally adjusting for autoimmune diseases, a potential risk factor for MI/stroke due to associated chronic inflammation; (2)

Table 1 Characteristics of allopurinol users

	All combined (%)	Allopurinol use (%)	
		Current‡	Previous‡
Total person days	3,724,768	2,053,185	1,671,583
Male gender	53.76	54.00	53.47
Age group			
≤ 50	7.55	6.54	8.79
51–60	12.86	11.66	14.33
61–65	9.70	9.32	10.17
66–70	24.00	24.68	23.16
71–75	19.73	20.12	19.26
76–80	14.16	14.41	13.86
> 80	12.00	13.27	10.44
Race			
Asian	4.49	4.29	4.73
Black	19.68	16.83	23.18
Hispanic	2.61	2.01	3.35
Other	1.87	1.78	1.98
Missing	4.89	4.26	5.67
White	66.46	70.83	61.09
Comorbidity			
Hypertension	85.57	85.35	85.85
COPD	9.12	9.00	9.27
Renal disease	26.11	27.71	24.14
PVD	8.12	8.17	8.05
Hyperlipidemia*	79.56	80.53	78.38

‡ Characteristics of individuals that contributed at least 1 person day to that column, and people could be represented in both columns, if they contributed to both current and previous allopurinol use; *Hyperlipidemia was defined as statin use or an ICD-9-CM code for hypercholesterolemia

Table 2 New Allopurinol use and Incident MI[a] or incident stroke[b] outcome

Allopurinol use	Total Person days (total person years)	Incident MI or Stroke	Per 100,000 PD (per 100 PY)
Current	2,053,185 person days (5621.3 person years)	158	7.70 (2.81 per 100 PY)
Previous	1,671,583 person days (4576.5 person years)	151	9.03 (3.30 per 100 PY)

PD person-days; *PY* person years

[a]For MI, the person days with baseline 410, 412, 430–438, 428.xx and 429.2X were removed. Also, the person days were censored at the occurrence of first MI or an outpatient diagnosis of 410.X1 or inpatient or outpatient diagnosis of 410 except 410.x1 and 412

[b]For stroke, the person days with baseline 410, 412, 430–438, 428.xx and 429.2X were removed. Also, the person days were censored at the occurrence of first stroke or an outpatient diagnosis of stroke or inpatient or outpatient diagnosis of 430–438 except for the dx codes for stroke. Stroke (430.xx, 431.xx, 433.x1 (433.01, 433.11, 433.21, 433.31, 433.81, 433.91), 434.xx excluding 434.x0 (434.01, 434.11, 434.91), 436.xx

additionally adjusting for the use of colchicine, a commonly used anti-inflammatory drug for gout that might have a cardio-protective effect [26]; or (3) using a prevalent user design, where we defined each day of follow-up as current, prior or never allopurinol use by adding never allopurinol users, defined as no allopurinol use (referent) from 2007 till the end of follow up.

Results

Patient demographic and clinical characteristics

We observed 2,053,185 person days of current allopurinol use and 1,671,583 person days of prior allopurinol use. Age distribution across groups was similar; 70.7% of current and 61.5% of prior allopurinol users were White (Table 1). Comorbidities were common in both groups: Hypertension, 85% each; hypercholesterolemia, 78–81%; and renal disease, 25–28% (Table 1).

Association of allopurinol use with incident MI or incident stroke

There were 158 and 151 incident acute cardiovascular events (MIs or strokes) in current and prior allopurinol users, respectively (Table 2). The crude rate of incident acute cardiovascular events (MI or stroke) in current and prior allopurinol users were 2.81 and 3.30 per 100 person-years, respectively. Association of allopurinol use with incident acute cardiovascular events (MI or stroke) in unadjusted and age-adjusted analyses including other significant correlates is shown in Table 3.

In multivariable-adjusted models that accounted for demographics and cardiovascular risk factors, compared to prior users, current allopurinol users had significantly lower hazard of incident stroke or MI, HR was 0.67 (95% CI, 0.53, 0.84) (Table 4). Other significant risk factors were older age and renal disease (Table 4).

Sensitivity analyses: adjustment for colchicine or immune disease and by prevalent use

Sensitivity analyses adjusting for colchicine revealed essentially the same results for current allopurinol use (yes/no) as in the main analyses above (Table 5). Colchicine was not significantly associated with the risk of incident MI or stroke, 0.80 (95% CI, 0.55, 1.18) (Table 5). Sensitivity analyses, additionally adjusted for immune disease confirmed the findings from the main analyses (Table 5); the presence of immune disease was not significantly associated, 1.04 (95% CI, 0.78, 1.37).

In multivariable adjusted analyses that used a prevalent user design analysis (not as robust as incident user design), we found that current allopurinol use was associated with similar hazard reduction of incident MI or stroke (as in the main analyses) when compared to: (1) prior allopurinol use, 0.84 (95% CI, 0.72, 0.98); and (2) never use, 0.86 (95% CI, 0.75, 0.99) (Additional file 2).

Table 3 Unadjusted and age-adjusted association of current allopurinol use with Incident acute cardiovascular event composite (MI or stroke) among patients with diabetes and gout

	Unadjusted		Age-adjusted	
	Hazard ratio (95% CI)	*p*-value	Hazard ratio (95% CI)	*p*-value
Allopurinol user				
Current	**0.71 (0.56, 0.89)**	**0.003**	**0.67 (0.53, 0.85)**	**0.0007**
Previous	Ref		Ref	
Male Gender	0.85 (0.68, 1.06)	0.14	1.01 (0.80, 1.27)	0.95
Age				
≤ 50	**0.40 (0.17, 0.92)**	**0.03**	-	-
51-60	0.86 (0.49, 1.50)	0.59	-	-
66-70	0.88 (0.54, 1.45)	0.62	-	-
71-75	**1.64 (1.03, 2.61)**	**0.04**	-	-
76-80	1.58 (0.97, 2.59)	0.07	-	-
> 80	**2.70 (1.70, 4.30)**	**<0.0001**	-	-
61-65	Ref		-	-
Race				
Asian	1.05 (0.62, 1.78)	0.85	0.95 (0.56, 1.60)	0.84
Black	0.90 (0.67, 1.21)	0.50	1.03 (0.77, 1.39)	0.84
Hispanic	1.35 (0.73, 2.47)	0.34	1.54 (0.84, 2.82)	0.16
Other	1.53 (0.79, 2.98)	0.21	1.59 (0.82, 3.10)	0.17
Missing	0.58 (0.30, 1.13)	0.11	0.73 (0.37, 1.43)	0.36
White	Ref		Ref	
Comorbidity				
Hypertension	1.08 (0.78, 1.50)	0.63	1.01 (0.73, 1.41)	0.93
Hyperlipidemia	0.90 (0.69, 1.17)	0.43	0.91 (0.69, 1.19)	0.49
COPD	1.10 (0.76, 1.59)	0.63	1.09 (0.75, 1.58)	0.66
Renal disease	**1.40 (1.11, 1.78)**	**0.005**	**1.34 (1.06, 1.70)**	**0.02**
Peripheral vascular disease	1.08 (0.73, 1.60)	0.70	0.96 (0.65, 1.43)	0.86
Immune diseases	1.05 (0.80, 1.39)	0.71	1.07 (0.81, 1.41)	0.62
Colchicine use	0.74 (0.51, 1.09)	0.13	0.77 (0.53, 1.12)	0.18

Significant odds ratios are in bold
COPD chronic obstructive pulmonary disease

Discussion

In this study, we found that current use of allopurinol was associated with a statistically significant and clinically meaningful reduction of the risk of acute cardiovascular events (incident stroke or MI) in patients with gout and diabetes. We also provided crude incident rates for acute cardiovascular events in patients with gout and diabetes, by current versus prior allopurinol use. Several findings in this study deserve further discussion.

Our finding of 33% hazard reduction of incident stroke or MI with current allopurinol use compared to prior allopurinol use in patients with gout and diabetes is novel. We are unaware of other large studies that have examined this question. We chose to study this patient population (gout and diabetes) due to a higher risk of cardiovascular events. The beneficial cardiovascular effect of allopurinol may be related to several potential mechanisms including: (1) allopurinol associated attenuation of intercellular adhesion molecule-1 levels noted in patients after a recent stroke [27]; (2) improvement in endothelial function and reduction of oxidative stress with allopurinol [28–33]; and (3) reduction in glycosylated hemoglobin (HbA1C) with high-doses of allopurinol [33]. The potential mechanisms of cardiovascular risk reduction with reduction of serum urate, including oxidative stress and inflammation, were recently reviewed [34]. The hazards were decreased by 29% in the prevalent user analyses. This is consistent with a greater risk reduction seen in the incident user vs. prevalent user design, and might explain the lack of finding an association if prevalent user design is used and the sample size is smaller or events fewer.

Table 4 Multivariable-adjusted associations of allopurinol use with incident composite outcome (MI and stroke)

	Incident MI or stroke	
	Hazard ratio (95% CI)	*p*-value
Allopurinol User		
Current	**0.67 (0.53, 0.84)**	**0.0006**
Previous	Ref	
Gender		
Male	1.00 (0.80, 1.26)	0.99
Female	Ref	
Age, in years		
≤ 50	**0.40 (0.17, 0.93)**	**0.03**
51–60	0.85 (0.49, 1.49)	0.57
66–70	0.88 (0.54, 1.45)	0.61
71–75	**1.64 (1.02, 2.62)**	**0.04**
76–80	1.59 (0.97, 2.60)	0.07
> 80	**2.70 (1.69, 4.34)**	**<0.0001**
61–65	Ref	
Race		
Asian	0.92 (0.54, 1.55)	0.74
Black	0.97 (0.72, 1.31)	0.84
Hispanic	1.41 (0.76, 2.59)	0.27
Other	1.55 (0.79, 3.03)	0.20
Missing	0.71 (0.36, 1.40)	0.32
White	Ref	
Comorbidity		
Hypertension	0.96 (0.69, 1.35)	0.83
Hyperlipidemia	0.91 (0.69, 1.20)	0.51
COPD	1.07 (0.74, 1.55)	0.73
Renal disease	**1.36 (1.07, 1.73)**	**0.01**
PVD	0.93 (0.63, 1.39)	0.74

Significant odds ratios are in bold

PVD peripheral vascular disease, *COPD* chronic obstructive pulmonary disease

Our findings must be interpreted in the context of current knowledge in this area. Most previous studies examined stroke as part of a composite cardiovascular outcome that included multiple cardiovascular outcomes, not just stroke and MI. In a 7-year follow-up of a 2-year RCT in patients with chronic kidney disease with glomerular filtration rate of < 60 ml/min, adjusted for race, sex and renal function, allopurinol use was associated with lower risk of 0.43 (95% CI, 0.21–0.88) of cardiovascular events (including CAD, cerebrovascular disease, heart failure and peripheral vascular disease) [35]. In an observational study of 187 patients with hypertensive nephropathy, allopurinol use was associated with a reduced hazard of 0.34 ($p = 0.04$) for cardiovascular disease (CAD, heart failure and stroke) [36]. In a study using Scottish database, allopurinol use was associated with no difference in adjusted hazards of cardiovascular events (non-fatal myocardial infarction, non-fatal stroke and cardiovascular mortality) compared to non-users 1.10 (95% CI, 0.95–1.26) [14]. Differences in the conditions included in the composite cardiovascular outcome, study populations and study designs, likely explain the differences in findings.

The three key studies examining the risk of MI reported that compared to non-use, allopurinol use was associated with a 48% decrease [13] vs. a 25% increase [14] vs. no significant change [12] in the risk of MI. The studies were similar in that they all used clinical databases, assessed non-fatal MI and controlled for several cardiovascular risk factors. However, several differences were evident. Two studies used prevalent-user design [12, 14], which puts them at the risk of adjusting for the mediating factors and missing early events. Thus, it was not surprising that the two studies that used prevalent design showed increased risk [14] or no difference in risk [12], while the only new user design study showed risk reduction for MI [13]. Our study, using a new user design, also shows statistically significant benefits of allopurinol for risk reduction of acute cardiovascular events, and these findings were confirmed in several sensitivity

Table 5 Sensitivity analyses with inclusion of colchicine in the main model or with immune disease in the model

	Main model[a] + colchicine		Main model[a] + immune disease	
	Incident MI or stroke			
	Hazard ratio (95% CI)	*p*-value	Hazard ratio (95% CI)	*p*-value
Allopurinol User				
Current	**0.68 (0.54, 0.85)**	**0.001**	**0.67 (0.53, 0.84)**	**0.0006**
Previous	Ref		Ref	
Immune disease	–	–	1.04 (0.78, 1.37)	0.81
Colchicine	0.80 (0.55, 1.18)	0.26	–	–

Significant odds ratios are in bold

[a]Main model was run without immune disease and without colchicine and included gender, age, race, hypertension, hyperlipidemia, peripheral vascular disease COPD and renal disease

analyses, including an analysis of prevalent allopurinol users (to allow comparability to the two previous studies). Our study is among the first to show allopurinol's protective effect on acute cardiovascular event, i.e., incident stroke or MI, in patients with gout and diabetes. However, our study differs in one important aspect from the previous cited studies, i.e., we focused on patients with both gout and diabetes. These patients likely have a higher risk of acute cardiovascular events than patients with only one of the two risk factors. This likely enriched our population for more acute cardiovascular events and likely made our study adequately powered, as intended.

This finding has a practical implication for patients and providers. For patients with both gout and diabetes, allopurinol has an added benefit of reduction of the risk of acute MI or stroke. The risk reduction is not only statistically significant, but also clinically meaningful (33% reduction). Patients should be informed of this potentially beneficial effect, when allopurinol is first prescribed. This risk reduction may potentially be even greater in patients with other cardiovascular disease risk factors.

Our study findings must be interpreted considering several limitations. The diagnosis of acute cardiovascular events, our study outcome, was based on the presence of ICD-9-CM codes, which may lead to misclassification bias. However, previous studies have shown the these codes for cardiovascular outcomes were accurate [24]. There is also evidence of a reasonable accuracy for codes used for covariates i.e., cardiovascular risk factors [23–25]. Serum urate levels were available for a small proportion of patients and therefore, we could not examine whether these associations were or were not mediated via the reduction of serum urate levels. The database also did not allow us to include other variables such as body mass index, smoking, diet and exercise, over the counter aspirin use, and family history of cardiovascular disease, important covariates/risk factors for MI and stroke. We had considered excluding patients with cancer, but decided to include them in our study to improve the generalizability of study findings. A very small proportion of patients on allopurinol (<0.5%) are usually receiving short-term allopurinol for prophylaxis against tumor lysis syndrome, since they are receiving chemotherapy [37]; we doubt that this study limitation influenced our results significantly. Examination of effect of allopurinol on other outcomes, including renal failure, dialysis or death, or rare side effects such as allergic reactions, was beyond the scope of current study. Future studies should examine these outcomes.

The contribution of healthy adherer effect to the observed allopurinol's beneficial effect for these outcomes can not be ruled out, since patients adherent to/using allopurinol may have other healthy behaviors, such as high adherence to other medications, healthier lifestyle, preventive care etc., which may all reduce the risk of stroke and MI. Whether these findings can be generalized to populations other than diabetes and gout is not known, and further study is needed in this area. Reasons for allopurinol discontinuation can be other than non-adherence, such as allopurinol cessation due to severe renal disease (which is not a contraindication for allopurinol use, since allopurinol can be used even in patients on severe kidney dysfunction and also dialysis), suspected or confirmed allergic reactions (which are extremely rare), the concomitant/new use of azathioprine for the rheumatic disease or organ transplantation (which is uncommon/rare), or switching to febuxostat, another xanthine oxidase inhibitor launched in 2009 (which would have likely decreased the observed difference, but likely did not have a major impact given the use of febuxostat in <7% patients with gout) [38]. These confounding biases would have likely reduced the differences, and likely made our current estimates conservative, since most of these conditions would likely increase the risk of MI and/or stroke in current allopurinol non-users.

Study strengths include a large sample size, the use of a sample that allows findings to be generalizable to cohorts with gout or diabetes in the U.S., the use of a new user design that reduces bias in observational studies [39–41], the inclusion of multiple risk factors for MI/stroke, and the robustness of estimates in sensitivity analyses.

Conclusions

In conclusion, in robust analyses of data from a representative sample of Americans, we found that current allopurinol use was independently associated with a lower risk of incident stroke or MI in patients with gout and diabetes. Our findings provide evidence for a potential cardiovascular protective effect of allopurinol in patients with gout and diabetes, a group of patients at high risk for cardiovascular events. Future studies need to explore the factors that mediate this protective effect, and examine what proportion of variability in this protective effect is explained by serum urate reduction and/or anti-oxidant effect of allopurinol.

Additional files

Additional file 1: International Classification for Diseases, Ninth revision, Clinical Modification (ICD-9-CM) Diagnostic Codes for each condition used for outcome, cohort eligibility, and covariate definitions. This file provides the ICD-9-CM codes for underlying conditions, study outcomes and covariates. (DOC 43 kb)

Additional file 2: Multivariable-adjusted associations of allopurinol use with composite outcome (MI or stroke) for prevalent allopurinol users* with gout and diabetes, with previous allopurinol users as the reference category. This file provides the results of sensitivity analyses, repeating the main analysis in prevalent allopurinol users, instead of incident allopurinol users. (DOC 31 kb)

Abbreviations

COPD: Chronic obstructive pulmonary disease; CV: Cardiovascular; ICD-9-CM: International Classification of Diseases, ninth revision, clinical modification; MI: Myocardial infarction; MI: Myocardial infarction; MPCD: Multi-Payer Claims Database; STROBE: Strengthening of Reporting in Observational studies in Epidemiology; UAB: University of Alabama at Birmingham

Acknowledgements

We thank the Actuarial Research Corporation for providing us with these data.

Funding

This study was supported by the Actuarial Research Corporation (on behalf of the Department of Health and Human Services) and resources and use of facilities at Birmingham Veterans Affairs medical center.

Authors' contributions

JAS developed the study protocol. JAS, RR and JC participated in finalization of the study protocol. RR and SY performed the data analyses. JAS wrote the first draft of the paper. All authors made critical revisions to the manuscript, read, and approved the final manuscript.

Author's information

JAS served as the co-chair of the gout working group of the Outcomes in Rheumatology trials (OMERACT).

"The views expressed in this article are those of the authors and do not necessarily reflect the position or policy of the Department of Veterans Affairs or the United States government."

Competing interests

JAS has received research grants from Takeda and Savient and consultant fees from Savient, Takeda, Regeneron, Merz, Bioiberica, Crealta and Allergan pharmaceuticals, WebMD, UBM LLC and the American College of Rheumatology. JAS serves as the principal investigator for an investigator-initiated study funded by Horizon pharmaceuticals through a grant to DINORA, Inc., a 501 (c)(3) entity. JAS is a member of the executive of OMERACT, an organization that develops outcome measures in rheumatology and receives arms-length funding from 36 companies; a member of the American College of Rheumatology's (ACR) Annual Meeting Planning Committee (AMPC); Chair of the ACR Meet-the-Professor, Workshop and Study Group Subcommittee; and a member of the Veterans Affairs Rheumatology Field Advisory Committee. JRC has received research grant funding to the university and consulting monies for unrelated work from Abbvie, Amgen, BMS, Janssen, Pfizer, Roche, and UCB. The other authors have no relevant disclosures. None of the authors have any other non-financial disclosures.

Author details

[1]Medicine Service, VA Medical Center, 700 19th St S, Birmingham, AL 35233, USA. [2]Department of Medicine at School of Medicine, University of Alabama at Birmingham, 510, 20th street South, Faculty office tower (FOT), Birmingham, AL 35294, USA. [3]Division of Epidemiology at School of Public Health, University of Alabama at Birmingham, 1720 Second Ave. South, Birmingham, AL 335294-0022, USA. [4]Department of Orthopedic SurgeryMayo Clinic College of Medicine, 200 1st St SW, Rochester, MN 55905, USA.

References

1. Krishnan E, Baker JF, Furst DE, Schumacher HR. Gout and the risk of acute myocardial infarction. Arthritis Rheum. 2006;54(8):2688–96.
2. De Vera MA, Rahman MM, Bhole V, Kopec JA, Choi HK. Independent impact of gout on the risk of acute myocardial infarction among elderly women: a population-based study. Ann Rheum Dis. 2010;69(6):1162–4.
3. Seminog OO, Goldacre MJ. Gout as a risk factor for myocardial infarction and stroke in England: evidence from record linkage studies. Rheumatology (Oxford). 2013;52(12):2251–9.
4. Johnson RJ, Kang DH, Feig D, Kivlighn S, Kanellis J, Watanabe S, Tuttle KR, Rodriguez-Iturbe B, Herrera-Acosta J, Mazzali M. Is there a pathogenetic role for uric acid in hypertension and cardiovascular and renal disease? Hypertension. 2003;41(6):1183–90.
5. Kim SY, Guevara JP, Kim KM, Choi HK, Heitjan DF, Albert DA. Hyperuricemia and risk of stroke: a systematic review and meta-analysis. Arthritis Rheum. 2009;61(7):885–92.
6. Kim SY, Guevara JP, Kim KM, Choi HK, Heitjan DF, Albert DA. Hyperuricemia and coronary heart disease: a systematic review and meta-analysis. Arthritis Care Res (Hoboken). 2010;62(2):170–80.
7. Feig DI, Kang DH, Johnson RJ. Uric acid and cardiovascular risk. N Engl J Med. 2008;359(17):1811–21.
8. Pacher P, Nivorozhkin A, Szabo C. Therapeutic effects of xanthine oxidase inhibitors: renaissance half a century after the discovery of allopurinol. Pharmacol Rev. 2006;58(1):87–114.
9. Harrison D, Griendling KK, Landmesser U, Hornig B, Drexler H. Role of oxidative stress in atherosclerosis. Am J Cardiol. 2003;91(3A):7A–11.
10. Struthers A, Shearer F. Allopurinol: novel indications in cardiovascular disease. Heart. 2012;98(21):1543–5.
11. Kelkar A, Kuo A, Frishman WH. Allopurinol as a cardiovascular drug. Cardiol Rev. 2011;19(6):265–71.
12. Grimaldi-Bensouda L, Alperovitch A, Aubrun E, Danchin N, Rossignol M, Abenhaim L, et al. Impact of allopurinol on risk of myocardial infarction. Ann Rheum Dis. 2015;74:836–42.
13. de Abajo FJ, Gil MJ, Rodriguez A, Garcia-Poza P, Alvarez A, Bryant V, Garcia-Rodriguez LA. Allopurinol use and risk of non-fatal acute myocardial infarction. Heart. 2015;101(9):679–85.
14. Wei L, Mackenzie IS, Chen Y, Struthers AD, MacDonald TM. Impact of allopurinol use on urate concentration and cardiovascular outcome. Br J Clin Pharmacol. 2011;71(4):600–7.
15. Ray WA. Evaluating medication effects outside of clinical trials: new-user designs. Am J Epidemiol. 2003;158(9):915–20.
16. Zhu Y, Pandya BJ, Choi HK. Comorbidities of gout and hyperuricemia in the US general population: NHANES 2007–2008. Am J Med. 2012;125(7):679–87. e671.
17. Kamath CC, Kremers HM, Vanness DJ, O'Fallon WM, Cabanela RL, Gabriel SE. The cost-effectiveness of acetaminophen, NSAIDs, and selective COX-2 inhibitors in the treatment of symptomatic knee osteoarthritis. Value Health. 2003;6(2):144–57.
18. STROBE Statement. Strengthening the reporting of observational studies in epidemiology. Link: http://www.strobe-statement.org/fileadmin/Strobe/uploads/checklists/STROBE_checklist_v4_cohort.pdf. Accessed 28 Feb 2017.
19. Singh JA, Hodges JS, Toscano JP, Asch SM. Quality of care for gout in the US needs improvement. Arthritis Rheum. 2007;57(5):822–9.
20. Miller DR, Safford MM, Pogach LM. Who has diabetes? Best estimates of diabetes prevalence in the Department of Veterans Affairs based on computerized patient data. Diabetes Care. 2004;27 Suppl 2:B10–21.
21. Singh JA. Accuracy of veterans affairs databases for diagnoses of chronic diseases. Prev Chronic Dis. 2009;6(4):A126.
22. Solberg LI, Engebretson KI, Sperl-Hillen JM, Hroscikoski MC, O'Connor PJ. Are claims data accurate enough to identify patients for performance measures or quality improvement? The case of diabetes, heart disease, and depression. Am J Med Qual. 2006;21(4):238–45.
23. Birman-Deych E, Waterman AD, Yan Y, Nilasena DS, Radford MJ, Gage BF. Accuracy of ICD-9-CM codes for identifying cardiovascular and stroke risk factors. Med Care. 2005;43(5):480–5.
24. Kiyota Y, Schneeweiss S, Glynn RJ, Cannuscio CC, Avorn J, Solomon DH. Accuracy of Medicare claims-based diagnosis of acute myocardial infarction: estimating positive predictive value on the basis of review of hospital records. Am Heart J. 2004;148(1):99–104.
25. Thigpen JL, Dillon C, Forster KB, Henault L, Quinn EK, Tripodis Y, Berger PB, Hylek EM, Limdi NA. Validity of international classification of disease codes to identify ischemic stroke and intracranial hemorrhage among individuals with associated diagnosis of atrial fibrillation. Circ Cardiovasc Qual Outcomes. 2015;8(1):8–14.
26. Crittenden DB, Lehmann RA, Schneck L, Keenan RT, Shah B, Greenberg JD, Cronstein BN, Sedlis SP, Pillinger MH. Colchicine use is associated with decreased prevalence of myocardial infarction in patients with gout. J Rheumatol. 2012;39(7):1458–64.
27. Muir SW, Harrow C, Dawson J, Lees KR, Weir CJ, Sattar N, Walters MR. Allopurinol use yields potentially beneficial effects on inflammatory

indices in those with recent ischemic stroke: a randomized, double-blind, placebo-controlled trial. Stroke. 2008;39(12):3303–7.

28. Kanbay M, Huddam B, Azak A, Solak Y, Kadioglu GK, Kirbas I, Duranay M, Covic A, Johnson RJ. A randomized study of allopurinol on endothelial function and estimated glomular filtration rate in asymptomatic hyperuricemic subjects with normal renal function. Clin J Am Soc Nephrol. 2011;6(8):1887–94.
29. Yiginer O, Ozcelik F, Inanc T, Aparci M, Ozmen N, Cingozbay BY, Kardesoglu E, Suleymanoglu S, Sener G, Cebeci BS. Allopurinol improves endothelial function and reduces oxidant-inflammatory enzyme of myeloperoxidase in metabolic syndrome. Clin Res Cardiol. 2008;97(5):334–40.
30. Kanbay M, Siriopol D, Nistor I, Elcioglu OC, Telci O, Takir M, Johnson RJ, Covic A. Effects of allopurinol on endothelial dysfunction: a meta-analysis. Am J Nephrol. 2014;39(4):348–56.
31. Melendez-Ramirez G, Perez-Mendez O, Lopez-Osorio C, Kuri-Alfaro J, Espinola-Zavaleta N. Effect of the treatment with allopurinol on the endothelial function in patients with hyperuricemia. Endocr Res. 2012;37(1):1–6.
32. Kao MP, Ang DS, Gandy SJ, Nadir MA, Houston JG, Lang CC, Struthers AD. Allopurinol benefits left ventricular mass and endothelial dysfunction in chronic kidney disease. J Am Soc Nephrol. 2011;22(7):1382–9.
33. Dogan A, Yarlioglues M, Kaya MG, Karadag Z, Dogan S, Ardic I, Dogdu O, Kilinc Y, Zencir C, Akpek M, et al. Effect of long-term and high-dose allopurinol therapy on endothelial function in normotensive diabetic patients. Blood Press. 2011;20(3):182–7.
34. Biscaglia S, Ceconi C, Malagu M, Pavasini R, Ferrari R. Uric acid and coronary artery disease: an elusive link deserving further attention. Int J Cardiol. 2016; 213:28–32.
35. Goicoechea M, Garcia de Vinuesa S, Verdalles U, Verde E, Macias N, Santos A, Perez de Jose A, Cedeno S, Linares T, Luno J. Allopurinol and progression of CKD and cardiovascular events: long-term follow-up of a randomized clinical trial. Am J Kidney Dis. 2015;65:543–9.
36. Terawaki H, Nakayama M, Miyazawa E, Murata Y, Nakayama K, Matsushima M, Miyazaki M, Sato H, Sato M, Sato T, et al. Effect of allopurinol on cardiovascular incidence among hypertensive nephropathy patients: the Gonryo study. Clin Exp Nephrol. 2013;17(4):549–53.
37. Rashid N, Coburn BW, Wu YL, Cheetham TC, Curtis JR, Saag KG, Mikuls TR. Modifiable factors associated with allopurinol adherence and outcomes among patients with gout in an integrated healthcare system. J Rheumatol. 2015;42(3):504–12.
38. Hatoum H, Khanna D, Lin SJ, Akhras KS, Shiozawa A, Khanna P. Achieving serum urate goal: a comparative effectiveness study between allopurinol and febuxostat. Postgrad Med. 2014;126(2):65–75.
39. Johnson ES, Bartman BA, Briesacher BA, Fleming NS, Gerhard T, Kornegay CJ, Nourjah P, Sauer B, Schumock GT, Sedrakyan A, et al. The incident user design in comparative effectiveness research. Pharmacoepidemiol Drug Saf. 2013;22(1):1–6.
40. Schneeweiss S. A basic study design for expedited safety signal evaluation based on electronic healthcare data. Pharmacoepidemiol Drug Saf. 2010; 19(8):858–68.
41. Solomon DH, Massarotti E, Garg R, Liu J, Canning C, Schneeweiss S. Association between disease-modifying antirheumatic drugs and diabetes risk in patients with rheumatoid arthritis and psoriasis. JAMA. 2011;305(24):2525–31.

25

Renal denervation improves cardiac function by attenuating myocardiocyte apoptosis in dogs after myocardial infarction

Li Wang[1,2†], Lijun Song[3†], Chao Li[2], Qiaoli Feng[1], Mengping Xu[1], Zhuqing Li[1] and Chengzhi Lu[2*]

Abstract

Background: Myocardial apoptosis is important in the pathogenesis and progression of myocardial infarction-induced heart failure (MI-HF). Renal sympathetic denervation (RDN) has become a promising therapeutic strategy for the treatment of HF. Previous studies have shown that RDN could improve heart function Yao et al. (Exp Ther Med 14: 4104-4110, 2017). However, whether and how RDN regulates myocardial apoptosis in MI-HF is unclear. This study sought to evaluate the effects of RDN on cardiac function and apoptosis-related gene expression in MI-HF dogs.

Methods: Eighteen healthy mongrel dogs were randomly divided into control group($n = 6$), model group($n = 6$) and treatment group($n = 6$). MI-HF was established in model group and treatment group by anhydrous alcohol embolization, after heart failure dogs in the treatment group and model group proceeded bilateral renal artery ablation and bilateral renal arteriography, respectively. The cardiac function parameters were evaluated by echocardiographic; the serum NT-BNP level was detected by ELISA; the degree of myocardial fibrosis was observed through masson staining; the expression of MMP-2, MMP-9 in the cardiac were got by immunohistochemistry. TUNEL method was used to observe cardiomyocyte apoptotsis and calculate the apoptosis index (AI). Relative expression of Bcl-2 and Bax, Caspase3 and GRP78 were detected using RT-PCR and Western Blot. Renal artery H&E staining and serum creatinine were conducted to access the efficacy and safety of RDN.

Results: Four weeks after RDN, the LVEDD, LVESD and LVEDP decreased, and the LVEF and LVSP increased in the treatment group compared with those in the control group (all $P < 0.05$). Moreover, NT-BNP, an indicator of cardiac function was decreased. Additionally, MMP-2 and MMP-9 levels in the myocardium decreased significantly in the treatment group. Furthermore, the levels of Bax, and caspase 3 decreased, while the level of Bcl-2 increased. Thus, myocardial apoptosis was attenuated in RDN treated dogs. We also found that the level of GRP78 which is activated in response to endoplasmic reticulum (ER) stress, was decreased. However, serum creatinine levels were not significantly different between the RND-treated dogs and the control dogs.

Conclusion: Cardiac function was improved by RDN treatment through regulating apoptosis and ER stress in cardiomyocytes in dogs after MI.

Keywords: Renal denervation, Heart failure, Myocardial infarction, Myocardial apoptosis

* Correspondence: lucz8@126.com
†Equal contributors
[2]Department of Cardiology, Tianjin First Center Hospital, Tianjin, China
Full list of author information is available at the end of the article

Background

Myocardial infarction is a leading cause of death in the world [1]. Heart failure (HF) is a common complication of acute myocardial infarction (AMI) and is characterized by cardiac dysfunction along with autonomic imbalance. HF is a serious condition with poor survival rates. Myocardial apoptosis is important in the pathogenesis and progression of MI-induced HF. The local adverse stimulus after MI induces myocyte apoptosis [2] and promotes the deterioration of cardiac function and ventricular remodeling. Loss of myocardial cells is associated with impaired heart function.

A previous study suggested that sympathoexcitation plays a critical role in the pathogenesis and progression of HF after MI. Thus, inhibiting the adverse stimulus of sympathetic overactivity after MI may attenuate myocyte apoptosis and improve cardiac function, which may have clinical significance in the treatment of HF. Catheter-based renal sympathetic denervation (RDN) selectively reduces both renal sympathetic efferent and afferent nerve activity, which has become a hot topic in the field of HF treatment [3, 4]. Whether and how RDN regulates apoptosis in MI-HF is unclear. Thus, the aim of the study was to evaluate the effects of RDN on cardiac function and apoptosis-related gene expression in MI-HF dogs.

Methods

Animal model

Mongrel dogs (male = 7, female = 11) weighing between 15 and 18 kg were purchased through the Experimental of Animal Care Center of Tianjin Medical University, there was no gender difference observed in our study. All the experiments were conducted in accordance with the guide for the Care and the Use of Laboratory Animials and were approved by the ethical committee of Tianjin Medical University.

Experimental groups

All experimental dogs were randomly assigned into three groups: (1) control group ($n = 6$) received only a coronary angiogram; (2) model group ($n = 6$) that underwent an established procedure to induce MI and four weeks later underwent a renal arteriogram; (3) treatment group ($n = 6$) first underwent MI-inducing procedure and then underwent RDN four weeks later.

Establishment of MI model

Dogs in model and treatment groups were anesthetized with sodium pentobarbital (30 mg/kg IV), intubated, and ventilated using a respirator with room air supplemented with oxygen. Continuous ECG monitoring was carried out. After femoral artery access was established and 1000 IU of heparin was injected, 0.2 ml of anhydrous alcohol was injected distally to the first diagonal of the left anterior descending coronary (LAD) as described in a previous study, resulting in left ventricular (LV) damage.

Renal sympathetic denervation

In the treatment group dogs, the ablation electrode (6F saline irrigated catheter tip) was inserted into each artery via the fermoral artery under fluroscopy, and radiofrequency (RF) energy was applied to the endothelial lining with an irrigation flow rate of 12 ml/min. The temperature and power of the radiofrequency ablation instrument was set at 43 °C and 10 W.The target sites were in different directions,lasted for at least 90 s.The catheter was then retreated1–2 cm to generate another ablation location. This procedure was repeated four times in each renal artery, and then, the similar RF energy was applied to the contralateral renal artery.

Transthoracic echocardiography

All of the dogs underwent transthoracic ecchocardiography at baseline, 4 weeks after MI and 4 weeks after RDN (CX50, Philips, Netherlands). The left ventricular ejection fraction (LVEF), left ventricular end-systolic dimension (LVESD), left ventricular end-diastolic dimension (LVEDD), left ventricular systolic pressure (LVSP) and left ventricular end-diastolic pressure(LVEDP) were recorded. Three consecutive cardiac cycles were observed, and the average values were recorded as the final cardiac parameters. The LVEF was calculated by the formula: (LVVmax- LVVmin) / LVVmax.

Evaluation of plasma NT-BNP and creatinine level

Venous blood were collected in vacutainers for the NT-BNP and Cr assays. Samples for the NT-BNP and Cr assays were centrifuged at 3000 g for 10 min at 4 °C, and the plasma was separated kept in microtubes and stored at − 70 °C until assay. NT-BNP and Cr levels were examined by using enzyme-linked immunosorbent assay (ELISA). All assays were performed twice.

Histological evaluation

After perfusion with ice-cold PBS, the hearts were cut and fixed in 4% phosphate buffered formalin for 48–72 h at 4 °C, subsequently, the tissues were then dehydrated and embedded in paraffin. Infarcted myocardial tissue was flash-frozen by liquid nitrogen then stored at − 80 °C. Masson's trichrome staining were performed to detect cardiac fibrosis.Connective tissue was differentiated on the basis of its color. Immunohistochemical staining was performed using the Power VisionTM two-step method. The sections were stained with MMP-2(polyclonal rabbit anti-MMP-2 antibody,Abcam, USA) and MMP-9(polyclonal rabbit anti-MMP-9 antibody Santa Cruz, USA). Immunohistochemical score (IHS) was utilized. This method has been shown to approximate data generated from image analysis-based scoring systems as described in a previous study [5]. HE staining was used to detect the renal artery.

TUNEL staining

TUNEL staining was performed using a commercial kit (In Situ Cell Death Detection FITC Kit or TMR red, Roche). Myocardial tissues were fixed in 4% paraformaldehyde and dehydrated with ethyl alcohol. Paraffin sections were incubated with anti-α-actin in antibodies (1:200 dilution; Sigma-Aldrich) in a humidified chamber. The cells that exhibited condensed nuclei with an irregular form or nuclei split into green particles were considered to be TUNEL-positive cells. The apoptotic index (AI) was calculated according to the following formula: AI = (number of apoptotic cells/total number of nuclei) × 100%.

Western blot

Protein expression levels of Bcl-2 (MDL, China), Bax (MDL, China), caspase 3 (MDL, China), and GRP78 (MDL, China) were assessed by western blotting. All antibodies were applied according to the manufacturer's instructions. The integrated optical densities of the protein bands were obtained by an imaging system.

RT-PCR

mRNA levels were assessed by using quantitative real-time reverse transcription polymerase chain reaction (RT-PCR). Total RNA was extracted from myocardial tissue. Purified RNA was quantified, and cDNA was synthesized using an I-script cDNA synthesis kit (Bio-Rad).

TaqMan primers from Life Technologies were used in the quantitative real-time RT-PCR. The sequences for the primers are summarized in supplemental Table 1. The values were corrected based on ß-actin levels, and the final mRNA level was calculated using the formula $x=2^{-\Delta\Delta CT}$, where x is the fold change relative to the control.

Statistical analysis

The data were presented as the mean ± SD. Group comparisons were subjected to analysis of variance (ANOVA), followed by the least significant difference (LSD) test to identify differences among various groups,and a probability value < 0.05 was required for statistical significance(version 20.0 SPSS).

Results

One dog in the treatment group died 1 day after AMI because of ventricular fibrillation, and one dog in the model group died of HF 30 days after AMI; there were no deaths in the normal group.

Baseline parameters

Dogs in each group underwent assessment of the LVEDD, LVESD, LVEF, LVEDP, LVSP and HR before MI (shown in in supplemental Table 2), and no significant baseline differences were found among the three groups (all $P > 0.05$).

RDN improved the function of failing hearts

Four weeks after MI, and compared to baseline data, the LVEDD, LVESD and LVEDP were significantly increased (all $P < 0.05$) while the LVEF and LVSP values were both reduced in the model and treatment groups (both $P < 0.05$). Importantly, 4 weeks after RDN, parameters such as LVEDD, LVESD, LVEF, LVEDP and LVSP were significantly improved in the treatment group compared with those in the model group (all $P < 0.05$), but the LVEDD, LVESD, and LVEDP in the treatment group were still higher than the baseline parameters (all $P < 0.05$), and LVEF lower than baseline group (all P < 0.05) (shown in Table 1).

At baseline, there were no differences in NT-BNP levels among the normal group, model group and treatment group. After myocardial infarction, NT-BNP levels in the model and treatment groups were significantly higher than those in the normal group ($P < 0.05$). However, after ablation, the NT-BNP level was significantly decreased in the treatment group compared with that in the model group ($P < 0.05$) (shown in Fig. 1).

RDN suppressed cardiac fibrosis

Following Masson's trichrome staining, the sections presented different colors in different regions, with the blue color indicating fibrosis. As shown in Fig. 2A, staining for collagen showed an increase in intercellular space in both the model and treatment groups. After RDN, the level of myocardial fibrosis in the treatment group was significantly improved compared with the model group, and the arrangement of the myocardial cells was neat,

Table 1 Data on cardiac function before and after RDN

	Model group ($n = 5$)		Treatment group ($n = 5$)	
	Pre-sham	Post-sham	Pre-RDN	Post-RDN
LVEDD (mm)	38.17 ± 1.92*	39.54 ± 1.89*	37.70 ± 3.04*	35.36 ± 2.63*#
LVESD (mm)	29.80 ± 1.42*	32.64 ± 4.51*	28.60 ± 3.21*	26.08 ± 3.89*#
LVEF (%)	41.13 ± 2.88*	36.78 ± 3.44*	39.86 ± 3.47*	43.80 ± 2.66*#
LVEDP (mmHg)	17.67 ± 6.50*	22.40 ± 5.90*	20.20 ± 6.54*	13.20 ± 3.19*#
LVSP (mmHg)	103.80 ± 12.70*	93.18 ± 6.96*	102.40 ± 14.36*	109.8 ± 14.53#

Note: pre-RDN denotes 4 weeks after MI; values are presented as the mean ± SD. *$P < 0.05$ vs. baseline data; #$P < 0.05$ denotes the comparison between the model group and the treatment group

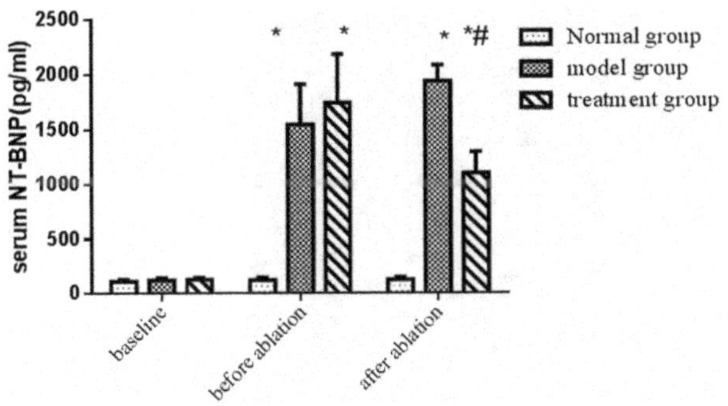

Fig. 1 Changes in NT-BNP. Note: * $P < 0.05$ vs. baseline data; # $P < 0.05$ indicates the post-RDN comparison between the model group and the treatment group

however there was still fibrotic change compared with the normal group. Similar to the result observed with Masson's staining, the MMP-2 (Fig. 2B) and MMP-9 (Fig. 2C) expression levels in the treatment group were significantly decreased compared with those in the model group but were still higher than those in the normal group, as shown in Fig. 2D.

RDN suppressed cardiomyocyte apoptosis and reduced ER stress in cardiomyocytes

The apoptosis index (AI), calculated as apoptotic cell/normal cell× 100, was used to estimate the degree of cardiomyocyte apoptosis, The AI in the normal, model and treatment groups was 2.30 ± 1.59, 30.26 ± 6.94 and 20.20 ± 4.00, respectively. Representative TUNEL staining is shown in Fig. 3. Compared with normal group, the optical density of TUNEL-positive cells was markedly increased in model and treatment groups ($P < 0.01$). and compared with the model group, RDN treatment significantly attenuated cardiomyocyte apoptosis ($P < 0.01$).

The western blotting and RT-PCR analysis of Bcl-2, Bax, caspase 3 and GRP78 is presented in Fig. 4. Quantitative analysis showed that the model group had significantly increased expression levels of caspase 3, Bax, and GRP78 compared with the normal group ($P < 0.01$), whereas the level of Bcl-2 decreased markedly($P < 0.05$). RDN significantly suppressed the upregulation of caspase 3, Bax and GRP78 and the downregulation of Bcl-2 protein and mRNA expression compared with the model group ($P < 0.01$).

The safety of RDN

After RDN in the treatment group, no damage in the intima of the vessel wall was detected,

but the adventitial nerve fibers were destroyed, as shown in Fig. 5.

No change in Cr levels before and after RDN

At baseline, there were no significant differences in Cr levels among the three groups. After building MI induced heart failure, there were still no markedly differences among three groups. Besides, there was no significant change after RDN in the treatment group, as shown in Fig. 6.

Discussion

Increased sympathetic nerve activity is a primary characteristic of patients with chronic heart failure (CHF). Increases in sympathetic nerve activity enhance the release of catecholamines, such as norepinephrine, in the heart. Stimulation of β-adrenergic receptors induces cardiac myocyte apoptosis and fibrosis in the heart [6].Prolonged stimulation of the β-adrenergic neurohormonal axis has been shown to contribute to the progression of CHF and mortality in both animal models and humans. Amount of studies, whether clinical studies or animal studies showed that RDN could improve cardiac function in heart failure patients or animals by decreasing sympathetic nerve activity [7–11]. Our research group also showed that RDN improved cardiac function by decreasing cardiac oxidative stress [12]. Besides, previous study demonstrated that RDN leads to a significant improvement of cardiac function by shifting cardiac apoptosis to autophagy in diabetic rabbits [13].Another study showed that RDN could decrease cardiomyocyte apoptosis in canines with prolonged atrial pacing [14]. However, how RDN and by what mechanisms regulates apoptosis in MI-HF is still unclear. Our study aimed to clarify the effect of RDN on cardiac function, and fibrosis, apoptosis-related factors and ER stress associated factors in HF dogs.

The present study in our lab demonstrated that RDN improved the deterioration of LV function.

and LV dilatation post-MI, including a significant increase in LVEF and a significant decrease in LVEDd compared with those in the model group. We further demonstrated that RDN decreased the level of NT-BNP, improved myocardial fibrosis, and decreased the expression of MMP-2 and MMP-9. Meanwhile, decreased Bax and caspase-3 mRNA and protein levels, and increased Bcl-2 mRNA and protein levels, led to an increase in the ratio of Bcl-2/Bax. Moreover, RDN significantly decreased the expression of GRP78 in HF dogs.

Myocyte apoptosis has been shown to commonly occur in HF, and the severity of myocardial apoptosis is closely associated with cardiac function. Numerous studies showed that ER stress (ERS) is an important pathway in cardiac myocyte apoptosis during the progression of HF [15]. GRP78, as a chaperone in the ER, plays a critical role in the regulation of ER dynamic balance, and is a key marker for the ER response. Our results show that RDN decreased GRP78 levels, indicating that RDN could reduce ER stress. Caspase, and the BCL-2 family of proteins are key factors in the apoptotic pathway [16].

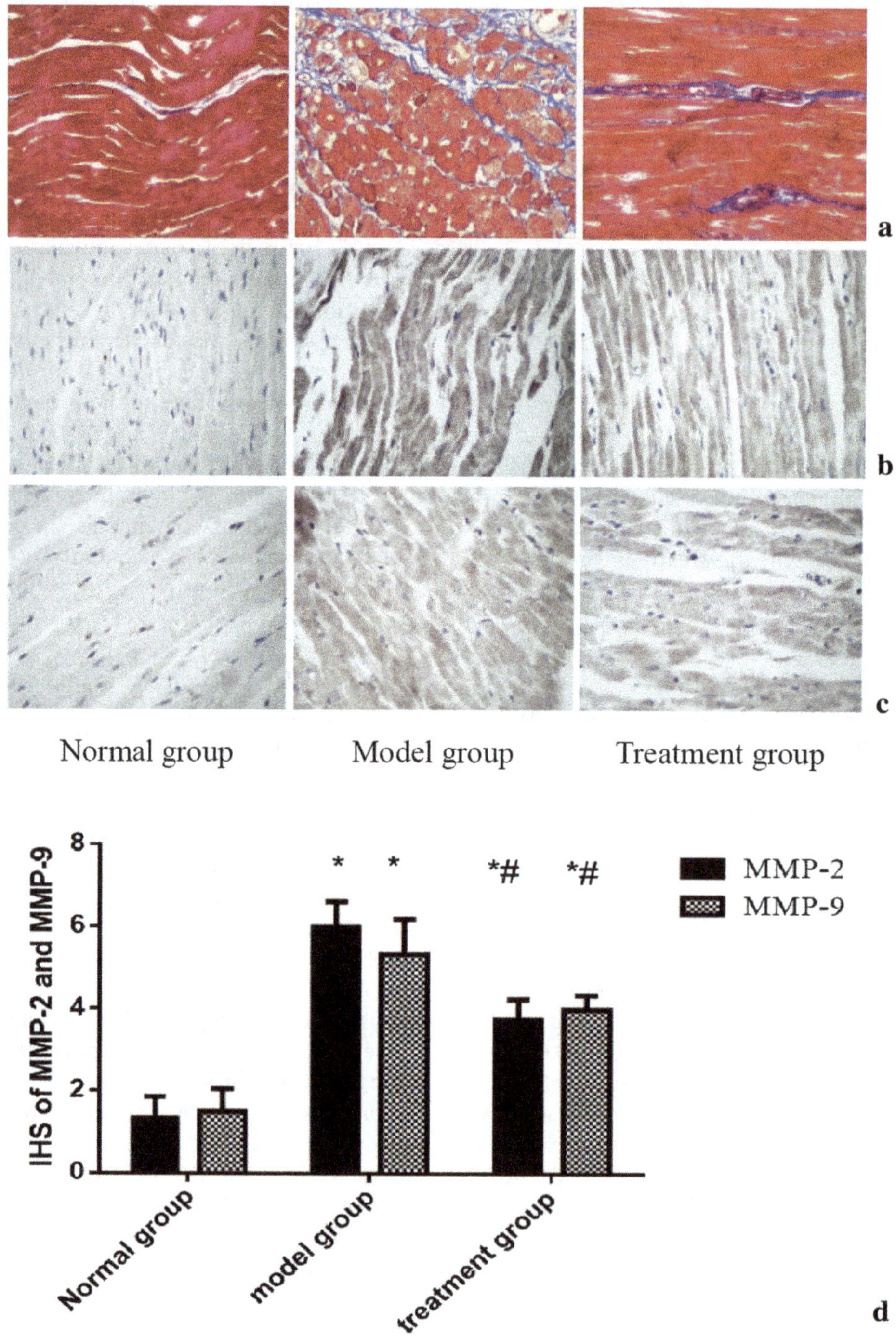

Fig. 2 a Heart sections underwent Masson's trichrome staining (magnification 400 X) to distinguish myocardial tissue (red) from fibrotic tissue (blue). In the normal group, the size of the myocardial cells was normal, and the muscle fibers were regular and no significant pathological changes were observed. In the model group, the cardiomyocytes were looser and the collagen fibers were significantly thickened and exhibited a net-like shape, and were infiltrated with a small amount of inflammatory cells. In the treatment group, the arrangement of myocardial cells was ordered, but there were still fibrotic changes compared with the normal group. **b** MMP-2 immunohistochemical staining of the infarct zone (400×). **c** MMP-9 immunohistochemical staining of the infarct zone (400×). **d** IHS of MMP-2 and MMP-9. Note: * $P < 0.05$ vs. the normal group; # $P < 0.05$ indicates the comparison of pre- and post-RDN between the model group and the treatment group

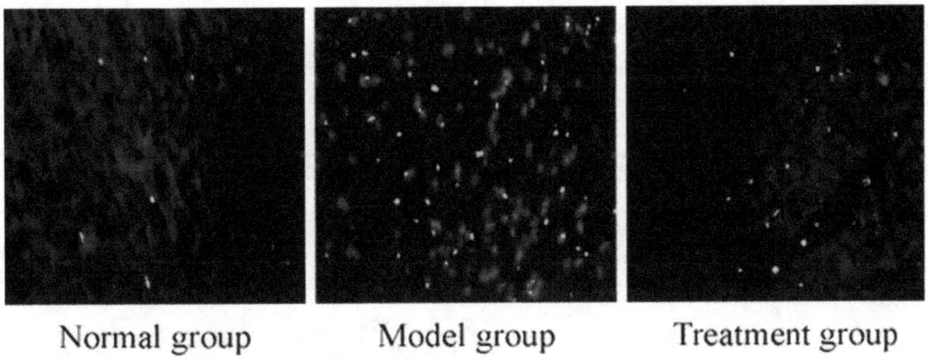

Fig. 3 The AI in the normal, model and treatment groups was 2.30 ± 1.59, 30.26 ± 6.94 and 20.20 ± 4.00, respectively. Compared with the normal group, the optical density of TUNEL-positive cells was markedly increased in the model group and the treatment group. Compared with the model group, RDN treatment significantly attenuated cardiomyocyte apoptosis

Caspase 3 is one of the major caspases involved in apoptosis, which is regulated by the Bcl-2 family proteins. Bcl-2 can inhibit cell death, whereas Bax promotes apoptosis. Sympathetic nerve overactivity plays a critical role in ERS and cardiomyocyte apoptosis after MI. Norepinephrine (NE), an important neurotransmitter of the sympathetic nerve system, specifically stimulates the ß1-adrenergic receptor (AR), which induces ERS and apoptosis in cardiac myocytes in vitro and in vivo [17, 18]. Wang HJ et al. found that cardiac sympathetic afferent denervation attenuates cardiac remodeling and apoptosis and improves cardiovascular dysfunction in rats with HF [19]. Results of our TUNEL staining and apoptosis-associated protein and gene expression analyses also suggested that RDN treatment markedly reduced MI-induced cardiomyocyte apoptosis. Thus, we speculate that RDN improves cardiac function by reducing ERS and ERS mediated cardiomyocyte apoptosis.

Both myocyte apoptosis and non-myocyte apoptosis are involved in MI-induced HF [20]. Extracellular signals

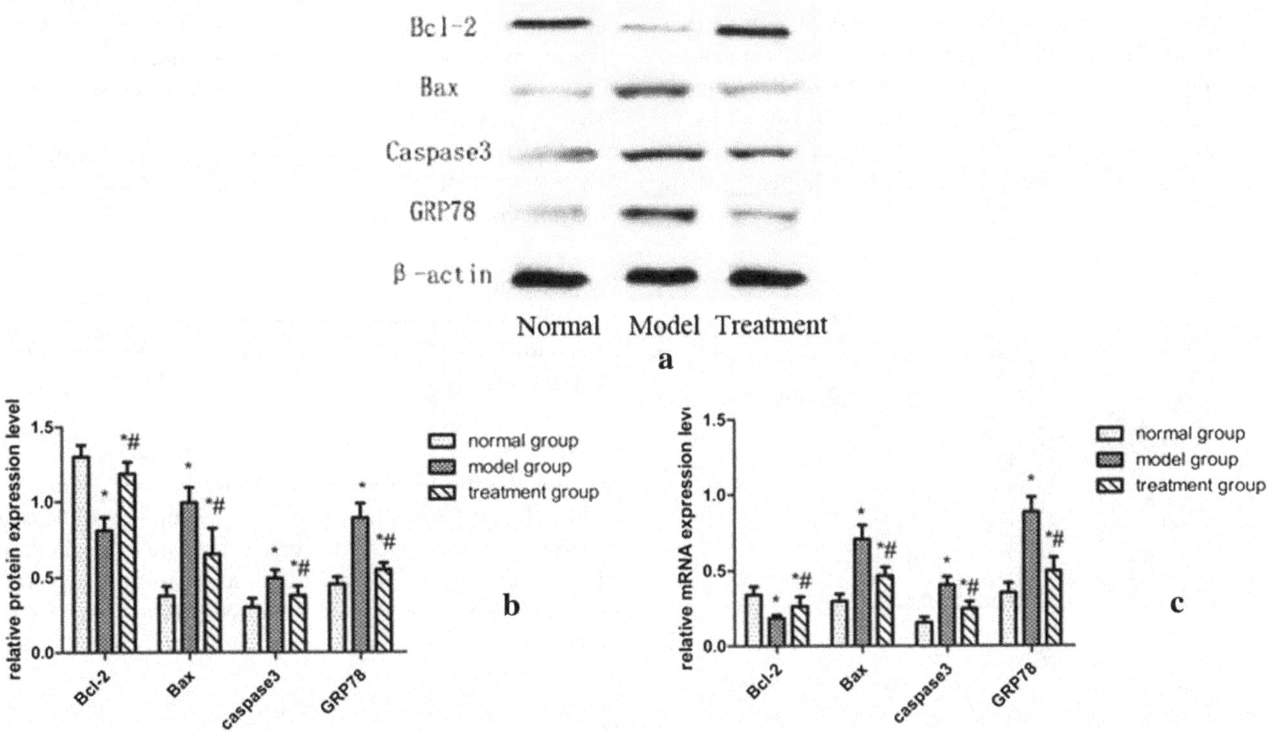

Fig. 4 Effect of RDN on cardiomyocyte apoptosis and ER stress. **a**. Western blotting analysis of Bcl-2, Bax, caspase 3, and GRP78. **b** Quantitative analysis of the western blots. **c** mRNA expression levels of Bcl-2, Bax, caspase 3 and GRP78. Note: * $P < 0.05$ vs. the normal group; # $P < 0.05$ indicates the post-RDN comparison between the model group and the treatment group

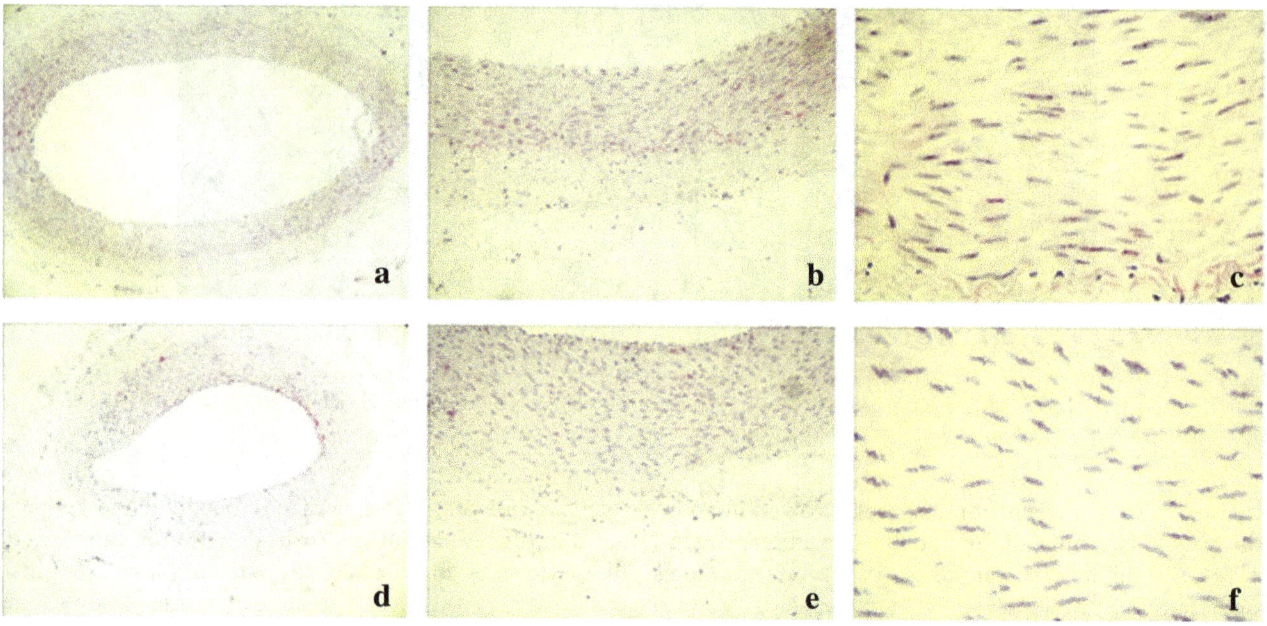

Fig. 5 HE staining of the renal artery. Normal group (**a-c**): no damage to the vascular wall, intima or media, or to adventitial nerve fiber integrity (**a**: 40 X; **b**: 100 X; **c**: 400 X). Treatment group (**d-f**): no damage to the intima of the vessel wall, but the adventitial nerve fibers were destroyed (**d**: 40 X; **e**: 100 X; **f**: 400 X)

also modulate apoptosis in the myocardial matrix. Matrix metalloproteinases (MMPs), which are key substances in the cardiac interstitial matrix, increase after MI, and MMP levels correlate with the extent of cardiac dysfunction in HF patients [21]. MMPs regulate the remodeling process by facilitating extracellular matrix turnover and, therefore, play a fundamental role in tissue remodeling, including remodeling of the heart [22]. Two of the most widely studied cardiac MMPs are MMP-2 and MMP-9. The involvement of MMP-2 and MMP-9 is considered to be important, as MMP-2 and MMP-9 are capable of degrading interstitial fibrillar collagen and causing non-myocyte apoptosis, ultimately leading to systolic and diastolic impairment in the heart. In our study, we found that RDN significantly decreased cardiac MMP-2 and MMP-9 expression. Given the close relationship between MMPs and non-myocyte apoptosis, MMP-2 and MMP-9 may play a role in decreasing cardiac non-myocyte apoptosis.

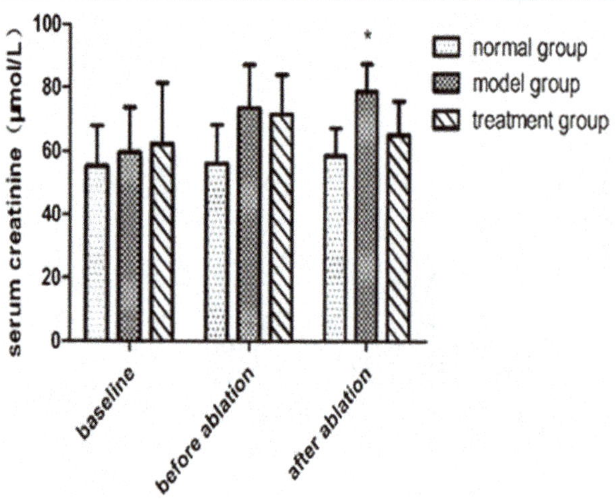

Fig. 6 Change in Cr levels in different groups. Note: * $P < 0.05$ vs. the normal group

Conclusion

RDN improves cardiac function, possibly by reducing ERS, inhibiting cardiomyocyte apoptosis and decreasing MMPs levels.

Limitations

The small sample size is a limitation of our study, We will further expand the experimental sample size to confirm our conclusion and further explore the effect of RDN on the ERS pathway. In addition, multicenter, randomized, controlled, double-blinded studies may be required to validate the efficacy and safety of RDN in patients with HF.

Abbreviations

AI: Apoptotic index; AMI: Acute myocardial infarction; ELISA: Enzyme-linked immunosorbent assay; ERS: Endoplasmic reticulum stress; HF: Heart failure; HR: Heart rate; IHS: Immunohistochemical score; LVEDD: Left ventricular end-diastolic dimension; LVEDP: Left ventricular end-diastolic pressure; LVEF: Left ventricular ejection fraction; LVESD: Left ventricular end-systolic dimension; LVSP: Left ventricular systolic pressure; MMPs: Matrix metalloproteinases; NT-BNP: N-terminal pronatriuretic peptide; RDN: Renal sympathetic denervation; RT-PCR: Real-time reverse transcription polymerase chain reaction

Acknowledgments
We thank all the researchers who participated in this work.

Author contributions
(1) Study design and model: CL1, and LW. (2) Data collection: LS and LW. (3) Data analysis: QF, CL2, and LW. (4) Manuscript writing: LW, MX and LS. (5) Final approval of the manuscript: CL1.

Funding
This work was supported by the research plan of the Tianjin Application Foundation and Advanced Technology (NO.14JCYBJC26100) and the Science and Technology Foundation of Tianjin Health and Family Planning Committee (NO.15KG131 and NO.2014KY11).

Competing interests
All authors declare that they have no competing interests.

Author details
[1]First Center Clinic College of Tianjin Medical University, Tianjin First Center Hospital, 24 Fukang Road, Nankai District, Tianjin 300192, China. [2]Department of Cardiology, Tianjin First Center Hospital, Tianjin, China. [3]Department of Digestion, Tianjin First Center Hospital, Tianjin, China.

References
1. Compostella L, Lakusic N, Compostella C, Truong LV, Iliceto S, Bellotto F. Does heart rate variability correlate with long-term prognosis in myocardial infarction patients treated by early revascularization. World J Cardiol. 2017;9(1):27–38.
2. Teringova E, Tousek P. Apoptosis in ischemic heart disease. J Transl Med. 2017;15(1):87.
3. Yao W, Wang N, Qian J, et al. Renal sympathetic denervation improves myocardial apoptosis in rats with isoproterenol-induced heart failure by downregulation of tumor necrosis factor-α and nuclear factor-κB. Exp Ther Med. 2017;14(5):4104–10.
4. Hu J, Ji M, Niu C, et al. Effects of renal sympathetic denervation on post-myocardial infarction cardiac remodeling in rats. PLoS One. 2012;7(9): e45986.
5. Soslow RA, Dannenberg AJ, Rush D, Woerner BM, Khan KN, Masferrer J, Koki AT. Cox-2 is expressed in human pulmonary, colonic, and mammary tumors. Cancer. 2000;89:2637–45.
6. Fu Y, Xiao H, Zhang Y. Beta-adrenoceptor signaling pathways mediate cardiac pathological remodeling. Front Biosci (Elite Ed). 2012;4:1625–37.
7. Chen W, Ling Z, Xu Y, et al. Preliminary effects of renal denervation with saline irrigated catheter on cardiac systolic function in patients with heart failure: a prospective, randomized, controlled. Pilot Study Catheter Cardiovasc Interv. 2017;89(4):E153–61.
8. Gao JQ, Xie Y, Yang W, Zheng JP, Liu ZJ. Effects of percutaneous renal sympathetic denervation on cardiac function and exercise tolerance in patients with chronic heart failure. Rev Port Cardiol. 2017;36(1):45–51.
9. Patel HC, Rosen SD, Hayward C, et al. Renal denervation in heart failure with preserved ejection fraction (RDT-PEF): a randomized controlled trial. Eur J Heart Fail. 2016;18(6):703–12.
10. Liu Q, Zhang Q, Wang K, et al. Renal denervation findings on cardiac and renal fibrosis in rats with isoproterenol induced cardiomyopathy. Sci Rep. 2015;5:18582.
11. Li JD, Cheng AY, Huo YL, et al. Bilateral renal denervation ameliorates isoproterenol-induced heart failure through downregulation of the brain renin-angiotensin system and inflammation in rat. Oxidative Med Cell Longev. 2016;2016:3562634.
12. Feng Q, Lu C, Wang L, Song L, Li C, Uppada RC. Effects of renal denervation on cardiac oxidative stress and local activity of the sympathetic nervous system and renin-angiotensin system in acute myocardial infracted dogs. BMC Cardiovasc Disord. 2017;17(1):65.
13. Liu Y, Li B, Li M, Yu Y, Wang Z, Chen S. Improvement of cardiac dysfunction by bilateral surgical renal denervation in animals with diabetes induced by high fructose and high fat diet. Diabetes Res Clin Pract. 2016;115:140–9.
14. Wang X, Zhao Q, Huang H, et al. Effect of renal sympathetic denervation on atrial substrate remodeling in ambulatory canines with prolonged atrial pacing. PLoS One. 2013;8(5):e64611.
15. Zhang C, Tang Y, Li Y, et al. Unfolded protein response plays a critical role in heart damage after myocardial ischemia/reperfusion in rats. PLoS One. 2017;12(6):e0179042.
16. Li Y, Song P, Zhu Q, et al. Liguzinediol improved the heart function and inhibited myocardial cell apoptosis in rats with heart failure. Acta Pharmacol Sin. 2014;35(10):1257–64.
17. Krishnamurthy P, Subramanian V, Singh M, Singh K. Beta1 integrins modulate beta-adrenergic receptor-stimulated cardiac myocyte apoptosis and myocardial remodeling. Hypertension. 2007;49(4):865–72.
18. Amin P, Singh M, Singh K. β-Adrenergic Receptor-Stimulated Cardiac Myocyte Apoptosis: Role of β1 Integrins. J Signal Transduct. 2011;2011: 179057.
19. Wang HJ, Wang W, Cornish KG, Rozanski GJ, Zucker IH. Cardiac sympathetic afferent denervation attenuates cardiac remodeling and improves cardiovascular dysfunction in rats with heart failure. Hypertension. 2014;64(4):745–55.
20. Jose CJ, Vatner DE, Vatner SF. Myocardial apoptosis in heart disease: does the emperor have clothes. Basic Res Cardiol. 2016;111(3):31.
21. DeLeon-Pennell KY, Meschiari CA, Jung M, Lindsey ML. Matrix metalloproteinases in myocardial infarction and heart failure. Prog Mol Biol Transl Sci. 2017;147:75–100.
22. Scofield SL, Amin P, Singh M, Singh K. Extracellular ubiquitin: role in myocyte apoptosis and myocardial remodeling. Compr Physiol. 2015;6(1): 527–60.

Permissions

All chapters in this book were first published in CD, by BioMed Central; hereby published with permission under the Creative Commons Attribution License or equivalent. Every chapter published in this book has been scrutinized by our experts. Their significance has been extensively debated. The topics covered herein carry significant findings which will fuel the growth of the discipline. They may even be implemented as practical applications or may be referred to as a beginning point for another development.

The contributors of this book come from diverse backgrounds, making this book a truly international effort. This book will bring forth new frontiers with its revolutionizing research information and detailed analysis of the nascent developments around the world.

We would like to thank all the contributing authors for lending their expertise to make the book truly unique. They have played a crucial role in the development of this book. Without their invaluable contributions this book wouldn't have been possible. They have made vital efforts to compile up to date information on the varied aspects of this subject to make this book a valuable addition to the collection of many professionals and students.

This book was conceptualized with the vision of imparting up-to-date information and advanced data in this field. To ensure the same, a matchless editorial board was set up. Every individual on the board went through rigorous rounds of assessment to prove their worth. After which they invested a large part of their time researching and compiling the most relevant data for our readers.

The editorial board has been involved in producing this book since its inception. They have spent rigorous hours researching and exploring the diverse topics which have resulted in the successful publishing of this book. They have passed on their knowledge of decades through this book. To expedite this challenging task, the publisher supported the team at every step. A small team of assistant editors was also appointed to further simplify the editing procedure and attain best results for the readers.

Apart from the editorial board, the designing team has also invested a significant amount of their time in understanding the subject and creating the most relevant covers. They scrutinized every image to scout for the most suitable representation of the subject and create an appropriate cover for the book.

The publishing team has been an ardent support to the editorial, designing and production team. Their endless efforts to recruit the best for this project, has resulted in the accomplishment of this book. They are a veteran in the field of academics and their pool of knowledge is as vast as their experience in printing. Their expertise and guidance has proved useful at every step. Their uncompromising quality standards have made this book an exceptional effort. Their encouragement from time to time has been an inspiration for everyone.

The publisher and the editorial board hope that this book will prove to be a valuable piece of knowledge for researchers, students, practitioners and scholars across the globe.

List of Contributors

Casper H Jørgensen, Gunnar H Gislason, Ole Ahlehoff, Charlotte Andersson, Christian Torp-Pedersen and Peter R Hansen
Department of Cardiology, Copenhagen University Hospital Gentofte, Niels Andersens Vej 65, Copenhagen 2900, Denmark

Christian Torp-Pedersen
Department of Health Science and Technology, Aalborg University, Niels Jernes Vej 12, Aalborg 9220, Denmark

Chao-Feng Lin and Ju-Chi Liu
Division of Cardiology, Department of Internal Medicine, Shuang Ho Hospital, Taipei Medical University, New Taipei City, Taiwan

Ya-Hui Chang
Pharmacy Department of Mackay Memorial Hospital, Taipei, Taiwan

Ming-Tsang Chuang
School of Public Health, College of Public Health and Nutrition, Taipei Medical University, Taipei, Taiwan

Li-Nien Chien
School of Health Care Administration, College of Management, Taipei Medical University, Taipei, Taiwan

Chao-Feng Lin
Division of Cardiology, Department of Internal Medicine, MacKay Memorial Hospital, Taipei, Taiwan
Department of Medicine, Mackay Medical College, New Taipei, Taiwan

Ingrid Brænne, Benedikt Reiz, Anja Medack, Mariana Kleinecke and Jeanette Erdmann
Institute for Integrative and Experimental Genomics, University of Lübeck, 23562 Lübeck, Germany

Ingrid Brænne, Benedikt Reiz, Anja Medack, Mariana Kleinecke and Jeanette Erdmann
DZHK (German Research Centre for Cardiovascular Research), partner site Hamburg/Lübeck/Kiel, 23562 Lübeck, Germany

Marcus Fischer
Klinik und Poliklinik für Innere Medizin II, Universitätsklinikum Regensburg, 93053 Regensburg, Germany

Hengstenberg
Deutsches Herzzentrum München and Medizinische Klinik, Klinikum rechts der Isar, Technische Universität München, 80636 München, Germany
DZHK (German Centre for Cardiovascular Research), partner site Munich Heart Alliance, 80636 Munich, Germany

Panos Deloukas and Salih Tuna
Wellcome Trust Sanger Institute, Wellcome Trust Genome Campus, Hinxton CB10 1SA, UK

Panos Deloukas
William Harvey Research Institute, Barts and The London School of Medicine and Dentistry, Queen Mary University of London, London, UK
Princess Al-Jawhara Al-Brahim Centre of Excellence in Research of Hereditary Disorders (PACER-HD), King Abdulaziz University, Jeddah 21589, Saudi Arabia

Liu-wei Zhang, Fang-fang Duan, Zhi-ke Liu, Si-yan Zhan, Yong-hua Hu and Da-fang Chen
Department of Epidemiology and Biostatistics, School of Public Health, Peking University Health Science Center, Beijing 100191, China

Jian-ping Li, Jie Jiang, Yan Zhang and Yong Huo
Department of Cardiology, Peking University First Hospital, Beijing 100034, China

Luís Leite, Joana Moura Ferreira, João Silva Marques, Elisabete Jorge, Vítor Matos, Jorge Guardado, João Calisto and Mariano Pego
Departament of Cardiology, Centro Hospitalar e Universitário de Coimbra, Praceta Prof. Mota Pinto, Coimbra 3000-075, Portugal

Tao Song, Xiu Fen Qu, Wei Cao, Bai He Han, Yang Li, Jing Yan Piao and Lei Lei Yin
Department of Cardiology, the First Affiliated Hospital of Harbin Medical University, No.23 Youzheng Street, Nangang District, Harbin City 150001, Heilongjiang Province, China

Ying Tao Zhang
School of Computer Science and Technology, Harbin Institute of Technology, Harbin, China

Heng Da Cheng
Department of Computer Science, Utah State University, Salt Lake City, UT, USA

Gunnar Nilsson and Lars Söderström
Department of Public Health and Clinical Medicine, Unit of Research, Education and Development - Östersund, Umeå University, Umeå, Sweden

Thomas Mooe and Eva Samuelsson
Department of Public Health and Clinical Medicine, Umeå University, Umeå, Sweden

Lars Söderström
Unit of Research, Education and Development, Östersund Hospital, Region Jämtland Härjedalen, Östersund, Sweden

Annina Kelloniemi, Jani Aro, Elina Koivisto, Erja Mustonen, Heikki Ruskoaho and Jaana Rysä
Research Unit of Biomedicine (Pharmacology & Toxicology), University of Oulu, Oulu, Finland

Juha Näpänkangas
Department of Pathology, Institute of Diagnostics, Oulu University Hospital, University of Oulu, Oulu, Finland

Heikki Ruskoaho
Division of Pharmacology and Pharmacotherapy, Faculty of Pharmacy, University of Helsinki, Helsinki, Finland

Jaana Rysä
School of Pharmacy, Faculty of Health Sciences, University of Eastern Finland, Kuopio, Finland

Sigrun Halvorsen
Department of Cardiology, Oslo University Hospital Ulleval and University of Oslo, Postboks 4956, Nydalen 0424, Oslo, Norway

Jarle Jortveit
Department of Cardiology, Sørlandet Hospital, Arendal, Norway

Pål Hasvold
AstraZeneca NordicBaltic, Södertälje, Sweden

Marcus Thuresson
Statisticon, Uppsala, Sweden

Erik Øie
Department of Internal Medicine, Diakonhjemmet Hospital and Center for Heart Failure Research, University of Oslo, Oslo, Norway

Elizabeth H Bradley, Heather Sipsma, Amanda L Brewster, Harlan M Krumholz and Leslie Curry
Department of Health Policy and Management, Yale School of Public Health, 60 College Street, New Haven, CT 06520-8034, USA

Elizabeth H Bradley, Harlan M Krumholz and Leslie Curry
Robert Wood Johnson Clinical Scholars Program, Department of Medicine, Yale University School of Medicine, New Haven, CT, USA

Harlan M Krumholz
Center for Outcomes Research and Evaluation, Yale-New Haven Hospital, New Haven, CT, USA

Harlan M Krumholz
Section of Cardiovascular Medicine, Department of Medicine, Yale University School of Medicine, New Haven, CT, USA

Karine Pernet, Fiona Ecarnot, Romain Chopard, Marie-France Seronde, Philoktimon Plastaras, Francois Schiele and Nicolas Meneveau
Department of Cardiology, EA3920, University Hospital Jean Minjoz, Boulevard Fleming, Besançon 25000, France

Martin Kirk Christensen and Jan Ravkilde
Department of Cardiology, Aalborg University Hospital, Aalborg, Denmark

Hui Huang
General Hospital of Ningxia Medical University, Yinchuan, China and Visiting Doctor at Department of Cardiology, Aalborg University Hospital, Aalborg, Denmark

Christian Torp-Pedersen
Department of Health Science and Technology, Aalborg University, Aalborg, Denmark

Torleif Trydal
Department of Clinical Biochemistry, Aalborg University Hospital, Aalborg, Denmark

Barbara Eržen and Mišo Šabovič
Department of Vascular Disease, University Clinical Centre, Ljubljana 1000, Slovenia

Mira Šilar
Laboratory for Clinical Immunology & Molecular Genetics, University Clinic of Respiratory and Allergic Diseases, Golnik, Slovenia

Anil Vaidya
Department of Clinical Epidemiology and Medical Technology Assessment (KEMTA), Maastricht University Medical Centre, Maastricht 6202 AZ, The Netherlands

Anil Vaidya
School for Public Health and Primary Care (CAPHRI), Maastricht University, Maastricht, The Netherlands

Johan L Severens
Institute of Health Policy and Management, Erasmus University Rotterdam, Rotterdam, The Netherlands

Johan L Severens
iMTA - Institute of Technology Assessment, Erasmus University Rotterdam, Rotterdam, The Netherlands

Brenda WC Bongaerts, Kitty BJM Cleutjens and Erik AL Biessen
Department of Pathology, Cardiovascular Research Institute Maastricht (CARIM), Maastricht University Medical Centre, Maastricht, The Netherlands

Leonard Hofstra
Cardiology Center Netherlands, Utrecht, The Netherlands

Marja van Dieijen-Visser
Department of Clinical Chemistry, Maastricht University, Maastricht, The Netherlands

Patty J Nelemans
Department of Epidemiology, Maastricht University, Maastricht, The Netherlands

Shengyu Zhang
Department of Internal Medicine, Peking Union Medical College Hospital, Chinese Academy of Medical Sciences, Beijing, China

Jing Yang, Xiaofeng Jin and Shuyang Zhang
Department of Cardiology, Peking Union Medical College Hospital, Chinese Academy of Medical Sciences, Beijing, China

Konstantinos E Farsalinos, Dimitris Tsiapras, Stamatis Kyrzopoulos, Maria Savvopoulou and Vassilis Voudris
Department of Cardiology, Onassis Cardiac Surgery Center, Sygrou 356, Kallithea 17674, Greece

Per-Ola Forsberg, Xinjun Li and Kristina Sundquist
Center for Primary Health Care Research, Clinical Research Centre (CRC), Lund University, building 28, floor 11, Jan Waldenströms gata 35, SE-205 02 Malmö, Sweden

P. K. B. Mahesh and S. M. Arnold
Office of Regional Director of Health Services, Colombo, Sri Lanka

M. W. Gunathunga
Department of Community Medicine, Faculty of Medicine, University of Colombo, Colombo, Sri Lanka

S. Jayasinghe
Department of Clinical Medicine, Faculty of Medicine, University of Colombo, Colombo, Sri Lanka

S. V. Mallawarachchi
Non Communicable Disease Unit, Ministry of Health, Colombo, Sri Lanka

D, S. K. Perera
Post Graduate Institute of Medicine, University of Colombo, Colombo, Sri Lanka

U. A. D. Wijesinghe
Cardiology Unit, National Hospital Sri Lanka, Colombo, Sri Lanka

Olga Gruzdeva, Evgenya Uchasova, Yulia Dyleva, Vera Matveeva, Victoria Karetnikova, Alexander Kokov and Olga Barbarash
Federal State Budgetary Institution "Research Institute for Complex Issues of Cardiovascular Disease", Kemerovo, Russia

Olga Akbasheva
Federal State Budget Educational Institution of Higher Professional Education "Siberian State Medical University" of the Ministry of Healthcare of the Russian Federation, Tomsk, Russia

Shuai Xu
Department of Stomatology, Xinqiao Hospital, Third Military Medical University, 400037 Chongqing, China

Mingbao Song, Xi Liu, Yongming He and Zhexue Qin
Department of Cardiology, Xinqiao Hospital, Third Military Medical University, 183 Xinqiaozhengjie St., Shapingba District, 400037 Chongqing, China

Yu Xiong
Department of Stomatology, Southwest Hospital, Third Military Medical University, 400038 Chongqing, China

W. D. Jayamali, H. M. M. T. B. Herath and Aruna Kulathunga
National Hospital, Colombo, Sri Lanka

Rony Oosterom-Calo and Wim Stut
Philips Research, Eindhoven, The Netherlands

Rony Oosterom-Calo and Saskia J. te Velde
EMGO Institute for Health and Care Research and the Department of Epidemiology and Biostatistics, VU University Medical Center, Amsterdam, The Netherlands

Yaacov Drory
Department of Rehabilitation, Sackler School of Medicine, Tel Aviv University, Tel Aviv, Israel

Johannes Brug and Yariv Gerber
Department of Epidemiology and Preventive Medicine, School of Public Health, Sackler Faculty of Medicine, Tel Aviv University, Tel Aviv, Israel

Johannes Brug
AmsterdamSchool for Communication Research, University of Amsterdam, Amsterdam, The Netherlands

Ettore Ambrosioni, Claudio Borghi, Stefano Bacchelli and Daniela Degli Esposti
Unit of Internal Medicine, Policlinico S. Orsola, University of Bologna, Bologna, Italy

Stefano Omboni
Clinical Research Unit, Italian Institute of Telemedicine, Varese, Italy

Giorgio Reggiardo
Mediservice S.r.l., Agrate Brianza, Italy

Claudio Borghi
Divisione di Medicina Interna, Policlinico S.Orsola, Via Massarenti 9, 40138 Bologna, Italy

Jasvinder A. Singh
Medicine Service, VA Medical Center, 700 19th St S, Birmingham, AL 35233, USA

Jasvinder A. Singh, Rekha Ramachandaran, Shaohua Yu and Jeffrey R. Curtis
Department of Medicine at School of Medicine, University of Alabama at Birmingham, 510, 20th street South, Faculty office tower (FOT), Birmingham, AL 35294, USA

Jasvinder A. Singh and Jeffrey R. Curtis
Division of Epidemiology at School of Public Health, University of Alabama at Birmingham, 1720 Second Ave. South Birmingham, AL 335294-0022, USA

Jasvinder A. Singh
Department of Orthopedic Surgery Mayo Clinic College of Medicine, 200 1st St SW, Rochester, MN 55905, USA

Li Wang, Qiaoli Feng, Mengping Xu and Zhuqing Li
First Center Clinic College of Tianjin Medical University, Tianjin First Center Hospital, 24 Fukang Road, Nankai District, Tianjin 300192, China

Li Wang, Chao Li and Chengzhi Lu
Department of Cardiology, Tianjin First Center Hospital, Tianjin, China

Lijun Song
Department of Digestion, Tianjin First Center Hospital, Tianjin, China

Index

www.ingramcontent.com/pod-product-compliance
Lightning Source LLC
LaVergne TN
LVHW080653210926
848485LV00003B/373